The U.S. Navy Medical Department in the Civil War

Also by Guy R. Hasegawa
and from McFarland

The Confederate Navy Medical Corps: Organization, Personnel and Actions (2024)

The U.S. Navy Medical Department in the Civil War

GUY R. HASEGAWA

Foreword by
Neil P. Chatelain

McFarland & Company, Inc., Publishers
Jefferson, North Carolina

Library of Congress Cataloging-in-Publication Data

Names: Hasegawa, Guy R. author | Chatelain, Neil P. writer of foreword
Title: The U.S. Navy Medical Department in the Civil War / Guy R. Hasegawa ; foreword by Neil P. Chatelain.
Other titles: United States Navy Medical Department in the Civil War
Description: Jefferson, North Carolina : McFarland & Company, Inc., Publishers, 2026 | Includes bibliographical references and index.
Identifiers: LCCN 2026016807 | ISBN 9781476658735 paperback ♾ ISBN 9798368601441 ebook
Subjects: LCSH: United States—History—Civil War, 1861-1865—Medical care | United States—History—Civil War, 1861-1865—Health aspects | United States. Navy Department. Bureau of Medicine and Surgery—History—19th century | BISAC: HISTORY / United States / Civil War Period (1850-1877) | MEDICAL / History
Classification: LCC E621 .H339 2026 | DDC 973.775—dc23/eng/20260430
LC record available at https://lccn.loc.gov/2026016807

ISBN (print) 978-1-4766-5873-5
ISBN (ebook) 979-8-3686-0144-1

Front cover images: Officers associated with the temporary naval hospital in Memphis, also known as Pinkney Hospital. *Standing, left to right*: Acting Assistant Surgeon Abner Thorp and Acting Assistant Paymaster Hugh Nott. *Seated, left to right*: Assistant Surgeon Gustavus H. E. Baumgarten, Surgeon William Grier, and Acting Assistant Surgeon Joseph B. Parker (Naval History and Heritage Command, Washington, DC [NHHC], image NH 53388). Naval hospital ship *Red Rover*, which served on the Mississippi River. The vessel's chief medical officer was Acting Assistant Surgeon George H. Bixby (NHHC, image NH 60501).

Printed in the United States of America

McFarland & Company, Inc., Publishers
Box 611, Jefferson, North Carolina 28640
www.mcfarlandpub.com

Contents

Foreword

Neil P. Chatelain

On October 22, 1861, Andrew A. Henderson, the surgeon assigned to the United States steam-sloop *Richmond*, sat in his small cabin to compose a letter. He was a career officer, having spent years at sea, including duty during the United States war with Mexico and long cruises to the far sides of the world. When not treating the sick or healing the injured, Henderson avidly collected flora and birds, a regular naturalist in the style of Charles Darwin or Patrick O'Brian's character Stephen Maturin. Taking pen in hand, Henderson gathered his thoughts, knowing that the words he put to paper would end the career of his commanding officer, Captain John Pope.

Richmond, and other ships blockading the Mississippi River, had recently suffered an embarrassing defeat at the Battle of the Head of Passes. This boosted Confederate morale and made the Federal blockade of the Mississippi River more precarious. Pope commanded blockading forces in that fleet action, which saw his ship run aground under enemy fire. The battle, during which Henderson stood ready with instruments laid out and sand poured on the deck to prevent slipping while treating wounded sailors, stretched Pope to the breaking point. Both the captain and surgeon agreed that Pope needed to return north, relinquishing command of *Richmond* in the process.

Henderson's letter, written to the Gulf Squadron commander, Flag Officer William W. McKean, detailed how Pope had a "slow and weak pulse" and "had vertigo," "could sleep but little," and "had no appetite." More alarmingly, Henderson noted Pope had "inertness of mind" and was "suffering from nervous exhaustion," causing "mental anxiety and loss of sleep." The symptoms hinted that Pope was suffering from post-traumatic stress and was on the verge of a mental breakdown that was further inflaming an "affection of the liver," which had developed years before while he cruised China's coastline.[1] The letter had its effect, and Pope was supplanted, returning north to never hold another command again. The surgeon's signature had essentially brought a 45-year career to a halt.

Henderson's letter demonstrates the vast array of responsibilities that U.S. Navy medical officers had to contend with during the Civil War. Surgeons and surgeons' stewards held a plethora of duties that each required different skills and competencies. Service afloat was most common and brought forth numerous responsibilities, often when no other medical expert was present, and support could be miles—or thousands of miles—away. Treating the wounded amidst raging battles put medical officers to the test, caring for sailors and Marines while waiting for an enemy shell to smash the hull and launch fragments and splinters into the room where they operated. They also handled noncombat injuries and treated illnesses, both physical and mental, while spending multiple continuous years at sea.

Ashore, surgeons maintained hospitals, where they treated those severely sick and injured. They inspected new recruits for fitness, ensuring they could handle arduous duties at sea, and they saw that applicants for admission to the U.S. Naval Academy were medically qualified. Medical officers also procured the needed medicines and supplies to keep everyone fit to fight and evaluated one another for appointments and promotions.

The growing blockade and expanding Federal naval forces created a consistent need for more doctors who could adjust to the rigors of sea life while treating patients. The antebellum service was minuscule compared with the wartime navy, and as such, hundreds of medical officers were needed to man ships deployed on waters within and surrounding the continent, and indeed the globe. Efforts paid off, and surgeons and stewards volunteered to fill gaps and keep ships operating. Without these medical personnel, many ships would have been unable to remain on station for prolonged periods, especially in the humid Gulf and the tropics amidst disease-prone summers. The Anaconda Plan itself was at stake, and these surgeons and their enlisted counterparts ably did their part to keep the Federal navy on station, properly manned, and ready to fight.

Much was at stake for these surgeons and stewards beyond their reputations as medical practitioners. Lives, and careers, could be saved or lost based on their treatments, prescriptions, methodology, and recommendations. Few naval officers not commanding their own ship at sea held as much sway as senior-ranking surgeons, who throughout the war continued fighting their own interdepartmental struggles for recognition and parity in rank.

Guy R. Hasegawa's *The U.S. Navy Medical Department in the Civil War* explores all these themes and more. Hasegawa details the U.S. Navy's medical corps' organizational and leadership structure, how it expanded to meet wartime needs, and how it kept supplies flowing. Included are descriptions of common and uncommon treatments and of locations where medical activity occurred, both ashore and afloat. Hasegawa's long interest in Civil War medicine and his decades of experience as a pharmacist and as an editor of a pharmacy journal combine to make him both knowledgeable in the field of Civil War medical studies and able to articulate both the statistical side of medical history and the human stories that connect each element.

Hasegawa has already written extensively on medical programs in the U.S. Civil War. His *Matchless Organization: The Confederate Army Medical Department* explored how the Confederate army built a medical program while simultaneously fighting for its own existence, and his *The Confederate Navy Medical Corps: Organization, Personnel and Actions* did the same for nascent Rebel naval forces. Now with *The U.S. Navy Medical Department in the Civil War*, that macrosurvey of wartime medical programs continues, expanding it to include explorations of how Federal medical officers and enlisted sailors kept the U.S. Navy healthy so the combat bluejackets and Marines could help crush the rebellion by manning the blockade, assaulting ports, hunting raiders, and patrolling inland rivers.

Biographies have been written about medical officers from the Civil War era. Several naval surgeons wrote their own memoirs. Letters and correspondence of others have also been preserved in archives. However, not until Hasegawa's *The U.S. Navy Medical Department in the Civil War* has there been a top-down, comprehensive exploration and analysis of the entire Federal navy's medical organization. Navalists and medical historians will find great value within, as will anyone with an interest in the naval, medical, or bureaucratic elements of the U.S. Civil War.

Neil P. Chatelain is an associate professor of history at Lone Star College–North Harris; historian for Emerging Civil War; and author of Treasure and Empire in the Civil War: The Panamá Route, the West and the Campaigns to Control America's Mineral Wealth *(McFarland, 2024).*

Preface

Among the vast literature on the fighting forces of the American Civil War, the largest portion is naturally devoted to the armies. The navies receive a fair amount of attention, but descriptions of naval medical care are relatively uncommon. Modern histories offer occasional summaries of medical activities, and there are letters, journals, or reminiscences of persons who provided care during the war. As a rule, participants' accounts describe activities that were not medically focused, such as blockade duty, shore excursions, and interactions with crewmates—understandably so, since naval life was new to so many of them. The organization of medical care has not been described in detail, even though such information would provide useful context for understanding other aspects of naval activity.

The publication of my book *The Confederate Navy Medical Corps: Organization, Personnel and Actions* (McFarland, 2024) was one step toward addressing that situation. Now, in *The U.S. Navy Medical Department in the Civil War,* I have tried to provide a behind-the-scenes look at medical care in the Union navy—how and why things were done as they were, who determined the course of action, and so forth. Not only does this book examine decision-making at the headquarters of the Bureau of Medicine and Surgery (BUMED) in Washington, but it also describes the activities of medical officers and their assistants, since an appreciation of the entire medical hierarchy aids in understanding any of its particular levels. Because BUMED did not operate in isolation, *The U.S. Navy Medical Department in the Civil War* also discusses how the bureau interacted with the secretary of the navy, with the Navy Department's other divisions, and with the army. My hope is that this book will give readers more perspective than is currently available about the Union navy's medical activities and furnish researchers with a springboard for further investigation.

This book is presented thematically, rather than strictly chronologically, to facilitate understanding. The latter approach would have been problematic because many factors of importance to the medical department, some of them having diverse reasons and implications, could be in play at the same time. The necessary explanations would have been distracting and disruptive to readers' train of thought. The thematic approach, however, necessitates some redundancy, because certain events were relevant to more than one theme and bear repeated mention.

To provide a book of reasonable length, I have included only as much background information about the naval war as I believe necessary for adequate understanding. Readers desiring additional context are referred to the numerous fine histories of the Civil War and the war's navies. With rare exceptions, I have not compared the medical services of the Union navy with those of the Union army or the Confederate navy or army. Such comparisons would undoubtedly be interesting, but any one of them would be a considerable undertaking. Because of the vast differences among the organizations in their missions and available resources, the comparisons would likely be of an apples-to-oranges nature.

There were other federal entities with men serving at sea, such as the U.S. Coast Survey and the Revenue Cutter Service, both under the direction of the U.S. Treasury Department. Although the organizations cooperated with the navy, the medical aspects of those relationships are not described here.

My desire to understand the workings of the medical department as a whole led me to rely heavily on its management by the wartime chief of BUMED, Surgeon William Whelan. BUMED's records at the National Archives and Records Administration (NARA) in Washington, D.C., were particularly helpful, with the most important being letters received and sent by the bureau. Whelan's letters were especially enlightening because of the precision of his wording and the full explanations that he offered. I was assisted by the online availability of some NARA records originating from BUMED and other naval divisions. Also available online, and of immense importance, were the annual reports of BUMED, including those of the years immediately after the war, and the Navy Department's registers of officers for the Civil War era.

I am not aware of a diary or collection of private letters left by Whelan. Although such a source might have provided further insight into his behavior or his personal views of naval medical matters, he does not appear to have been an enigmatic figure. Whelan's candid opinions sometimes appear in correspondence and memoranda kept by BUMED, and from all indications, his official actions were rarely, if ever, influenced by anything other than a commitment to leadership and duty.

There is still much to be learned about Union naval medicine, and there is probably enough archival material available for in-depth investigations of many topics in this book, such as volunteer medical officers, surgeons' stewards, and temporary hospitals. My intention in this work is to strike a balance between presenting a useful and readable big-picture view and including enough detail to convey a sense of the complexity of issues. For future researchers enticed by any of those issues, this book's thorough documentation of sources should prove a good starting point.

I am grateful for the generosity of numerous associates and experts. Among the most helpful was Gary McQuarrie, PharmD, MBA, who encouraged my interest in the Civil War navies, provided valuable advice throughout the project, and commented on the book's manuscript. Neil P. Chatelain, who teaches history at Lone Star College–North Harris and works with Emerging Civil War, also critiqued the manuscript and honored me by contributing the foreword. Experts in Civil War medicine who reviewed all or part of the manuscript or provided valuable information or advice include Jonathan O'Neal, MD; F. Terry Hambrecht, MD; Bruce A. Evans, MD; and Kevin M. Bair, MA and PhD candidate. Staff members at NARA were always helpful in helping me find the materials I needed. I am grateful to McFarland and editor Elizabeth Foxwell for seeing the value in this project and guiding it through publication.

My wife, Betsy, first urged me about 30 years ago to become involved in Civil War medicine. None of my efforts in the field would have occurred without her constant support and without the encouragement of our sons, David and Stephen.

Introduction

IN LATE 1861, WITH THE CIVIL WAR not even a year old, U.S. Secretary of the Navy Gideon Welles described the duty that lay ahead of the navy as "more arduous, it is believed, in some respects, than has before been demanded from the maritime power of any government." Indeed, what had already started, and would continue, was a huge augmentation of naval personnel, vessels, and responsibility. That growth, said Welles after the war, took place in a "navy reduced during fifty years of peace to a low standard of efficiency." Between the commencement and end of the war, the number of men serving in the U.S. Navy (USN) grew from 7,600 to 51,500, and the number of vessels increased from 42 to nearly 700, including those under construction.[1]

The tasks described by Welles affected all of the navy's administrative divisions, including the Bureau of Medicine and Surgery (BUMED), which was responsible for all aspects of medical care for naval personnel, including Marines. The navy's health was vitally important to its mission. A flag officer might have vessels at his disposal to perform a certain assignment, but he still needed enough healthy men to operate them. Even with fairly intact crews, illness or injury of key officers could seriously impair efficiency. Throughout history, many more men in the armed services had died from disease than from combat injuries. Unhealthy sailors would not only reduce the navy's fighting effectiveness, but their care would also consume time and resources.[2]

Having more sailors, with the potential for large numbers of sick and wounded, meant that many more medical officers would be needed, but recruiting them was not as simple as printing announcements and waiting for responses. The USN had a long tradition of requiring that candidates for the medical corps pass a rigorous examination, which was meant to ensure that sailors received a high quality of care. Unfortunately, the inducements to join the medical corps, in salary and prestige, were not such as to ensure a rush of applicants, let alone those who would prove qualified. Furthermore, a large number of USN medical officers left the service to join the Confederate navy, so BUMED faced a deficit of officers in addition to a need to augment its rolls well beyond prewar levels. Newly recruited medical officers would, for the most part, have limited clinical experience and be unaccustomed to navy practices. They were likely to be thrown into situations they could not have imagined.

Also required were more enlisted men to serve as surgeons' stewards (assistants to medical officers) and nurses, who could markedly improve the efficiency and availability of care. Efforts were required to enhance the compensation for such individuals because qualified men were not easy to find and retain.

By May 1861, the Pensacola and Norfolk Naval Hospitals had been captured by Confederate forces, a setback that left the USN with no hospitals in the South. The bulk of Union naval personnel served in blockading squadrons patrolling the Confederate coastline, or on rivers, particularly the Mississippi. Not all sailors needing hospital care could be easily or quickly transported to a naval facility in the North, so expedients, such as establishing temporary hospitals in Union-controlled portions of seceding states, were needed.

The formation and operation of new naval squadrons would present BUMED with administrative, supply, and other concerns. The units of primary concern were known through most of the war as the North Atlantic Blockading Squadron (NABS), South Atlantic Blockading Squadron (SABS), East (or Eastern) Gulf Blockading Squadron (EGBS), West (or Western) Gulf Blockading Squadron (WGBS), and the Mississippi Squadron (or Mississippi River Squadron). Medical officers and enlisted assistants had to be distributed among the squadrons, and new models of supply had to be improvised. The urgency of some needs and the impossibility of quick communication with BUMED headquarters in Washington forced the senior medical officers of squadrons, called fleet surgeons, to make on-the-spot decisions that might not, in normal times, be allowed. Granting such responsibility required faith in those officers' judgment and BUMED's willingness to be something other than an all-controlling entity.

Although BUMED had a robust and centralized prewar medical-supply system, it faced the task of obtaining adequate stores of medicines, instruments, and other necessities for a vastly expanded navy and transporting them where needed. The wide distribution of forces, their frequently critical need for supplies, and the inconvenient presence of the enemy pointed to the need for flexibility in the stockpiling and delivery of medical goods.

Certain types of naval service—such as blockade duty and

patrolling rivers—and the introduction of ironclad vessels came with their particular mix of illnesses. Medical officers had to seek ways to mitigate the problems through alerting their superiors about their concerns, improving the environment in which sailors served, and other means.

The navy, whose size and expenditures were dwarfed by those of the army, seemed to draw relatively little attention from federal lawmakers. Nevertheless, dealing with legislators regarding actions that might affect medical personnel and the public good was part of the job of BUMED's chief and required persistence, tact, and political acumen.

Handling such issues required sound decision-making on the part of BUMED and its medical officers. It necessitated that BUMED act to optimize its own performance, maintain a healthy and cooperative relationship with the secretary of the navy, collaborate with other naval bureaus and government departments, and exercise leadership in steering medical officers—those with command authority and novices alike—toward a course most advantageous to patients, the bureau, the navy, and the war effort. How the USN medical department, led by Surgeon William Whelan and comprising medical officers and their enlisted assistants, dealt with the many challenges before it is examined here.

Chapter 1

The Bureau of Medicine and Surgery

At the beginning of the Civil War, the Navy Department's administrative structure included the Office of the Secretary of the Navy, Marine Corps headquarters, and five bureaus established in 1842: the Bureau of Yards and Docks; Bureau of Construction, Equipment, and Repairs; Bureau of Provisions and Clothing; Bureau of Ordnance and Hydrography; and BUMED. The chief of each bureau was appointed by the president, with Senate approval, to serve an indefinite term.[1]

BUMED was charged with the "general control of every thing relating to the treatment of the sick and wounded of the navy, whether at hospitals, navy yards, or on board of public vessels." Included in that charge were medical personnel, including attendants, and medical and surgical supplies. The bureau was to "keep a record of the services of all medical officers, and to nominate them for duty of every description." The actual duty assignments were made, in consultation with BUMED, by the Office of Detail within the Office of the Secretary of the Navy. Official communications between medical officers and the Navy Department were to be routed through BUMED.[2]

Surgeon William Whelan served as BUMED chief throughout the Civil War. Whelan, who was born in Philadelphia in 1808, graduated as a doctor of medicine from the University of Pennsylvania in 1828 and was commissioned as surgeon's mate (assistant surgeon) in the USN on March 25, 1828, to date from January 3 of that year. He was promoted to surgeon in 1837 and served at various hospitals and twice as fleet surgeon of the Mediterranean Squadron.[3]

Whelan evidently assumed the role of BUMED chief in September 1853 but was officially nominated by President Franklin Pierce in December of that year and confirmed by the Senate in January 1854. At the time, a common expectation would have been for such a position—comparable to that of army surgeon general—to be filled by the officer with the most seniority. In fact, the two most senior naval surgeons, William P.C. Barton and Thomas Harris, had already served in the role before Whelan, and many of the other senior officers were sickly or otherwise unfit to serve. When nominated by Pierce, Whelan—who was about 22 and 24 years younger than Barton and Harris, respectively—stood 25th in seniority among 69 surgeons yet still boasted a quarter century of naval service.[4]

Less than two years into his term, in late August 1855, Whelan was riding in a train that derailed, with one of the cars running completely through and killing most of the occupants of the next car. He was among about 70 injured passengers. According to one account, Whelan never completely recovered from the severe injury he sustained, yet his official correspondence reveals no hint that the accident impaired his ability to work.[5]

When the number of naval bureaus was increased in 1862, President Abraham Lincoln renominated Whelan, certainly at the suggestion of Secretary of the Navy Gideon Welles, for the post of BUMED chief for a term of four additional years. After Senate confirmation, Whelan expressed to Welles his sincere appreciation for the Navy Department's "renewed manifestation of its confidence." At that time, Whelan ranked sixth in seniority among 80 surgeons. Throughout all or most of his service as BUMED chief, Whelan lived in Washington, D.C., with his wife, Adeline, and their five children: Ellen, William, Mary, Frances, and Albert.[6]

Whelan's years of service accounted for his acquaintance with many senior line officers. In June 1863, when Rear Admiral Andrew Hull Foote was dying of kidney disease in New York, Secretary Welles sent Whelan there to comfort him. Whelan, wrote Welles, was "an old and intimate friend and shipmate of Foote ... has been his daily companion for years in different climes.... His presence, even, will be cheering and pleasant to Foote." The rear admiral died a few days after Whelan's arrival; up to that time, Whelan had kept Welles updated by telegram on Foote's condition.[7]

Starting in 1842, the bureau was allowed a staff (other than the chief) of one assistant surgeon, two clerks, and a messenger. At the time, passed assistant surgeons—assistant surgeons who had passed an examination qualifying them for promotion to surgeon—were considered a subset of assistant surgeons, and for most or all of the time between 1842 and the Civil War, the bureau's assistant-surgeon position was indeed filled by a passed assistant surgeon. In 1853, the position came to be called that of a "class number four" clerk, and appropriations legislation ceased referring to BUMED's assistant surgeon.[8]

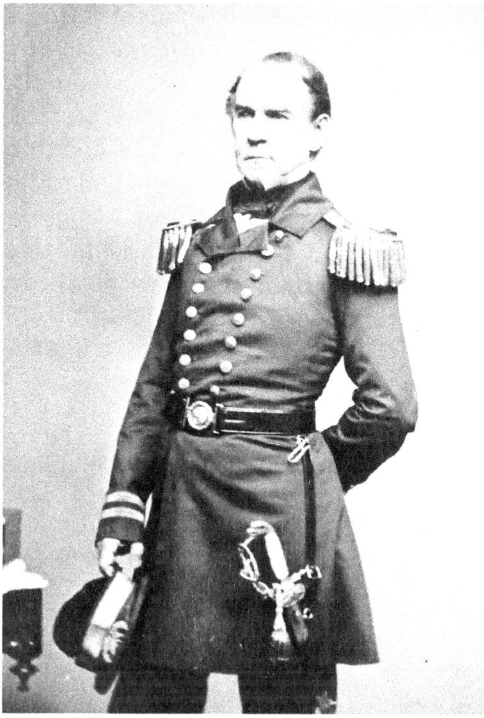

Surgeon William Whelan, chief of BUMED from 1853 until his death in 1865. His uniform reflects regulations in effect during the first 15 months of the Civil War (Library of Congress, control no. 2011647850).

Starting in mid–1859, that spot was occupied by Passed Assistant Surgeon Phineas J. Horwitz, who was promoted to surgeon in April 1861. Fearing that Horwitz's promotion would result in his being transferred out of the BUMED office, Whelan asked Secretary Welles to keep him there on "temporary special duty" because of the difficulty of finding a replacement and of "the greater importance of his services amid our pressure of business than those of an inexperienced officer." In mid–1862, the secretary of the navy was authorized to transfer clerks from one bureau to another and to detail a commissioned medical officer of any grade to the bureau. That legislation seems to have resulted in Horwitz being the detailed officer, which removed any question about his continuing to assist the bureau chief. Horwitz, who had been in the navy since 1847, served in the BUMED office throughout the war as did clerks Chester Tuttle and Wythe Denby and messenger March B. Clark. With the possible exception of a civilian laborer, the office's staff never numbered more than five throughout the war.[9]

Whelan was proud of his staff's ability to handle great quantities of paperwork despite his never being given, or asking for, additional office personnel. For the first nine months of 1864, he estimated that this office wrote close to 9,000 letters, each of which was copied twice—once in a letterpress book, and once transcribed by hand into a ledger—and received about 8,000 letters, each of which was classified and filed. (In the letterpress copy method, a freshly written letter, with damp ink, was inserted between translucent pages in a bound book. When the book was pressed, some of the letter's ink was transferred to the page that had been on top of the letter. Although the copy was a mirror-image, it could be read from the opposite side of the page because of its translucency.) There were also several thousand reports, requisitions, bills, and vouchers to record, tabulate, or otherwise handle, plus communications from the Pension Office.[10]

BUMED's office staff spent considerable time dealing with incorrectly prepared paperwork submitted by medical officers. Documents from officers serving in squadrons were usually gathered by their fleet surgeon, who checked them before submitting them to the BUMED office. Fleet Surgeon George Clymer of the SABS described his experience:

> I have spared no pains to collect the returns from the medical officers of the squadron in order that I might forward them promptly to the Bureau. But, with few exceptions, they have come to me so defective that I have returned them and rereturned them for correction. Directions the most explicit, and reiterated, in the Book of Instructions [the Navy Department's *Instructions for the Government of Medical Officers*] appear to have been unheeded, and I have made it my especial duty to tutor the young medical officers in their duties in this respect; and I wish that I could say that the necessity for this tutoring had been limited to the volunteer element in our corps [acting assistant surgeons], that portion of which, being only temporarily connected with the service, might perhaps (if any might) be excused for indifference to its forms.[11]

Clymer urged that acquaintance with all the *Instructions*' forms and directions be evaluated in the examination for promotion of assistant surgeons. Such familiarity, in fact, was already a stated requirement for passing that examination. Whelan agreed with Clymer and explained, "The correspondence of the office is vastly increased by the inattention of the young officers to the subjects to which you invite attention; and tho' letters are daily written, explanatory of errors, in the hope of making the system more intelligible, we are very unsuccessful in reducing our labor." Whelan patiently explained to one acting assistant surgeon the defects in his report and suggested, "You might confer with some Surgeon in the Navy who will take pleasure in giving you any requisite information."[12]

Young officers were not alone in creating paperwork problems. Whelan reminded Fleet Surgeon Ninian Pinkney of the Mississippi Squadron that he had failed to respond to three requests to submit quarterly reports of sick, without which Whelan could not complete his annual report to the secretary of the navy.[13]

Managing paperwork was problematic enough, but Whelan had

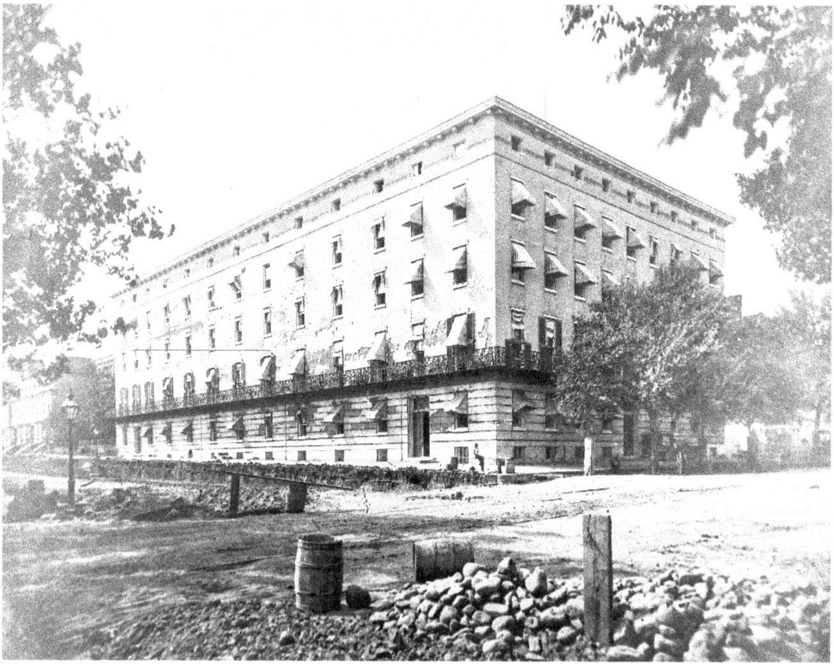

The Winder Building in Washington, D.C., photographed during the Civil War era. The structure housed the BUMED office and was across the street from most other Navy Department offices (Library of Congress, control no. 2005687014).

manifold other concerns. They included recruiting new medical officers, making officers' assignments, establishing new hospitals, obtaining and distributing medicines and other supplies, and generally improvising ways to handle issues that arose in a greatly expanded navy that was performing unfamiliar roles while dispersed over a large geographic range. Indeed, the charge of controlling everything related to the care of the navy's sick and wounded was a huge responsibility, especially for Whelan's meager staff.

BUMED's office was in the Winder Building, at the northwest corner of 17th and F streets NW, in Washington, D.C. Office hours, as dictated by Secretary Welles, were from nine o'clock to four o'clock, with no absences permitted unless approved by Whelan. No person, unless on public service, was permitted in the office, and clerks behind in their assignments were required to work after hours until they were done. Most or all of the other Navy Department offices were across the street in the Navy Department building, which itself was just south of the War Department building. All three structures were just outside the western boundary of the White House grounds. The Winder Building still stands and currently houses the Office of the U.S. Trade Representative.[14]

For BUMED to succeed, it had to operate efficiently and exhibit flexibility in managing new situations. That challenge would test Whelan's leadership and the resourcefulness of the navy's medical officers. Having enough such officers, with the requisite skills, was a concern throughout the war.

Chapter 2

Commissioned Medical Officers

At the commencement of the Civil War, the USN had three grades of commissioned medical officer: assistant surgeon, passed assistant surgeon, and surgeon. Commissioned medical officers—or simply *medical officers*—were those nominated by the president and confirmed by the Senate. The title of surgeon of the fleet (or fleet surgeon) was assumed by the commanding medical officer of a squadron, usually or always the most senior, while he held that position and was not a separate grade per se. Men entered the service as assistant surgeons and were eligible, after two years of sea service, to be examined for suitability for promotion to surgeon. Satisfactory performance on the examination carried with it a promotion to passed assistant surgeon, an internal process that did not involve the president or Senate. When an opening occurred at the grade of surgeon, a passed assistant surgeon was promoted—subject to presidential nomination and Senate confirmation—to full surgeon. (Army and navy physicians were often called *surgeons* collectively, without regard to grade or whether they performed surgical procedures. The term *full surgeon* is used here when necessary to distinguish men at the grade of surgeon from assistant or passed assistant surgeons.)[1]

Grade indicated a tier in the army or navy hierarchy and was indicated by a title such as captain, lieutenant, or assistant surgeon. *Rank*, on the other hand, referred to an officer's standing in relation to other officers. Because the grade of surgeon was higher than that of assistant surgeon, all surgeons outranked all assistant surgeons. Within a grade, however, rank was determined by seniority, the date of appointment to that grade. For assistant surgeons appointed on the same date—a common occurrence during the war—rank was determined by their score on the admission examination. The highest-ranking officer in a grade was typically entitled to be the first promoted to the next-higher grade or appointed to a prestigious posting. If two officers of the same grade served at the same post, the higher-ranking one would take precedence in the command structure. In informal contexts, *rank* was often used to mean *grade*, so a man could say that he held the rank of assistant surgeon. He could also be more specific by saying that his rank was, say, 12th among 100 assistant surgeons.

The allowed number of surgeons and assistant surgeons (including passed assistant surgeons) was established by law. If all of the allowed slots at the grade of surgeon were filled, a passed assistant surgeon could not be promoted until a surgeon died, resigned, or was dismissed. Although promotion was traditionally granted to the highest-ranking officer within a grade, an officer's poor performance or other impediment could result in his being bypassed for promotion by lower-ranking officers at his grade.[2]

Officers who were elderly or infirm—and presumably incapable of performing expected tasks, especially during duty afloat—accumulated among the longest-serving surgeons and passed assistant surgeons, and there was no effective way to remove them. This situation put more responsibility on younger and healthier officers and, at the same time, made promotion to surgeon agonizingly slow. In January 1861, the five highest-ranking surgeons had been at that grade for at least 25 years, and the five lowest-ranking surgeons had served in the navy for at least 13 years before attaining that grade.[3]

There was no limit specified for the number of passed assistant surgeons other than that assigned for assistant and passed assistant surgeons combined. Thus, if there were enough passed assistant surgeons to fill the number of openings thought to be imminent among surgeons—usually the case before the war—then, as long as the examination was passed, promotion to passed assistant surgeon, with its higher salary, might simply be a reward for faithful service. Prewar opportunities for promotion to passed assistant surgeon were far from automatic after two years of sea service, a qualification held in January 1861 by more than half of assistant surgeons. Those men would await an order from the Navy Department to appear for the examination. Failure to present oneself before an examining board, in the absence of an acceptable explanation, or performing poorly enough on the examination to be deemed "not qualified" by the board, resulted in the officer being dropped from the rolls of naval officers. Reexamination of assistant surgeons who failed the promotion examination was not allowed, but BUMED's practice was to allow those officers to resign rather than face the humiliation of "the more stringent decision of the department" (dismissal).[4]

The number of young men allowed to become assistant surgeons during a year approximated the number of slots—typically 10 or fewer before the war—anticipated to open among surgeons, passed assistant surgeons, and assistant surgeons. Eight, 10, and 5 men were appointed assistant surgeon in 1858, 1859, and 1860, respectively.[5]

Legislation enacted in August 1842 capped the number of medical officers to the number serving on January 1 of that year. For surgeons, the limit was 69, which was in effect and generally met until changed by legislation enacted in July 1861. For assistant and passed assistant surgeons combined, the cap, which was originally 65 or 67 (depending on the source), somehow became 80 by 1848, where it remained—and was generally met—until July 1861.[6]

Increasing the Number and Efficiency of Medical Officers

Although the BUMED chief consistently asked, without success, for more medical officers in the years leading up to the war, the secession crisis and outbreak of hostilities forced actions to bolster the medical corps' manpower. Not only were more medical officers needed to staff the numerous vessels being acquired by the navy and to care for new enlistees, the Navy Department in 1861 accepted the resignation of or dismissed 38 medical officers, 34 of whom joined the medical service of the Confederate States Navy. (Starting in spring 1861, dismissal, which implied shame, was commonly applied to officers thought to have Southern sympathies who tendered their resignation or refused to sign a loyalty oath.) That loss amounted to about a quarter of medical officers on the rolls. The effort to augment the USN's medical officer corps, in number and efficiency, took various forms. One followed BUMED chief Whelan's June 16, 1861, suggestion to Secretary Welles to raise the allowed limits on numbers of medical officers to 80 surgeons and 120 assistant and passed assistant surgeons, a total increase of 51 men over the current limits of 69 and 80 officers at those grades. Legislation enabling that change was enacted on July 31, 1861.[7]

Another step, allowed by three pieces of 1861 legislation, was to remove selected officers from the line of promotion—and cease including them in the numerical limits—by relegating them to a "retired list." That process created vacancies among the ranks of remaining officers, who were said to be on the "active list." Officers eligible for the retired list included those who were proved "permanently incapable, from physical or mental infirmity, of further services at sea" (act of February 21), those with 40 years of naval service who requested placement on the list or those found to be incapable of performing the duties of their office

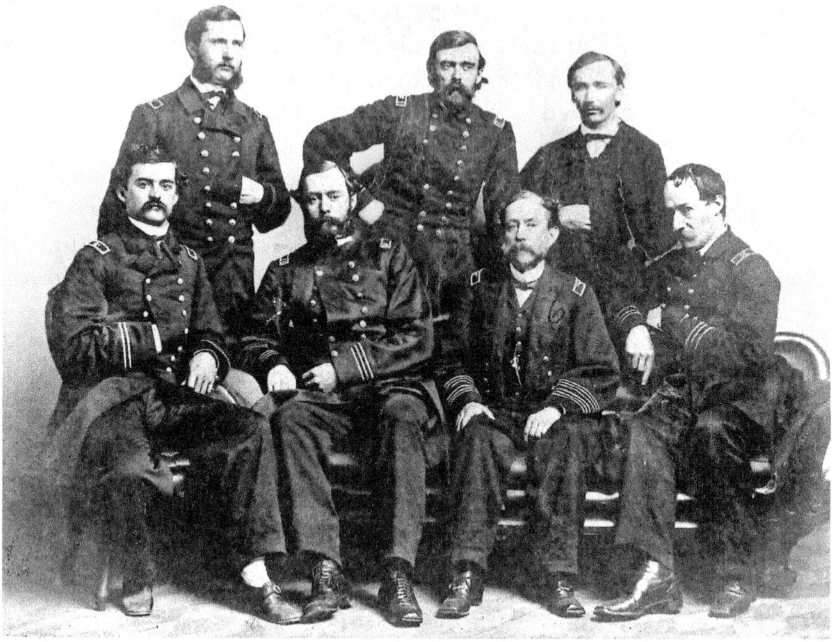

Officers of the Mississippi Squadron, probably in late 1864 or early 1865, including various grades of regular and volunteer medical officers. Standing, from left: Acting Assistant Surgeon Jacob F. Field, Acting Assistant Paymaster Alexander W. Pearson, and George Lawrence (not further identified). Seated, from left: Acting Assistant Surgeon George H. Bixby, Passed Assistant Surgeon James S. Knight, Fleet Surgeon Ninian Pinkney, and Passed Assistant Surgeon Michael Bradley (Naval History and Heritage Command, Washington, D.C. [NHHC], image NH 45613).

(act of August 3), and those with 45 years of naval service or who had reached the age of 62 years (act of December 21). Officers affected by the December 21 act could be assigned to shore duty at full shore pay; otherwise, placement on the retired list carried reduced pay. Determination of inability to perform one's duties was made by a board of five to nine officers, two-fifths of whom were medical officers.[8]

The first medical officer to be retired, on April 25, 1861, was Surgeon William Swift, who requested that distinction on the grounds of physical infirmity. Swift, a veteran of the War of 1812, was in his 83rd year, "which alone," remarked Whelan, "would permanently disqualify him for active service, if to it were not superadded many of the infirmities incident to longevity."[9]

Whelan was quick, in communications dated as early as March 11, 1861, to suggest other candidates for the retired list. Officers suffering from debility were present not only among full surgeons. Whelan informed Secretary Welles in April 1861 of two passed assistant surgeons "whose mental, or physical, disqualifications for service of any description, are so manifest as to render them proper subjects for the Retired List." Whelan reported that John B. Elliott, a passed assistant surgeon since 1836, "is now, and has been, insane for more than 20 years." Passed Assistant Surgeon Frederick Horner, Jr., had also been considered insane for the past eight years. Both men resided at the Government Hospital for the Insane in the District of Columbia. Edward H. Van Wyck, an assistant surgeon since 1838, sustained an attack of paralysis that year, had been unable to perform duty of any kind since then, and was considered incurable. All three, and others, were retired because of infirmity. By the end of 1861, 14 medical officers had been retired for physical or mental incapacity, with 2 of them subsequently joining the Confederate States Navy after resigning or being dismissed from the USN. By January 1, 1865, 19 surgeons, 6 passed assistant surgeons, and 5 assistant surgeons had been placed on the retired list. At least 5 of those officers would have been removed from the active list for another reason—resignation, dismissal, or death—before that date. Whelan himself remained on the active list, in spite of contending with chronic "pain and debility" from the 1855 train accident.[10]

The allowance of 51 more medical officers, plus additional wartime openings in the active list—created by resignation, dismissal, death, or placement on the retired list—accounted for vacancies to be filled, after promotions, through more active recruitment of men to be assistant surgeons. Those additions numbered 48 in 1861, 73 in 1862, 17 in 1863, and 17 in 1864 and failed at times to fill all of the available slots, especially in the latter part of the war (Appendix A). Whelan found the late-war shortage of assistant-surgeon applicants alarming and advocated for higher pay and rank for such officers to attract good applicants. On the other hand, starting in late 1862 and extending through the war, the new limit for full surgeons was filled because there were enough passed assistant surgeons—or assistant surgeons, with the requisite sea duty, who could be quickly examined—waiting for vacancies to occur. Progression from civilian life to full surgeon was, for some men, drastically shortened. It was not unusual before the war for that process to take more than 20 years, but on January 1, 1864, the newest surgeon had been in the navy for only 30 months. At least four assistant surgeons—Jonathan C. Bertolette, Benjamin F. Gibbs, William M. King, and Thomas W. Leach—passed the surgeons' examination in May 1862. About four weeks later, the Senate confirmed their promotion to full surgeon, retroactive to the date of passing the examination. (It was common for the

Senate to confirm promotions long after officers assumed duties and began receiving salaries associated with those promotions.) Thus, those men appear never to have held the intermediate grade of passed assistant surgeon.[11]

Appointments in the Volunteer Navy

Addressing the medical-manpower shortage by hiring a large number of civilian physicians was apparently never considered. Such employees might have been assigned to hospitals ashore and freed naval surgeons for duty elsewhere. Although there may have been rare instances of private physicians assisting in temporary hospitals during emergencies, large-scale employment of civilian doctors, even those deemed medically qualified, would have been disruptive. Their likely failure to adapt quickly to naval regulations, discipline, and accountability would have been especially problematic at sea, where additional physicians were most needed and where replacing unsatisfactory performers was most difficult.

The most effective means of increasing the number of medical officers was appointing temporary or volunteer assistant surgeons—officially called "acting assistant surgeons"—an action initially taken as a necessity and without direct authorization of law. The USN also appointed volunteer (acting) line officers and nonmedical staff officers (acting engineers and acting paymasters). Men applying for appointment as an acting assistant surgeon underwent an expedited and much less stringent examination than those hoping to enter the regular or permanent medical corps. (In Whelan's parlance, *medical corps* usually referred to officers in the regular or permanent navy only. *Medical department* could refer to BUMED or to all naval medical personnel, whether regular or volunteer.) Acting assistant surgeons were originally envisioned as serving on vessels chartered or purchased by the USN. Such appointments, which began in May 1861, were ratified and confirmed by legislation enacted on July 24, 1861, and were to be in effect until the vessels employing the appointees returned from cruises or until "the suppression of the present insurrection." The temporary officers were considered, for the sake of classification, to be commissioned, even though individual presidential nomination and Senate confirmation were lacking. By January 1, 1865, the so-called volunteer or temporary navy had welcomed at least 426 acting assistant surgeons, who received the same pay as their regular-navy counterparts, although only 245 were serving on that date. In comparison, 159 assistant surgeons were appointed in the regular navy in 1861 through 1864. Losses among acting assistant surgeons before 1865 were most commonly due to resignation, although 26 had died and 31 had received appointments as assistant surgeons in the regular navy.[12]

The status of the USN's acting assistant surgeons differed from that of men who held the identical title in the Union army or the Confederate army or navy. In those other branches, acting assistant surgeons, also known as contract surgeons, were civilians and were not considered to be commissioned officers.[13]

Interest in the USN's temporary appointments was keen in the latter part of 1861. Whelan wrote in mid–October 1861 that the Navy Department had so many applicants for acting assistant surgeon that he could not say when a new applicant might expect an appointment. The final several months of the war saw fewer appointments of acting assistant surgeons and more resignations, perhaps as potential and actual appointees sensed that the war would soon end or realized that the compensation was inadequate. In late March or early April 1865, the Navy Department, in fact, decided not to accept the resignation of any medical officer until he had served at least two years and not at all if he was under orders for duty, was currently attached to a vessel or a vessel's station, or was on his way thereto. Whelan had objected in January 1865 to such a decision because general knowledge of its implementation "would effectively estop the few applications now being made" for appointments as assistant surgeons. The department began issuing honorable discharges to acting medical officers in May 1865; the discharges numbered 129 in 1865 and 47 in 1866.[14]

Appointments of volunteer medical officers ceased shortly after the war but then resumed, a slow pace, during the first half of the 1870s. It was not until 1879 that legislation called for the 21 acting medical officers still on the rolls to be mustered out or transferred to the regular navy. Of those 21 men, 8 had originally been appointed during the war, and 6 of those 8 had left the service and were reappointed during the 1870s. The other 2 were Francis V. Greene, who entered the volunteer service in December 1862 and was promoted to acting passed assistant surgeon in August 1865, and Isaiah Dewling, who became an acting assistant surgeon in May 1864. Those two men served continuously until placed on the retired list in June 1879 as officers in the regular navy—Greene as a passed assistant surgeon, and Dewling as an assistant surgeon—as allowed by the 1879 legislation.[15]

Secretary Welles conceded that some temporary appointments—not just those of medical officers—had probably resulted from "improper recommendations" and that some men who were commendable in other traits had "been found addicted to intemperance," a habit considered "a disqualification in any officer" and grounds for immediate dismissal. Twenty-one acting assistant surgeons had their appointments revoked before 1865, but the reasons have not been determined.[16]

BUMED chief Whelan was less than enthusiastic about using acting assistant surgeons, characterizing them as "inexperienced persons whom our necessities compel us to employ." He noted that inadequate inducements offered to potential regular-navy medical officers forced BUMED to expend "all our exertions to provide, indifferently, for the temporary service." Whelan reasoned that young physicians of the highest ability and character were not, as a rule, attracted by the meager pay and status offered by the regular or volunteer navy. That left physicians of lower professional and personal quality, who sought appointment as volunteer assistant surgeons because better-paying army or civilian positions were unavailable to them. Nevertheless, the volunteer force helped to ease Whelan's manpower problem and contributed some qualified officers to the regular medical corps. Secretary Welles, in fact, decided by mid–1864 that all assistant-surgeon vacancies in the regular navy should be filled only by capable volunteer assistant surgeons. Such candidates still had to be of the requisite age and pass the examination used for permanent-navy assistant-surgeon candidates, but they had the benefit of some naval service and were probably invited to be examined only if recommended by regular-navy colleagues. Welles likely thought that closing the regular-navy vacancies to new medical graduates would encourage those graduates to take the expedited (volunteer)

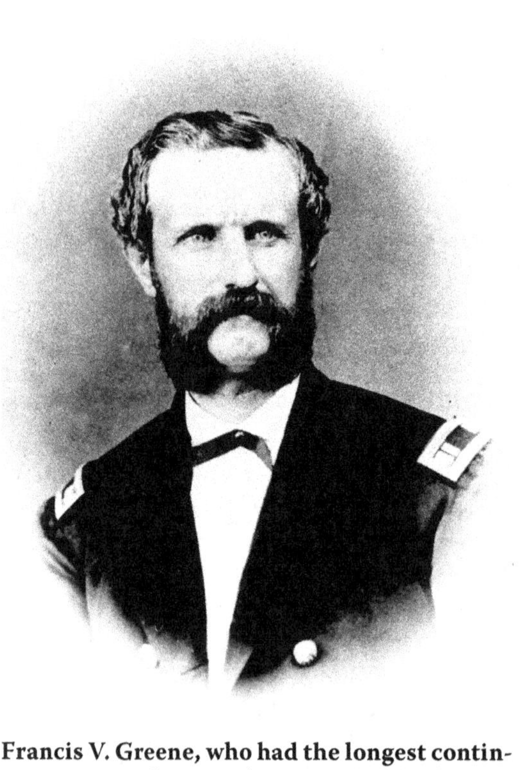

Francis V. Greene, who had the longest continuous service (1862-79) as a medical officer in the volunteer navy (NHHC, image NH 49386).

route into naval service, which would result in quicker appointments and fewer rejections. By late June 1865, the dramatic postwar downsizing of the navy made it unnecessary to admit new acting assistant surgeons, and BUMED began allowing new appointments into the regular navy only.[17]

Indeed, Whelan was grateful that volunteer medical officers could be appointed expeditiously. In 1864, when Congress was considering a bill mandating Senate confirmation of temporary appointments, he was quick to tell Representative Alexander H. Rice of Massachusetts, chairman of the House Committee on Naval Affairs, that such a requirement would slow the appointment process and hinder his ability to provide vessels with medical officers. Whether Whelan was convincing is not known, but the bill was not enacted.[18]

Despite Whelan's reservations about volunteer medical officers, he acknowledged that many were "men of much intelligence, culture, and most respectable social position" and should not be undervalued. Because the temporary appointments did not have "the advantage of permanence," he recommended in April 1864 creating an avenue for promotion, and legislation allowing the same was enacted in March 1865. Promotion would occur "in the same manner as acting assistant surgeons are now appointed." The Navy Department added the requirements that candidates for acting passed assistant surgeon could not be older than 40 years and must have accumulated two years of naval service, "except under peculiar circumstances, to be judged of by the Department." The service requirement contrasted with the two years *at sea* required for promotion of an assistant surgeon in the permanent navy, but because acting assistant surgeons spent most of their time at sea, the difference was more technical than practical.[19]

The late-war shortage of assistant surgeons in the regular navy, and the rate of resignation of regular and volunteer medical officers, prompted Whelan in March 1865 to begin encouraging volunteer officers who had served for at least two years to apply for examination for promotion to acting passed assistant surgeon or acting surgeon. A higher grade and salary, Whelan reasoned, might induce some of the best volunteer officers to remain in the navy. Only three acting assistant surgeons were promoted to acting passed assistant surgeon before May 1865. The end of the war and the rapid reduction of the naval force reduced the urgency to offer such promotions.[20]

The rapid expansion of the navy outpaced the medical department's ability to provide enough medical officers to meet the situation.

Whelan took advantage of the liberalized allowance in the number of officers and the advent of the retired list. Formation of a volunteer navy provided him with a large number of new medical officers, but he had doubts about their competence.

Chapter 3

Examinations for Appointment and Promotion of Medical Officers

The medical department had a long-standing tradition, backed by legislation, of requiring a rigid examination for appointment as an assistant surgeon and promotion to passed assistant surgeon. The professional aptitude and good character purportedly ensured by the examination process was a point of pride for the department. Examinations continued throughout the war but came to include more casual evaluations of candidates for acting assistant surgeon.

Examining Prospective Assistant Surgeons (Regular Navy)

In the years leading up to the Civil War, a medical board met yearly to examine civilian applicants for the position of assistant surgeon. The same board—which typically consisted of four surgeons, with one serving as president and the junior officer as recorder—would also examine assistant surgeons for promotion to passed assistant surgeon. During 1858–60, the board session started in early March at the Philadelphia Naval Asylum and Hospital. The time of year coincided with the usual graduation time for medical schools, and Philadelphia had two of the most prominent: Jefferson Medical College and the University of Pennsylvania. The city was also convenient to other schools in the Northeast.[1]

BUMED chief Whelan followed convention in calling for a board to meet in Philadelphia starting on March 1, 1861. That board was active for the usual duration of about two months and was dissolved on May 2, but Whelan quickly expanded the bureau's examination capacity by having another board meet at the New York Naval Hospital in Brooklyn starting on June 1, 1861; that board was not dissolved until January 26, 1862. Additional boards met in Philadelphia starting in March, August, and November 1862 and in March, September, and December 1863. With one exception, the 1862 and 1863 boards met for one to three months. The December 1863 board was not dissolved until February 1866. Whelan reported using "all sorts of publicity" about the examinations in hope of attracting candidates. Indeed, he placed announcements for the 1861 Brooklyn board in at least 10 newspapers and medical periodicals, mostly in the Northeast but including Washington (DC), Baltimore, Chicago, and Cincinnati. (Places of examination ideally had an available dispensary and hospital, in which part of the evaluation could be conducted.) At least one publication took the liberty to mention the "unprecedentedly large" number of openings available for assistant surgeons.[2]

Prewar Navy Department regulations stated that applicants for assistant surgeon could not be "under 21 or over 25 years of age." Whelan quoted that range in 1861. Whether men between their 25th and 26th birthday—being commonly considered 25 years old—were eligible was unclear; some newspapers stated that applicants must be under, or not over, 26. In 1862, Whelan began specifying the upper age as not more than 26—possibly a temporary change aimed at widening the applicant pool. In early 1863, Whelan, still quoting 26 years as the upper limit, said that the Navy Department was unlikely to expand the age range as long as vacancies were being filled, which was generally the case at that point of the war. Naval regulations, evidently established in 1864 but published in 1865, stated an upper limit of no more than 25 years.[3]

Candidates were to write the secretary of the navy for permission to be examined, state their place of residence and date and place of birth, and enclose "respectable testimonials of moral character." Whelan informed the president of a medical examining board of a standard, which had not publicized, for applicants to the medical corps: "None but American citizens by birth, or naturalization, will be received into the service." Whelan noted that many applicants were of foreign, especially German, birth or extraction. Because he did not want to discriminate, Whelan was quick to grant permission to apparently qualified men to be examined. He advised, though, against letting into the medical corps any man, regardless of his professional qualifications, whose command of English was insufficient to perform his duties "or even to such a degree as to make him an object of ridicule, instead of respect." He noted that the examination did not "embrace collegiate attainments"

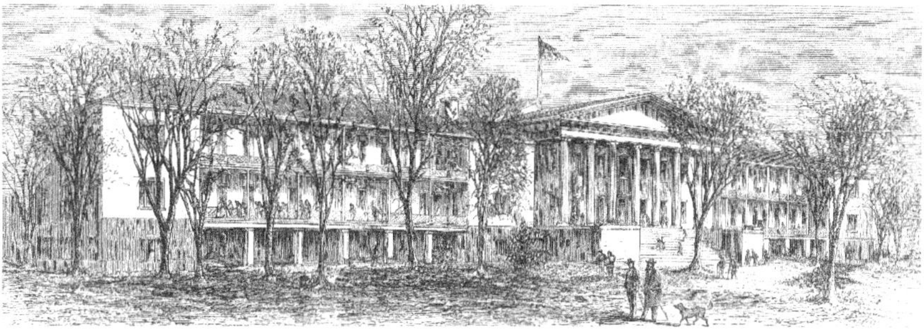

The Philadelphia Naval Asylum and Hospital, as the facility appeared in the late 1870s. Numerous examination sessions were held here for men seeking to become naval medical officers or to be promoted from assistant surgeon to passed assistant surgeon (*Harper's Weekly*, February 23, 1878).

per se but that candidates "should possess such preparatory scholastic education, as is essential to a respectable standing in our profession, in civil life." There was evidently no requirement in the initial communication for a candidate to describe his medical training.[4]

The USN and U.S. Army appear to have heavily favored candidates who had attended a school that taught allopathic (orthodox or regular) medicine rather than one of the many sectarian models that were popular at the time, such as homeopathic, botanical, or eclectic medicine. In general, sectarians favored what they characterized as gentler therapies over the supposedly harsh methods used by allopaths through the years, such as bloodletting and administering mercury compounds. Many allopaths, on the other hand, thought of sectarians as quacks. That BUMED favored allopathic practice is evident in the medicines and devices made available to its medical officers. One newspaper described the assistant-surgeon examination as "rigid, but fair, upon such branches of professional knowledge as are taught in respectable [probably meaning established allopathic] medical schools."[5]

Mentions of nonallopathic naval medical officers are rare. In one instance, Fleet Surgeon William Maxwell Wood of the NABS told Whelan of apparently improper ordering of supplies by a medical officer who, Wood was told, was a homeopath. Wood seems to have had no good reason to mention homeopathy other than to imply that the officer's medical beliefs made him less likely to abide by normal practices in requisitioning supplies.[6]

A medical-school term typically lasted from about October to March and consisted of a single series of lectures that changed little, if at all, from year to year. Graduation required studying under a preceptor, attendance at two terms of medical school—with the assumption that students would learn or remember more after hearing the same lectures a second time—and perhaps a final examination and thesis. Some students who attended two terms did so at different schools, but many students attended one term only, since the second would have been redundant and a diploma was not needed to practice medicine. Admission to a medical school depended primarily on an applicant's ability to pay the lecture and other fees.[7]

A candidate receiving permission to be evaluated for entry into the medical corps first underwent a physical examination by the board and attested in writing that he was in good health, that he did not have a chronic disease, and that his "organs of sense are without imperfection." Whelan asked the September 1863 board to be more rigid in conducting physical examinations. "Several of the younger members of the Department," observed Whelan, "are already unfitted for service by disease not manifestly contracted since their admission into the Navy."[8]

An examinee was required to submit a letter saying how far he had met BUMED's stated requirements, his age and place of birth, his educational accomplishments (including medical training and possible graduation), and his medical preceptor's name. If the letter's content was found acceptable, he completed an essay (called a dissertation or thesis), in private and within a specified time, on a medical topic selected by the board. If the essay was satisfactory—in literary and professional aspects, including grammar, orthography, and professional knowledge—he was allowed to proceed to the "professional examination."[9]

In that segment of the ordeal, the candidate wrote, in private, answers to 12 questions—3 from each board member—"embracing the leading features of the various departments of the profession." He then proceeded to the "object examination" in the hospital's laboratory (pharmacy or dispensary), which evaluated his knowledge of "the appearance, and physical properties, as well as the chemical composition, and therapeutic uses, of the various articles of the materia medica [medicinal agents], writing prescriptions, and the art of compounding medicines." Finally, the candidate would accompany at least one board member to a hospital ward to diagnose assigned cases and explain the reasoning used.[10]

If the opportunity presented itself, the candidate would also demonstrate his knowledge of anatomy and his ability to apply bandages and splints. Surgeon James M. Greene, president of the medical examining board convening at Philadelphia in December 1863, reported to Whelan that he had arranged with Dr. D. Hayes Agnew to use dissection rooms at the Philadelphia School of Anatomy. "In consequence of the high price of subjects [cadavers]," wrote Greene, "he will charge thirty dollars for each, which he furnishes, with the use of instruments, attendance &c &c." Greene considered the facilities ideal "for the purposes of carrying out the portion of the examination, in practical anatomy, and operations on the cadaver."[11]

In light of the urgent need to quickly appoint a large number of assistant surgeons, Whelan suggested to the board commencing in June 1861 that the traditional examination be streamlined by omitting the thesis and reducing the 12 written questions to 8 or 9 by having each board member submit 2, rather than 3, questions or by omitting the recorder as a questioner. Whelan favored retaining other parts of the examination. Still, for any particular candidate, the examination probably consumed at least two full days.[12]

The board rated candidates on a numerical scale, with a total score of at least 540, out of a possible 780, qualifying a candidate for appointment. Individual scores were determined in nine areas. For each of five areas (general aptitude, literary and scientific acquirements, anatomy and physiology, principles and practice of surgery, and principles and practice of medicine), a passing score was 80 out of 100. For two areas (materia medica and chemistry), a passing score was 50 out of 100, and for the other two (obstetrics and medical jurisprudence), a passing score was 20 out of 40. Candidates with the highest total scores during a particular board session were the first to be appointed assistant surgeon to fill available vacancies. For men appointed on the same date, their examination score determined their rank—the order in which they would ordinarily be considered for promotion if they had the requisite sea service. If a candidate with a satisfactory score was not appointed within a year of his examination, he would have to be reexamined if he still wished to enter the medical corps.[13]

During the Civil War years, about 400 men—spurred, perhaps by patriotism or by the hope of rapid promotion—began the examination process for appointment as an assistant surgeon. Although they had attended more than 50 medical schools, the University of Pennsylvania, the College of Physicians and Surgeons (New York City), and Jefferson Medical College together accounted for about 36 percent of applicants; about 9 percent of candidates reported not graduating from a medical school. Separate tabulations for 1861–63 and 1861–65 show about 37 percent and 42 percent of applicants, respectively, receiving a passing score. It is unclear whether wartime boards made it easier to achieve a passing score so that more appointments could be made. Before the war, however, the number of candidates with passing scores generally exceeded the number of open slots, and applicants with the lowest passing scores were not appointed. Late in the war, the shortage of assistant surgeons probably necessitated offering appointments to all candidates with a passing score. If so, the overall quality of incoming assistant surgeons may have dropped, at least as determined by examination scores.[14]

Whelan acted quickly to have assistant-surgeon appointments issued to candidates with passing scores. He urged Surgeon Samuel Barrington, president of the June 1861 Brooklyn board, to provide the names of candidates passing the examination as soon as that determination was made and then asked Secretary Welles to appoint them immediately. (The formality of presidential nomination and Senate confirmation could follow.) Ranking the new appointees according to their score would have to wait until the board's session was over. Consequently, 33 men were appointed assistant surgeon with a commission date of July 30, 1861, and their rank was later indicated by the order in which they appeared in the Navy Department's *Register.* Barrington's board was evidently considered to have met in two sessions, for another batch of 57 passed candidates received appointments in late January 1862, about the time that the board was officially dissolved.[15]

Examining Prospective Acting Assistant Surgeons (Volunteer Navy)

Some medical men were apparently attracted by the temporary nature of the volunteer navy. Perhaps they were driven by patriotic zeal and were willing to endure hardships and poor pay to assist the country, but only during the war. Some applicants may have thought themselves unable to pass the examination for admission to the regular navy's medical corps, while others may not have been able to find a better-paying position elsewhere. Whelan told one man in late 1861 that the department had an abundance of applications for volunteer positions but that he might consider applying for the permanent navy. Appointments with the latter, wrote Whelan, "can be relinquished as readily as acting appointments and have many advantages." Physician Ezra Pray applied in September 1861 for a volunteer appointment but made plans, in case that effort failed, to study in preparation for taking the examination for the regular navy.[16]

In rare instances—according to one source, just 10 times during the Civil War years—a candidate for assistant surgeon in the permanent navy who achieved a good, but not passing, score during his examination was given the opportunity to become an acting (volunteer) assistant surgeon without reexamination. That was the case for Samuel P.

Boyer, who missed a passing score by 15 points during his March 1862 examination and was invited by Whelan in June 1862 to accept an appointment as acting assistant surgeon. Another example was Lucian H. Kendall, whom Whelan described as having "a respectable examination though below our standard." On June 25, 1862, Kendall was appointed acting assistant surgeon, three days after Whelan suggested that possibility to Secretary Welles.[17]

The procedures and standards used in assessing candidates for acting assistant surgeon appear to have been inconsistent—or at least difficult to determine from existing records—but were certainly much less rigid than those applied for permanent medical appointments. Men aspiring to the temporary posts, suggested Whelan shortly before the commencement of such appointments, should present testimonials of good habits, should not be older than 28 years, and should be subject "to such examination as may be conducted by the Surgeons of the Stations where the vessel is to be fitted for sea." He suggested that commandants of naval stations be authorized to appoint a board of medical officers, not exceeding three men, to examine candidates. Evaluations, of course, could not be as thorough as those used for candidates for regular-navy assistant surgeon, but they should still be "sufficient to guard the lives and health of the ship's company from improper persons." Men who accepted appointments should be made to understand that appointment in the regular navy would require the type of examination routinely conducted for permanent appointments.[18]

An application for a temporary appointment was to be sent to the secretary of the navy and include "respectable testimonials of character and capacity." At least one applicant misconstrued the instructions and submitted testimonials from "non-professional gentlemen" only. Whelan informed him that because "the formalities of examination are dispensed with in making these temporary appointments, it is necessary the professional competence of the applicant should be certified by some respectable medical men." Whelan told another potential applicant that "appointments are made either upon such evidence [testimonials from medical men]" or after examination by a naval surgeon. Thus, evaluating candidates for temporary appointments was, at least in some cases, more casual than what Whelan originally envisioned. He told one surgeon that temporary appointments "are more dependent upon qualification than the possession of a [medical] diploma, and while the diploma is not considered to bestow any advantage, its absence is not to operate as a detriment."[19]

Having convincing testimonials was indeed enough, in some cases, to forgo an examination. When Surgeon John L. Fox, USN, stationed at the naval hospital in Chelsea, Massachusetts, found that Ezra Pray was interested in a temporary appointment, he offered to assist in and submit Pray's application. The paperwork probably included Fox's testimonial, and Pray was appointed a few weeks later. In at least one instance, a young physician was appointed as acting assistant surgeon and reported for duty before being examined. Daniel D.T. Nestell, was told that he had been placed on a list of accepted candidates on December 19, 1861, received his appointment dated January 25, 1862, and reported for duty on February 3. On February 19, Welles told him to report to Surgeon Benjamin F. Bache in Brooklyn for examination of his professional qualifications. Perhaps the relatively casual nature of such appointments resulted in the proper sequence of steps not being followed in Nestell's case.[20]

Boards for examining candidates for entry into, or promotion in, the regular navy sometimes evaluated candidates for temporary appointments, but whether boards were appointed at various stations specifically for the latter is unclear. In many cases, Secretary Welles simply ordered a pair of medical officers to examine candidates. Thus, Surgeon Bache and Surgeon Thomas J. Turner saw candidates at the navy's medical laboratory in Brooklyn, and Surgeons William S.W. Ruschenberger and Samuel F. Coues did the same at the Boston Navy Yard. Whelan asked Secretary Welles to authorize "any two medical officers of the Navy" stationed on the James River or at Hampton Roads, Virginia, to examine Loren R. Boyce, a yeoman on USS *Port Royal* of the Potomac Flotilla for appointment as a volunteer assistant surgeon. Should Boyce prove acceptable (which he did), Whelan asked that the commander of the Potomac Flotilla be directed to discharge Boyce from the service and assign him to duty on any flotilla vessel that lacked a medical officer; Boyce's reentry into the navy would come with his commission as acting assistant surgeon. In late 1864, Whelan reported that candidates for temporary appointments could be examined at Portsmouth, New Hampshire; Boston; New York; Philadelphia; Washington, D.C.; Chicago; Cairo, Illinois, and in various squadrons, but interest had waned by that time, and BUMED could not find enough qualified applicants to fill available openings.[21]

Whelan's initial suggested age limit of 28 years was certainly not applied, and age, he wrote, was "not of so much consequence" in the temporary as in the permanent navy. In 1863, he stated that the limit was 30 years, yet William Argyle Watson was 37 years old when appointed, and Samuel Clement Smoot was 43. Surgeons Bache and Turner reported that candidate James Kinnier, who gave his age as 53, was "excellently qualified." Kinnier appeared "much older but seems to be a healthy, able man." He was appointed acting assistant surgeon in July 1862.[22]

Whelan described the examination for acting appointments as "necessarily below the standard for permanent appointment, though it covers the same ground—a fair knowledge of business, sufficient educational attainments, and professional knowledge to discharge the ordinary duties of a medical officer." For the period spanning January 1, 1862, to November 4, 1864, Whelan reported that 86 (46%) of 188 candidates examined for acting appointments had been approved. His figures are suspect, since the number of appointees (not just examinees) for that period exceeded 300, but his point was that a minority of applicants were considered qualified for an appointment.[23]

Men seeking temporary appointments were not limited to those unqualified for the permanent navy. Indeed, the performance of some acting assistant surgeons—in their examination or on duty—was such that they were offered an opportunity to take the examination for a permanent appointment. One example was William Longshaw, Jr., who was appointed as acting assistant surgeon on June 25, 1862. He was examined for a permanent appointment in August 1862 and was appointed assistant surgeon in October 1862. Of 55 volunteer assistant surgeons so examined for the permanent navy in 1862–64, 16 passed and were appointed. As enthusiasm for serving abated late in the war, acting assistant surgeons were less interested in joining the permanent navy. In the latter half of 1864, 36 such officers were offered the chance to take the examination, but only 4 agreed to be examined, and 3 passed. During the war years, about 35 men made the switch from the volunteer to the permanent medical corps.[24]

Examining Assistant Surgeons for Promotion

The large number of medical-corps vacancies occurring early in the war created a need not only to appoint new assistant surgeons but also to promote officers to fill vacancies among surgeons. The list of available passed assistant surgeons was depleted by promotion, so Whelan expedited the promotion of assistant surgeons. Doing so replenished the list of passed assistant surgeons so that upcoming surgeon vacancies could be filled quickly. In some cases, as previously described, assistant surgeons were promoted directly to surgeon because not enough passed assistant surgeons were available to be promoted. During the war, Whelan preferred to have all assistant surgeons who had entered the service during a certain year (a class) examined for promotion at the same board session. Doing so simplified ranking those officers on the basis of their performance on the promotion examination.[25]

Assistant Surgeon James J. Magee, on learning in early 1862 that Whelan wanted him and other officers of similar rank to be examined for promotion, was concerned that he would not have adequate time to study. Given the circumstances, replied Whelan, BUMED could not accord the usual indulgence—in the form of detachment from current postings, and facilities for study—for candidates to prepare for the examination. However, because Magee and his peers had been appointed assistant surgeon relatively recently (in 1858), Whelan hoped that they had acquired enough professional knowledge during their service "as to dispense with the necessity of any prolonged preparation for a not unfamiliar event." Whelan suggested that if Magee and his peers would advise him of their preference for the time and place of examination, he would be glad to accommodate them to the extent possible. When other assistant surgeons appeared anxious about their preparedness for the promotion examination, Whelan reassured them that they were readier than they thought and that they should think twice about declining an opportunity that might not present itself again in the near future. Whelan was clearly reluctant to order unwilling assistant surgeons to be examined, because their refusal or failure in the examination would end their naval career.[26]

Examinations for promotion in the medical corps were conducted by the same boards that evaluated candidates for appointment as assistant surgeons. Candidates for promotion were to write the board a letter detailing their naval service and present "testimonials of correct deportment and habits of industry from the surgeons with whom they have been associated on duty." The board was also to examine a journal of practice or case book kept by candidates in their own handwriting. Candidates were to be familiar with medical officers' duties as specified in the Navy Department's booklet *Instructions for the Government of Medical Officers*. The board was to carefully scrutinize candidates' physical qualifications and to present them with written questions to be answered in writing. It is unclear whether promotion candidates were required to make and explain diagnoses, display pharmaceutical competence, or perform operations or dissections on cadavers.[27]

In at least one instance, an early opportunity to take the promotion examination was offered in recognition of meritorious service. In December 1863, Secretary Welles informed Assistant Surgeon William Longshaw, Jr., whose gallantry in action had been praised, that he would be allowed to take the examination as soon as his two years of sea service had been completed and not somewhat later when his class would ordinarily have been examined. Upon passing the examination, Longshaw would take rank as a passed assistant surgeon from the date of his examination without regard for his original appointment date or how well he performed compared with other examinees of his "date or class." At that time during the war, promotions to passed assistant surgeon were slowing down, so the opportunity offered by Welles might have given Longshaw enough of an advantage in rank to actually speed his eventual promotion to surgeon. Longshaw, who died in January 1865, appears not to have accumulated enough sea service to take advantage of Welles's reward.[28]

The examination for promoting acting assistant surgeons would have been cursory at best. On March 31, 1865, Whelan appointed two surgeons to constitute a board in New York to examine candidates for appointment to or promotion in the volunteer medical corps. "As these officers [applying for promotion] came into the service with a lower professional standard than is, and has been, required for the permanent Navy," Whelan instructed the board's president, "it is not proposed to conduct the examination for promotion with the rigid scrutiny that is enforced in the regular service. The manner of procedure, however, is left to your own judgment and discretion." Volunteer assistant surgeons, unlike their counterparts in the regular navy, were free to decline a promotion examination without detriment to their position. By the beginning of 1866 and 1867, 12 and 20 men, respectively, had been promoted to acting passed assistant surgeon, and only three such promotions occurred before May 1865. It is likely that the Navy Department saw such promotion as a reward for faithful service and a means, because of the higher salary, to retain such officers in the service.[29]

Whelan hoped that Acting Assistant Surgeon George H. Bixby, who had distinguished himself by his service on the hospital ship *Red Rover*, would apply for promotion to acting passed assistant surgeon. Whelan's intent, as expressed to Fleet Surgeon Ninian Pinkney of the Mississippi Squadron in late April 1865, was to recommend Bixby for further promotion to acting surgeon should he remain on that vessel. If he should leave the squadron, however, promotion to acting surgeon would be less likely, "as we have and shall have small occasion to employ acting surgeons elsewhere, owing to the probable early reduction of the navy." (It is unclear what sort of approval would have been needed for Whelan's recommendation to take effect.) Bixby evidently had health problems, resigned, and was not promoted. It appears that no promotion to acting surgeon ever occurred.[30]

The examination of candidates for admission to or promotion in the medical corps was a time-honored tradition meant to ensure that naval personnel received competent medical care. The urgent need for more assistant surgeons necessitated the lowering of standards when examining candidates for appointment as acting assistant surgeons. It is unclear whether the quality of men appointed as assistant surgeons in the regular navy fell during the war.

CHAPTER 4

The Standing of Medical Officers

WILLIAM WHELAN WAS CONVINCED THAT much of the difficulty in recruiting and retaining medical officers was attributable to the navy and legislators not fully recognizing their accomplishments and importance and thus failing to offer satisfactory inducements to join and stay in the navy. He spent considerable effort to raise the official status of medical officers and was frustrated when obstacles blocked the introduction of meaningful changes.

Assimilated Rank

Medical officers, like engineers and paymasters, were classified as staff or civil officers, as opposed to line officers. Staff officers lacked the authority to command outside their own corps, whereas officers of the line—comprising, at the start of the war and in descending order, captains, commanders, lieutenants, masters, second masters in line of promotion, passed midshipmen, midshipmen, boatswains, gunners, and warranted masters' mates—had command authority and filled the basic martial role of engaging the enemy. Many line officers considered staff officers to be beneath them and resented attempts to place staff and line officers on anything approaching an equal footing. "Line officers," confided Surgeon Benjamin F. Gibbs, stationed at Pensacola, to Whelan, "know little, and care little for our department & toward certain of them I feel peculiarly bitter in consequence of the arrogance I have patiently borne from them at this place."[1]

Where a staff officer stood relative to line officers affected factors such as the respect he was accorded, the place he occupied for ceremonies, where he sat at the dining table, and where his quarters were on a vessel; such standing was of vital importance to naval traditionalists.

Because the grades of medical officers differed from those of line officers, some authority had to define medical officers' place in the naval hierarchy—their *assimilated rank*.[2]

The 1841 naval regulations placed surgeons with lieutenants, passed assistant surgeons with masters, and assistant surgeons with passed midshipman. In 1846, Secretary of the Navy George Bancroft upgraded the status of medical officers such that fleet surgeons and surgeons who had been at that grade for more than 12 years ranked with commanders, newer surgeons ranked with lieutenants, passed assistant surgeons ranked next after lieutenants, and assistant surgeons ranked next after masters. Bancroft's decree was enacted into law in 1854.[3]

On July 16, 1862, Congress created four new grades of line officer by enacting the bill labeled H.R. 280. Rear admiral and commodore were the new top and second grades (respectively, above captain), lieutenant commander was placed between commander and lieutenant, and ensign was placed between master and midshipman. During the congressional debates preceding passage of H.R. 280, Whelan learned of an amendment that James W. Grimes, senator from Iowa, might propose regarding the assimilated rank of medical officers. The amendment called for surgeons with 20 years at that grade to rank with but junior to captains, surgeons with 15–20 years at that grade to rank with but junior to commanders, surgeons with 12–15 years at that grade to rank with but junior to lieutenant commanders, and newer surgeons to rank with but junior to lieutenants.[4]

The "with but junior to" phrase meant that the most experienced surgeons, for example, would outrank all line and staff officers at grades (or assimilated ranks) lower than captain but would be outranked by all captains who were line officers. Not only did the amendment reduce, compared with the status quo, the assimilated rank of many medical officers, the "with but junior to" provisions smacked of a caste system by presuming the navy's medical men to be inferior to the most junior line officer at their assimilated rank. As an example of unfairness, Whelan mentioned surgeons with less than 12 years at that grade. Those were "matured men educated out of their own pockets," a reference to the many hundreds of dollars typically spent to attain a medical degree. The amendment unfairly called for them to rank with but junior to lieutenants, whom Whelan characterized as "youths ... educated at the public expense," a probable allusion to their training at the U.S. Naval Academy. Whelan begged Senator Grimes to refrain from making matters worse by introducing the amendment but instead to consider another amendment (not found) that the medical corps endorsed. If the latter was impossible, Whelan implored the senator to "pray leave us in the condition of humble inferiority to which our necks have become accustomed." The senator appears never to have introduced the amendment.[5]

The addition of grades for line officers necessitated the redefining of assimilated rank of staff officers, a topic discussed among various officials, including Whelan; Rear Admirals Louis M. Goldsborough, Andrew H. Foote, and Charles H. Davis; and Assistant Secretary of the Navy Gustavus V. Fox. In November 1862, Whelan asked Goldsborough to remove any mention of medical officers from his written opinion because its provisions would not meet the expectations of the medical officers Whelan represented. Eventually, an agreement among Whelan, Foote, and Davis was presented to Secretary Welles, who accepted it and issued it as a general order on March 13, 1863. The BUMED chief now ranked with commodores; fleet surgeons and surgeons at that grade for more than 15 years ranked with captains; surgeons at that grade for 5–15 years ranked with commanders; newer surgeons ranked with lieutenant commanders; passed assistant surgeons ranked with lieutenants; and assistant surgeons ranked with masters. Medical officers' higher assimilated ranks did not change what they were paid, which was less than line officers with whom they now ranked. For example, for sea service, a surgeon starting his sixth year at that grade received $2,400 a year, whereas his commander counterpart received $2,800. For sea service, an assistant surgeon, regardless of his length of service, was paid $1,250 a year, while a master received $1,500.[6]

Welles recalled after the war doubting his order's legality and encouraging staff officers to present it to Congress to be enacted into law. Those officers, however, were not satisfied with the extent to which the order altered their standing and probably, thought Welles, would have opposed legislation that strengthened the order's legal standing.[7]

Whelan told Fleet Surgeon Jonathan M. Foltz, "You are not aware … of the months of untiring, and almost heart sickening importunity it required to obtain the modicum of rank" set forth in the general order. "If the subject had been within my control," continued Whelan, "the result would have been very different, but such as it is, it is gratifying to know that it is not wholly unacceptable to a great many worthy members of the corps." Whelan explained further: "No exertion was spared either to induce Congress to establish a higher grade in our corps; and we should have succeeded if other corps of the Navy, deeming themselves rightfully entitled to any, and every, concession made to the Medical Department, had not sought to attach amendments to our bill which rendered its defeat so probable, as to make it wiser to withdraw the proposition for the present." It is unclear whether Whelan was referring to H.R. 280.[8]

Even if some medical officers were satisfied with the general order of March 13, 1863, Whelan considered its changes inadequate and claimed that they effectively demoted surgeons with the longest service. Before the change, a senior surgeon ranked with a commander, the second-highest grade possible for a line officer. After the change, the same surgeon ranked with a captain, now the third-highest line grade, so that surgeon was now further from the top than he was before. Practically every captain on January 1, 1861, who remained on the active list had been promoted by the end of August 1862 to rear admiral or commodore. Similarly, most commanders remaining on the active list had been promoted to captain, with several promoted to rear admiral or commodore. At best, the March 1863 changes allowed senior surgeons to barely keep pace with line officers in assimilated rank but not in pay.[9]

Whelan could have cited the example of Surgeon William Johnson, who was assigned as fleet surgeon of the SABS in August 1863. By that time, Johnson, who had been in the navy since August 1826, had an assimilated rank of captain, two grades below that of Rear Admiral John A. Dahlgren, flag officer of the SABS. Johnson's total naval service was not even 7 months shorter than Dahlgren's, and by January 1865, he had 17 more months of sea service than the rear admiral. Dahlgren's annual sea-service salary at that time was $5,000 while Johnson's was $3,300. It was even difficult, at times, for the most experienced surgeons to maintain parity with other staff officers. In January 1865, Johnson had the same pay and assimilated rank as SABS Fleet Paymaster James H. Watmough and Fleet Engineer Robert Danby, both of whom had entered the navy about 18 years after Johnson.[10]

Whelan gave numerous examples of countries that were more generous than the United States in rewarding the service of medical officers and pointed out that some USN surgeons had more total and sea service than some of the highest-ranking officers of the line. His pleas to raise the status of medical officers beyond the changes that had already occurred were fruitless, yet he persisted. He considered it "not only a grateful office, but a positive duty, to bear testimony to the faithful and efficient services of medical officers of the navy" and to urge, as their representative, that they be accorded their deserved recognition. He confessed to Assistant Secretary Fox that he was lobbying about "a Subject that possesses, as I am painfully aware, but little interest for any but Medical Officers & their widely spread professional brethren." Whatever Secretary Welles believed about the rightful status of medical and officers, he was constrained because many line officers objected to sharing their privileges with staff officers.[11]

Whelan considered pay, which was related to assimilated rank,

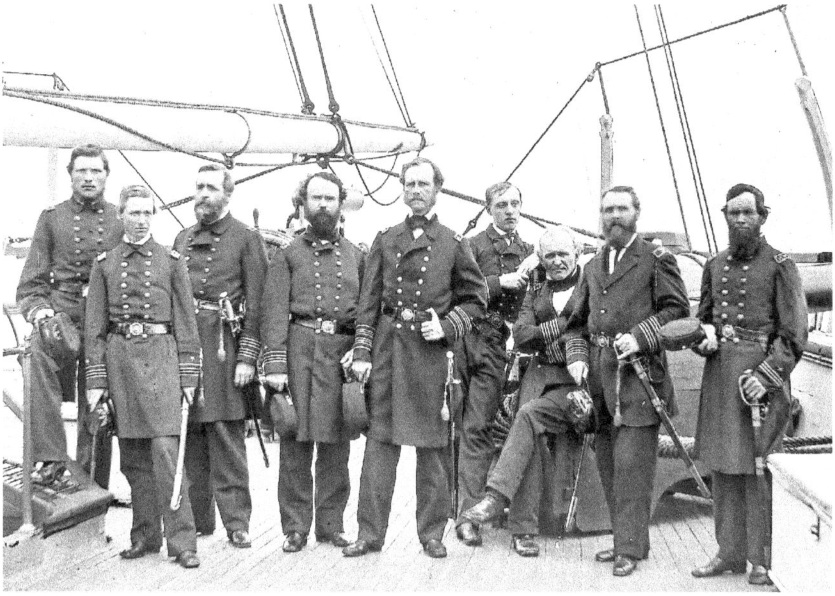

Officers of the SABS on USS *Pawnee* in 1864 or 1865. From left: Ensign Ernest J. Dichman, Lieutenant Commander E. Orville Matthews, Fleet Paymaster James H. Watmough, Lieutenant Commander Joseph M. Bradford, Rear Admiral John A. Dahlgren, Acting Ensign Walter Cooper, Fleet Surgeon William Johnson, Fleet Engineer Robert Danby, and Acting Lieutenant and Pilot William Heffords (identifications: Civil War Photograph Collection, vol. 64, Military Order of the Loyal Legion of the United States, Massachusetts Commandery [MOLLUS-MASS], U.S. Army Heritage and Education Center, Carlisle, Pennsylvania [USAHEC]; photograph: National Archives and Records Administration [NARA], identifier 524483).

a key factor in the continuing difficulty of attracting qualified men to become and remain medical officers. The compensation of naval medical officers, said Whelan, was little more than—if even equal to—the pay of "mechanical or clerical pursuits." That being the case, there was no reason "to expect that a man would give his education and time to the navy for such disproportioned compensation and position."[12]

For young physicians determined to serve in the armed forces, the navy offered no monetary advantage over the army. Whelan estimated that medical officers in the army received 33–50 percent more than their navy counterparts. Although some of his computations may have been based on extreme examples—using, for example, naval officers' pay while on leave or awaiting orders—he still had a point. A naval assistant surgeon with any length of service, for example, received $1,050 a year, and no ration, while on shore duty. (Naval officers at sea were entitled to one daily ration, which could be commuted to its value of 25¢ and added to their salary.) A new army assistant surgeon received a base pay of $53.33 per month and four rations a day (commutation value, $36 per month) and was allowed one servant (commutation value, $23.50 per month), for a total compensation of $112.83 per month, or $1,354 per year. Sea duty generally entitled naval medical officers to about the same compensation as their army counterparts with similar service, but service afloat was arduous, and even before the war, many assistant surgeons resigned "on account of the constant pressure for duty on shipboard." The army's "greater inducements," stated Whelan, referring to new assistant surgeons, were appropriating "nearly all the available medical talent," and better pay in the navy was needed "to give the navy a fairer opportunity for competition in recruiting that talent."[13]

Whelan's Final Effort

Whelan's last attempt to improve medical officers' standing occurred in early 1865. In January of that year, he presented Secretary Welles with the proposed wording of a bill "to reorganize the Medical Department of the Navy."[14] The key elements of the proposal were that the medical corps should consist of

- The BUMED chief, with the new grade of director general
- Twenty medical directors of fleets, with the rank and pay of a captain; after five years at that grade, the rank and pay of a commodore
- Eighty surgeons, with the rank and pay as specified in the general order of March 13, 1863
- Forty surgeons of the second class (replacing passed assistant surgeons), with the rank and pay of a lieutenant
- One hundred sixty assistant surgeons, with the rank and pay as specified in the general order of March 13, 1863

Furthermore,

- The director general and medical directors would be appointed by the president with Senate confirmation but only after a physical examination to determine their fitness for promotion
- Medical directors would supervise the sanitary and hygienic affairs of fleets or squadrons and perform other duties as ordered by the medical department

- Any medical officer would be placed on the retired list if found incapable of performing the duties of his station; those on the retired list could be promoted to medical director on the retired list
- Acting assistant surgeons could be promoted to surgeon of the second class after two years of service and satisfactory examination as prescribed by the medical department
- All acts and parts of acts in conflict with the above would be repealed

The major proposed changes to the status quo—other than a larger allowed number of medical officers, and pay matching that of line officers of the same assimilated rank—were the new grade of medical director and the five-years of service required for the assimilated rank of a medical director to be elevated from captain to commodore. Whelan believed that the five-year delay would allow time for the resolution of disagreements between line and staff officers about assimilated rank.[15]

The bill—whether it contained Whelan's original wording has not been determined—was introduced in the House of Representatives on January 24, 1865, and referred to the House Committee on Naval Affairs. Whelan's efforts to garner support for the bill included sending long letters to Congressman Alexander H. Rice, Congressman William D. Kelley, Senator James W. Grimes, and Senator Charles Sumner. Whelan decided against leaving Washington, in case his "personal exertions" were needed before Congress adjourned on March 3.[16]

Whelan usually argued that medical officers had great responsibility and were exposed to the same dangers as their line brethren and should therefore be granted similar rank and pay for similar durations of service. Whelan wrote to Kelley—who was born in Philadelphia, the putative center of American medical education at the time—that "an opportunity of winning the respect, and gratitude of a numerous, learned, and influential profession [medicine] has rarely, if ever, been accorded to an American legislator."[17]

Many of Whelan's arguments related to the difficulty of recruiting competent physicians of high character into the regular navy when the inducements to seek an appointment were inadequate. In the nearly 50 vessels of the Potomac Flotilla, Whelan told Rice on February 2, 1865, "there are but three medical officers of any kind." Sailors, said Whelan, deserved better medical care than what BUMED could provide. He sardonically suggested to Grimes that the legislation's title ("A bill to reorganize the medical department of the United States Navy") should actually be "A bill to protect the officers and men of the Navy engaged in suppressing the rebellion against the mediocrity of talent and professional acquisitions which alone finds inducements to enter the Navy, with present humble rank, and inadequate pay." To illustrate the character of men BUMED had been compelled to admit to the medical corps, Whelan cited, on February 13, examples from the past week. A lady reported a medical officer to Secretary Welles for "attempted seduction of her daughter, and other infamous conduct." Another woman reported a medical officer for theft of her deceased husband's watch. An addition officer, added Whelan, "is reported for wife desertion, bigamy, lying, &c." Yet another was allowed to resign "under charge of theft."[18]

Whelan gave recent examples of medical officers struggling to support their families with their current pay. Two who had recently returned from sea requested a return to sea duty because they could not support their families without the extra pay. Another, who had been wounded in battle, asked to resign so he could work elsewhere and earn enough for his family. One officer asked to be reassigned because his salary would not "defray the expense of living in a single room on the 5th floor of a third-rate hotel in a Western city."[19]

Some aspects of Whelan's proposal—possibly including the delayed, rather than immediate, elevation of medical directors to the assimilated rank of commodore—did not meet with Secretary Welles's approval, and a board of line officers met to discuss the matter. The board's final recommendations would have reduced the rank and pay of most medical officers, but Whelan was apparently successful in convincing Welles not to act on them.[20]

Line officers, in fact, seemed to be the problem. It was curious, said Whelan, that "a majority of line officers of the Navy consider their personal status assailed, their official dignity wounded by the rank of medical officers" at the same time that army medical officers were being promoted on the recommendation of the army's most distinguished field commanders. "If a live man be worth more than a dozen dead men," Whelan wrote to Senator Sumner, "he who contributes by his skill, and knowledge, to save a man to the Government, should be deemed not unworthy [of] some of the honor, and advantage awarded to he whose mission is to slay." It appears that the bill died in committee.

Various other bills dealing with assimilated rank were introduced after the war but were not passed. On March 29, 1869, U.S. Attorney General Ebenezer R. Hoar ruled that only Congress could establish assimilated rank. Three days later, the new secretary of the navy, Adolf E. Borie, revoked former Secretary Welles's general order of March 3, 1863, an action that confirmed Welles's fears about the order's legality. Assimilated rank thus reverted to what had been enacted by Congress in 1854, with most categories of medical officers being lowered in standing, compared with line officers.[21]

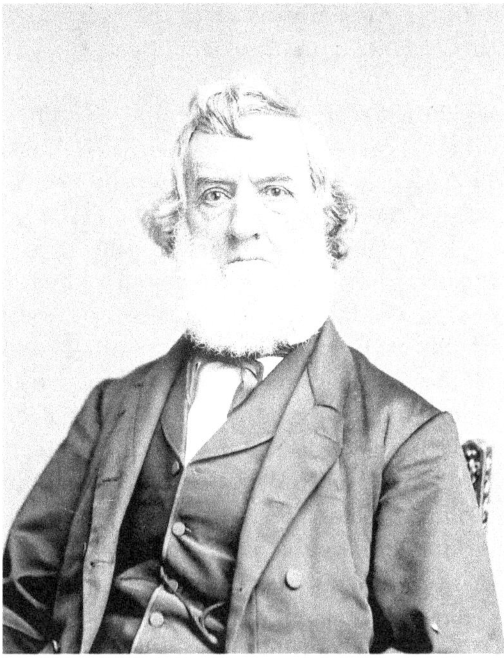

Gideon Welles, who served as secretary of the navy throughout and after the Civil War. Welles agreed with many suggestions of BUMED Chief Whelan but also had to weigh opposing sentiment by line officers (NARA, identifier 524418).

Other Aspects of Status

Relative rank was often used to mean *assimilated rank*, but when a user intended to differentiate between the terms, *relative rank* referred to how officers of the army and navy—an army colonel and a naval captain, for example—stood relative to each other. The topic was of common interest to naval line and staff officers because they wanted to be paid and respected as much as army counterparts who had similar responsibilities and service time. Relative rank could theoretically have implications about who would outrank whom in joint army–navy operations. Whelan seemed content to let others fight that battle, because improvements in the relative rank of naval line officers would also elevate the status of staff officers of equivalent assimilated rank.[22]

One of the consequences of Congress failing to approve Whelan's 1865 bill was the enactment in March 1865 of legislation allowing acting assistant surgeons to be promoted to acting passed assistant surgeon or acting surgeon. Whelan had actually advocated that possibility in 1864 and then included it in his failed 1865 bill. He denied that the March 1865 bill (concerning promotion of acting assistant surgeons) originated in BUMED—meaning, probably, that he did not push for this particular provision after his entire bill failed. Rather, said Whelan, it came from the Senate's Naval Committee, which "finding the necessity of some action for the advantage of the Medical Officers, contented itself with the measure ... instead of adopting the bill I had ventured to propose."[23]

One concern about precedence—for line as well as staff officers—was how permanent and temporary officers ranked in relation to each other. Assistant Surgeon George H. Cooke, for example, wrote in May 1863 on behalf of several officers on USS *Somerset*, to Rear Admiral Theodorus Bailey, flag officer of the EGBS, for a decision on "the relative rank of regular and volunteer officers of the same grade." In July 1863, the Navy Department agreed with a board of rear admirals that officers of a particular grade—regardless of whether in the permanent or volunteer navy—should rank according to their date of appointment. If a regular and volunteer officer of the same grade shared the same appointment date, the former would take precedence. Among volunteer officers of the same grade and appointment date, precedence would be based on the alphabetical order of their family name. The ruling had the potential for causing hard feelings among medical officers, because those with permanent appointments, having survived a vigorous entrance examination, would surely object to being outranked by acting assistant surgeons who had entered the service earlier but did so after only the most casual evaluation. Whelan could avoid creating such conflict by taking care not to assign regular and volunteer assistant surgeons to the same vessel or station unless the regular officer had the older appointment date. Since only three acting assistant surgeons were promoted to acting passed assistant surgeon before May 1865, it was unlikely that a temporary medical officer would outrank a permanent medical officer on the basis of grade.[24]

The addition of line-officer grades in 1862 and the adjustments of assimilated rank by Secretary Welles's March 3, 1863, general order necessitated changes in officers' uniforms. Whelan reminded Secretary Welles that during deliberations on the subject, "It was indulgently permitted to Medical Officers to express a preference in regard to some matters of detail." His officers, reported Whelan, desired black velvet, rather than the standard navy blue cloth, as the fabric on shoulder straps, "with the understanding it was to be the distinctive mark of the [medical] Corps." Other staff branches evidently objected to medical officers thus standing out, so black was considered for all staff officers, a development that Whelan said defeated medical officers' desire to "preserve the identity of their profession." Whelan also suggested that medical officers' cap ornaments include their insignia of grade, because the designs being contemplated for medical and other staff officers were so similar as to be indistinguishable at most distances. Whelan's efforts were futile. Uniform regulations issued later in 1863 continued to specify navy blue cloth for all officers' shoulder straps, and his recommendation for medical officers' cap ornaments was not followed.[25]

Whelan was tireless in his attempts to elevate the status and pay of medical officers. Such elevation would not only be just, he argued, it would help attract competent physicians of good character to the medical department and help ensure that the navy's fighting men received the care they deserved. That his attempts were largely thwarted stemmed, he believed, from the influence of line officers unwilling to share their status, from the meddling of other staff officers envious of benefits being considered for medical officers, and from legislators unwilling to act on behalf of the medical department.

Chapter 5

Stewards and Nurses

Medical officers could not, by themselves, perform all of the tasks required to care for patients and tend to all of the associated responsibilities. Among their most important assistants were petty officers called surgeons' stewards. The Navy Department, starting early in the war, also allowed enlisted men to serve as nurses.

Surgeons' Stewards

One surgeon's steward was allowed on any vessel having a commissioned medical officer. A surgeon's steward at sea was kept busy changing dressings, preparing medicines, helping with paperwork, and performing various other tasks. A surgeon's steward could function as a vessel's de facto medical officer if its assigned surgeon was absent or unable to perform his duties. During the war, many small vessels lacking a medical officer had a surgeon's steward as their only health practitioner.[1]

Until mid–1861, a man destined to be a surgeon's steward entered the service by enlisting at a naval rendezvous (recruiting station) and signing the usual shipping articles. He was then assigned to a ship and rated (selected) by the vessel's medical officer, with the consent of the commander, as a petty officer with the title of surgeon's steward. He could be disrated for unacceptable behavior or performance and was usually discharged from the navy at the end of his vessel's cruise. He received $24 a month, the same as a ship's cook and more than an ordinary seaman ($14). In choosing surgeons' stewards, medical officers were to "endeavor to select such as have some knowledge of pharmacy and ordinary accounts, and are of industrious and temperate habits." One surgeon noted that men possessing the qualities desired in a surgeon's steward could easily find a higher-paying job ashore. Surgeons' stewards were comparable in duties and desired attributes to army hospital stewards, whose monthly pay rose in April 1862 from $22 to $30.[2]

BUMED chief Whelan, believing the pay to be too low, suggested on June 12, 1861, to Secretary Welles that the salary of surgeons' stewards should reflect the amount of work they were expected to do. Whelan recommended monthly salaries of $25 for serving on vessels with a complement of less than 200 men, $35 for a complement of 200–400, and $40 for a complement of more than 400. He also suggested that a surgeon's steward be rated at the rendezvous rather than after being assigned to a ship. Whelan added that beyond the surgeon's steward on a vessel, any attendance upon the sick and wounded came from crewmembers, whose assistance could not be relied upon because of their other assigned responsibilities. He thus recommended the allowance of one (male) nurse on vessels with a complement under 200, and two nurses for vessels with more crewmembers. The nurses' exclusive duty would be attendance on the sick and wounded. They would be paid $14 a month and were not to be considered petty officers. Exactly what tasks were expected of nurses in unclear, although they probably assisted with moving and feeding patients, cleaned the sickbay, changed bedding, and saw to patients' general comfort. Nurses probably reported not only to medical officers but to surgeons' stewards as well.[3]

Welles consequently issued two general orders. The first, on June 19, 1861, showed his faith in Whelan's judgment by essentially repeating the bureau chief's suggestions about salary and the addition of nurses; the order also specified that nurses be appointed by the vessel's medical officer with concurrence of the commander. The second order, on November 11, 1861, removed the requirement that surgeons' stewards sign the ordinary shipping articles and substituted specific articles of agreement. The regular shipping articles, used for seamen and other enlistees, specified a term of service—for example, one or three years, unless curtailed by proper authority—a salary, and an agreement to comply with the navy's laws, regulations, and discipline. The new articles for a surgeon's steward differed in that the time commitment was the vessel's term of service, unless shortened by proper authority or by the provisions of the November 11 general order. That order stated that the steward was "subject to be discharged, in case of misbehavior, in any port, foreign or domestic, without claim for passage money," provided that the misbehavior was established by a summary court. A misbehaving surgeon's steward might previously have been disrated while at sea but could still complete the cruise at a lower rating. The new articles presented to the steward the prospect of being stranded at some port for poor behavior and constituted, in Whelan's words, an agreement "by which a surgeon's steward binds himself to a proper subordination to the laws and authorities of the Navy during service therein."[4]

Later in the war, Welles issued a general order that revised the pay table and introduced the new rating of surgeon's steward in charge. The table, effective on June 30, 1864, established pay for various personnel, including surgeons' stewards, on the basis of the type and tonnage of the vessel on which they served. Vessels were categorized into four rates, with first-rate vessels generally being the largest and fourth-rate the smallest. The monthly salary for surgeons' stewards was set at $40 for first-rate vessels, $33 for second-rate, and $25 for third- and fourth-rate; receiving ships were considered third-rate vessels.[5]

Even after the issuance of Welles's orders, surgeons consistently complained that wages for surgeons' stewards were too low to attract and retain high-quality applicants. To one, Whelan responded that it was impossible to raise the pay because the Navy Department was confident that "if the pay was increased in any one instance, however meritorious, the same consideration would be claimed by all others, irrespective of their qualifications, or usefulness."[6]

Because acting assistant surgeons were in short supply, it was often necessary to assign a surgeon's steward as the sole provider of care "on board vessels of small size, and complement; as store ships, sailing vessels, &c., to which it is impossible to provide other kind of medical aid." A man with such an assignment would be designated surgeon's steward in charge with a monthly salary of $40. (The steward could, if necessary, ask his ship's captain to request medical assistance from a nearby squadron vessel.) Whelan advised a fleet surgeon that if he had stewards "whose character, and capacity, justify the advancement," he could grant them the higher rating of surgeon's steward in charge, with the approval of the commanding officer, and transfer them to small vessels so that their acting assistant surgeons could be assigned elsewhere. In at least one instance, a surgeon's steward who had performed admirably during a yellow-fever crisis on USS *Tioga* was given the choice by Whelan of being examined for appointment as an acting assistant surgeon or being named a surgeon's steward in charge. It appears that Whelan intended the latter to provide a higher salary without mandatory assignment to another vessel as its only medical man.[7]

A few months after Welles's general order, Whelan suggested that surgeons' stewards serving on receiving ships receive $40 rather than $25. Receiving ships accommodated recruits for training and indoctrination—as well as men whose ships were being repaired—and the numbers of such men on board routinely exceeded the complements of the navy's largest ships. Welles compromised and allowed $33 monthly. The

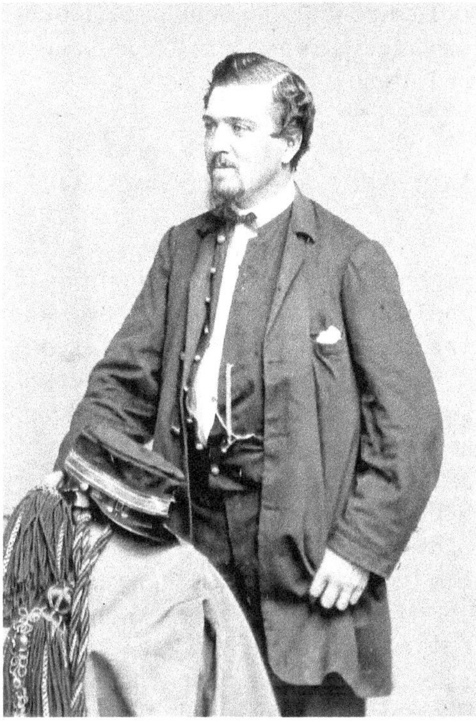

Cornelius S. Hale, who served as a surgeon's steward on USS *Isaac Smith* of the SABS and USS *Morse* of the NABS (Civil War Photograph Collection, vol. 119, MOLLUS-MASS, USAHEC).

Navy Department's reasoning, according to Whelan, was that the pay should be "based upon the permanent crew of the vessel, and not upon the fluctuating number of recruits that may be on board."[8]

Despite his belief that arguing for higher pay for surgeons' stewards was futile, Whelan could not resist the opportunity to do so to Congressman Alexander H. Rice in February 1865. "At this time," Whelan wrote, "there are at least seventy vessels in medical care of surgeons stewards in charge and surgeons stewards while exposed to all the contingencies of war; these people wear the uniform of a sailor and mess with the crew on the berth deck; the former receive $40 per month, the pay of a cabin servant to the commander in chief [of a squadron]; the latter $25 per month, or $10 per month less than the cabin cook of a commander in chief."[9]

A surgeon's steward's completed articles of agreement were to include an endorsement regarding his physical condition written by the vessel's medical officer or any medical officer on duty at the station. That endorsement was to either fully describe any physical defects that were present but did not disqualify the steward from performing his duties, or certify that the steward was free from any disease that was likely to be the basis of a future pension claim. A druggist who applied to be a surgeon's steward recalled having his competence assessed by "an examination of a decidedly technical and professional nature." Although no standardized examination was administered and no specific educational achievements were required, men with pharmacy training were particularly apt candidates because surgeon's stewards were often called upon to compound prescriptions and manage a vessel's supply of medicines. It is probable that surgeons' stewards also included men who had attended medical school.[10]

Stewards at Shore Facilities

A surgeon's steward was also allowed at all hospitals and navy yards. He ideally had the qualities of industriousness, temperance, and "some knowledge of pharmacy and ordinary accounts"—the same as those sought in a seagoing surgeon's steward—and presumably had duties similar to those performed at sea. Land-based surgeons' stewards signed the same articles of agreement as those required for surgeons' stewards afloat except that the formers' service ended when discharged rather than at the end of a vessel's service. A surgeon at a navy yard, with the approval of his station commandant, evidently had the option of designating his surgeon's steward as a surgeon's steward in charge so that he could receive the highest salary allowed ($40 a month).[11]

Hospitals were also entitled to a separate worker called a hospital steward. His duties were probably those first put forward in 1812, when the establishment of naval hospitals was being contemplated. Those proposed responsibilities were to take charge and be accountable for all hospital supplies and fixtures, purchase food for patients, keep accounts of purchases, keep track of patients and employees, and manage the hospital grounds; he was to "superintend generally the concerns of the hospital" under the surgeon's direction. Direct patient care was not included in his duties. A hospital steward was appointed by the hospital's surgeon with the concurrence of the commanding officer, and he signed articles of agreement similar to those required of surgeons' stewards serving ashore. The Navy Department fixed a hospital steward's monthly salary at $40. Local conditions, however, could necessitate higher salaries. Whelan told Surgeon William Grier, at the naval hospital at Mound City, Illinois, that "the Naval rates of pay are to be considered the rule for hospital employees, but where the sum is inadequate to procure the service desired, you are at liberty, with the concurrence of the commanding officer, to increase the amount, as a temporary expedient, to meet the necessity."[12]

It is probable that, at times, hospital stewards were erroneously called surgeons' stewards. The opposite was certainly true, as when Surgeon Phineas J. Horwitz at the BUMED office, wrote to Fleet Surgeon James C. Palmer about the "hospital steward" (meaning surgeon's steward) on USS *Tallahatchie*. When Du Fay Bowman was appointed hospital steward at the naval hospital at New Bern, North Carolina, his articles of agreement referred to him as a surgeon's steward. It is also possible that some civilians hired to perform the aforementioned duties were called hospital stewards, and that some bona fide naval hospital stewards were simply called stewards. Hospitals also hired civilian apothecaries, probably when the hospital steward, if present, lacked the time or expertise to compound prescriptions.[13]

Before mid–1864, annual cost estimates for navy yards and stations, including hospitals, were prepared by the Bureau of Yards and Docks and included surgeons' stewards at a monthly salary of $40; an exception was the navy yard at Mare Island, California, where the salary was $62.50 a month. After BUMED assumed responsibility for those estimates, surgeons' stewards were shown at $25 per month at all hospital locations but Mare Island, which was omitted. (Published pay scales appear not to have included surgeons' stewards at hospitals, but $25—allowed for service on third- and fourth-rate vessels—was probably appropriate for less-hectic shore service.) Stewards (not called hospital stewards in the estimates) at the same facilities were shown usually at $40 and once each at $50 and $60. Because the specified monthly salary for a hospital steward was $40, the men Whelan called stewards—and the ones whom the Bureau of Yards and Docks had called surgeons' stewards—were probably hospital stewards. The monthly salaries of $50, $60, and $62.50 probably reflected supply-and-demand conditions at their localities.[14]

Number of Stewards and Nurses

A BUMED compilation of appointment papers for surgeons' and hospital stewards contains about 650 names for 1861–65 but certainly understates the actual number of men who served in those roles during the war. Appointments made before November 1861 may not appear because there was not yet a requirement to sign specific articles of agreement, which constitute a large portion of the accumulated papers. Although a copy of each man's signed articles was to be submitted to BUMED, some documents were likely never submitted or were lost. The number also does not indicate how many men were serving at the same time. Any particular appointment could be short-lived, and some men may have been appointed multiple times.[15]

One example of a surgeon's steward with an early appointment—and missing from BUMED's compilation—is Cornelius S. Hale, who enlisted in New York on October 17, 1861, at the age of 25 years. Hale had been an apothecary and was rated at the rendezvous as a surgeon's steward. He served first on USS *Isaac Smith* of the SABS and later on USS *Morse* of the NABS.[16]

No summary statistics have been found on the number of nurses employed on vessels. Hospitals also employed nurses, but the extent to which they generally included civilians or women is unknown.

Surgeons' stewards assisted medical officers afloat and ashore. Because of the overall shortage of medical personnel, a surgeon's steward might be the only medical caregiver on a vessel. Nurses, drawn from the ranks of enlisted men, could also be appointed, but how many served is not known.

Chapter 6

Assignments

The navy's rapid wartime growth outpaced BUMED's ability to assign medical officers where they were needed. The bureau responded by making extensive use of volunteer medical officers and by expanding the responsibilities of selected surgeons' stewards, but it still had to allot their human resources in a way that would best serve the war effort.

Assignments to Vessels

At any moment during most of the war, the majority of regular and volunteer medical officers were assigned to war vessels. For example, the Navy Department's 1863 *Register*—published early in the year and undoubtedly based on incomplete returns—shows 253 medical officers in the regular and volunteer navy serving on 308 vessels. Those men comprised 33 of 80 surgeons, 92 of 120 assistant surgeons in the permanent navy, and 128 of about 141 assistant surgeons in the volunteer navy. (At that time, there were few or no passed assistant surgeons, and none were serving afloat. Their ranks had been depleted by promotions to surgeon, and their numbers had not yet begun to be replenished by the promotion of assistant surgeons.) At about the same time, December 1862, Secretary Welles reported that the navy had 427 vessels. Although many were being built, repaired, or fitted out, it is certain that many vessels in active service—perhaps 100 or more—did not have a medical officer.[1]

In December 1863, Welles reported that the number of naval vessels had increased to 588. Many large vessels required more than one medical officer, and dozens of medical officers were needed for shore assignments. Clearly, the total number of regular and volunteer medical officers at that time, about 400, was insufficient to allow at least one such officer per vessel.[2]

A vessel's rating—which could depend on its type, tonnage, armament, and complement—generally determined the grades of officers assigned to it. Which guidelines were used at the start of the war is unclear, but a set developed by 1858 divided ships into four classes or ratings. First class included ships of the line with more than 70 guns and steamers with a complement of more than 500. Fourth class embraced "small vessels," including all sailing vessels with up to 14 guns and steamers with a complement up to 75. The 1858 allowances showed the grade of officer suitable for command of vessels in each class but not the allowed number of commissioned, warrant, or petty officers or other crewmembers.[3]

That particular information—the allowance for personnel other than ships' commanders—was included in tables issued from time to time by the Navy Department. The advent of new types of vessels necessitated the development of more specific guidelines. The Navy Department, for example, issued in September 1861 an order specifying the complement allowed on "the new gunboats," and in October 1862, it did the same for the ironclad monitors "Nahant, Passaic, Catskill and vessels of that class." No table issued since 1838 allowed more than one full surgeon on a vessel, although the largest might have a surgeon and one or more assistant surgeons.[4]

In 1864, the department established the numbers of officers and crewmembers allowed on vessels, divided into those powered by wind and steam, depending on their complement. In most instances—and in all cases for medical personnel—the allowance of officers was identical for sailing vessels and steamers with the same complement. The department specified 10 ranges of complement, with the largest and smallest being 570–760 and 12–25 men, respectively. For a complement of 570–760, the allowance was one surgeon and three assistant surgeons; for complements of 225–375 and 375–570, one surgeon and two assistant surgeons; for complements of 100–175 and 175–225, one surgeon and one assistant surgeon; for a complement of 80–100, two assistant surgeons; and for complements of 25–40, 40–60, and 60–80, one assistant surgeon. In these allowances, assistant surgeons included passed assistant surgeons.[5]

The USN's largest squadrons, which accounted for the most assignments of medical officers, were the NABS, SABS, EGBS, WGBS, and the Mississippi Squadron. In 1864, the EGBS had about 24 vessels, while the other four had between 48 and 65.[6]

The NABS, formed by the October 1861 division of the Atlantic Blockading Squadron, was based for most of the war at Hampton Roads, Virginia—its base was moved to Beaufort, North Carolina, in

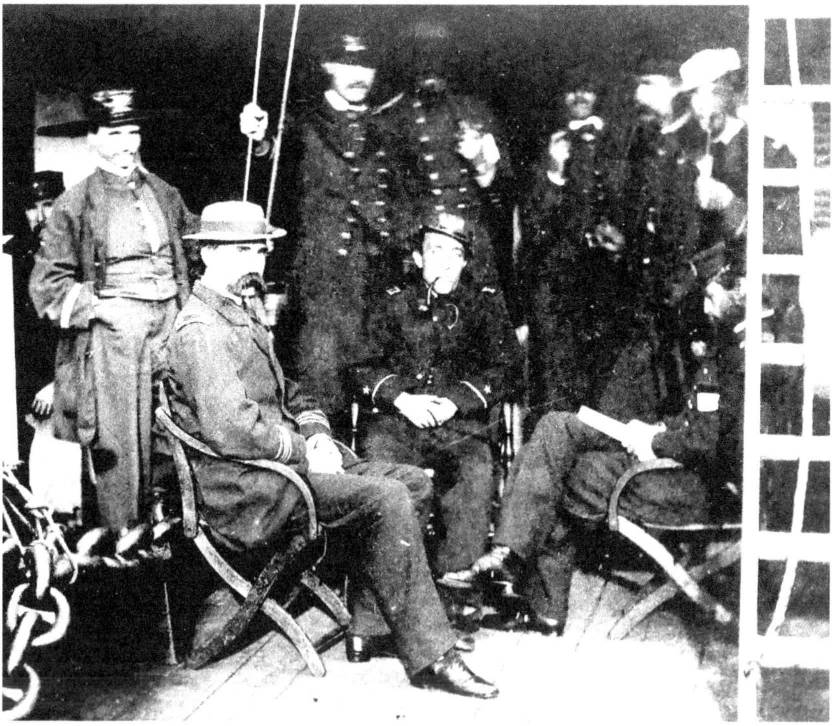

Officers of USS *Hartford* in the latter half of 1864. Seated, from left: Surgeon Philip Lansdale, Acting Ensign William H. Whiting, and Chief Engineer Thomas Williamson. Standing, from left: Assistant Surgeon William Commons, Paymaster William T. Meredith, Captain Charles Heywood (U.S. Marine Corps), Lieutenant Herbert B. Tyson, First Lieutenant John C. Kinney (Acting Signal Officer, U.S. Army), and Acting Ensign George D.B. Glidden. Extreme left, behind Commons: Acting Assistant Engineer T. Benton Brown. When *Hartford* was not a flagship, its official allowance of medical officers was one surgeon and two assistant surgeons (NHHC, image NH 47089).

July 1864—and covered the Virginia and North Carolina coasts. (There was also a Beaufort, South Carolina.) The James River Flotilla, which existed for about two months in 1862, was an independent command within the NABS.[7]

The SABS, also formed by the split of the Atlantic Blockading Squadron, was based at Port Royal, South Carolina, and was initially responsible for the South Carolina coast and the Atlantic coast of Florida to its southern extremity, including Key West. Its southernmost limit was later changed to Cape Canaveral, on Florida's Atlantic coast.[8]

The Gulf Blockading Squadron, formed in May 1861, was split in January 1862 into the EGBS and WGBS. The range of the EGBS, based at Key West, extended from Cape Canaveral to, and including, St. Andrew's Bay, Florida, which is east of Pensacola and the site of present-day Panama City. The Bahamas and Cuba were included within the EGBS's limits.[9]

The WGBS, based for most of the war at Pensacola, was responsible for blockading the Gulf Coast extending from, but not including, St. Andrew's Bay to the Rio Grande River. Also included within the squadron's limits were the coasts of Mexico and Yucatán. During much of the war, the WGBS's vessels were divided into those on blockade duty and those ascending the Mississippi River.[10]

The Mississippi Squadron was created when the Western Gunboat Flotilla—which had been controlled by the army but had USN officers commanding its vessels—was transferred to the navy. That transfer was mandated by a July 1862 act of Congress but not completed until September 30, 1862. The official change of command occurred on October 1. Before the transfer, acting medical officers for the flotilla were appointed by its successive flag officers: Commander John Rodgers, Captain Andrew H. Foote, and Captain Charles H. Davis. Such appointments were allowable with the approval of the secretary of the navy, but BUMED chief Whelan had apparently been kept in the dark about them. In August 1862, Surgeon Edward Gilchrist was named fleet surgeon of the Western Gunboat Flotilla and of the future Mississippi Squadron. At that time, Whelan told Gilchrist that because the navy was assuming control of the flotilla in its current state, "it is supposed Medical Officers—probably acting assistant surgeons—appointed by the War Department [actually, by naval commanders], will be retained, unless you should deem changes conducive to the public interests." The Mississippi Squadron, working out of Cairo and Mound City, Illinois, made its way down the Mississippi River while WGBS vessels ascended it.[11]

Among the remaining naval units was the Potomac Flotilla, which was based at Washington, D.C., kept the Potomac River open, and combatted smuggling between Maryland and Virginia. During the mid- to late-war years, the flotilla contained 17–25 vessels, with all or most rated as fourth class.[12]

Of other, smaller units, the Pacific Squadron, which existed before the war, had eight vessels in 1864 and probably occupied most of Whelan's attention because of plans to build a hospital at Mare Island, California, to care for the squadron's sick. Pacific Squadron vessels escorted ships, some carrying gold, traveling between California and the Isthmus of Panama and kept on the lookout for possible Confederate commerce raiders. The West India Squadron—which existed for a few months in 1861 and then from September 1862 to September 1864—consisted of six vessels in 1864 and worked largely out of Havana, Cuba, and Cape Haitien (Cap-Haïtien), Haiti. During most of its existence, the squadron searched for commerce raiders and escorted ships from Panama to New York. The Brazil, Africa, and Mediterranean Stations consisted of one or two ships each in 1864. Several ships on "special service" hunted the high seas for commerce raiders.[13]

It was common for Whelan to recommend that the Navy Department assign medical officers, especially regular and volunteer assistant surgeons, to squadrons rather than to specific vessels so that flag officers and fleet surgeons could place those officers where most needed. This practice sometimes made it necessary for Whelan to ask fleet surgeons to name the vessels to which medical officers were assigned.[14]

Assistant surgeons at sea saw that medicines were properly weighed, measured, and labeled; tended to duties as assigned; ensured the comfort and cleanliness of the sick; and saw that surgeons' stewards and nurses performed their duties. If no surgeon was assigned to his vessel, an assistant surgeon took on the addition duties of a surgeon. They included taking charge of medicines and medical supplies (including making requisitions), caring for patients and reporting their status to the commanding officer, being on the lookout for contagious diseases, examining men joining the crew, preparing for the care of the wounded, sending patients to hospitals, and keeping and submitting a multitude of paperwork.[15]

Being allowed medical officers did not guarantee having them assigned. In early 1863, for example, no medical officer was assigned to *Ceres*, a sidewheel steamer in the NABS, or to *Dragon*, a screw steamer in the Potomac Flotilla. Those fourth-class vessels had complements of 45 and 42, respectively, well above the minimum of 25 required to have an assistant surgeon. The magnitude of the staffing shortage, which grew worse as vessels were added to the navy and the appointment of new medical officers slowed, was demonstrated in early 1865 when Whelan pointed out that the large majority of vessels in the Potomac Flotilla did not have their own medical officer. Vessels without adequate medical personnel would seek assistance, when needed, from nearby squadron vessels carrying a medical officer or surgeon's steward.[16]

Whelan leaned heavily on acting assistant surgeons, who outnumbered permanent medical officers late in the war. He stated in 1863 that acting assistant surgeons "are never assigned to shore service; but are invariably employed in the smaller, and supplementary, vessels of the Navy." Although most such officers did indeed serve on fourth-class vessels, Whelan was not entirely accurate. Acting Assistant Surgeon A. Shirk, for example, served on USS *St. Lawrence*, flagship of the EGBS, and Acting Assistant Surgeon J.J. Brownlee served on USS *Quaker City* of the SABS; both vessels were rated as second class. A small number of acting assistant surgeons also served at hospitals on shore.[17]

In September 1863, Fleet Surgeon Ninian Pinkney reported from Cairo, Illinois, that the Mississippi Squadron had 69 vessels. Included were two receiving ships—at Cairo, with an acting assistant surgeon, and at Cincinnati, with no medical officer—and hospital ship *Red Rover*, on which Pinkney served with a pair of acting assistant surgeons. Among the other 66 vessels, there were 8 assistant surgeons and 35 acting assistant surgeons, with no vessel carrying multiple medical officers. Thus, 23 squadron vessels were left without a medical officer. At least one of those, USS *Covington*, did not even have a surgeon's steward in late August 1863, when its crew, excluding officers, numbered 37.[18]

Shore facilities associated with the squadron included Pinkney Hospital in Memphis, with a surgeon and a pair of acting assistant surgeons; a naval rendezvous in Cincinnati, with an acting assistant surgeon; and the Marine barracks and naval station at Cairo, with an acting assistant surgeon. After Rear Admiral David D. Porter, the squadron's flag officer, divided his command into eight districts, Whelan recommended that Pinkney assign an assistant surgeon to each district "to look after the forms, accounts &c of the acting officers."[19]

Before 1864, allowance tables rarely if ever showed a vessel type that was not entitled to at least a surgeon's steward. The 1864 tables allowed one surgeon's steward on any vessel with at least 25 crewmembers; vessels with a smaller complement were not entitled to a medical officer or surgeon's steward. The tables showed no situation in which a surgeon's steward would serve afloat in the absence of a medical officer, but exactly that circumstance was allowed by creating the grade of surgeon's steward in charge and assigning men at that grade as the sole providers of medical care on some small vessels. In early 1865, Whelan claimed that at least 70 vessels had a surgeon's steward as their only medical caregiver.[20]

Being assigned to a vessel or squadron did not guarantee that all of a medical officer's duties would be performed on that ship or on missions associated with that ship only. Surgeons could, for example, accompany shore expeditions whose personnel comprised men from numerous vessels. They sometimes established or worked at temporary hospitals serving multiple ships, and they occasionally assisted army surgeons at army hospitals.

Fleet Surgeons

A fleet surgeon, the administrative medical officer of a squadron—analogous to a medical director in the army—was appointed at BUMED's suggestion and was that squadron's most senior surgeon, a convention that Whelan carefully observed (Appendix B). Although Surgeon Edward Gilchrist was originally assigned early in the war to the flagship *Minnesota* as fleet surgeon of the Atlantic Blockading Squadron, that squadron's rapid growth—it was later divided into the NABS and the SABS—meant that it would soon be assigned additional surgeons, at least one of whom might be senior to Gilchrist. Thus, Whelan requested on May 3, 1861, that Gilchrist's assignment as fleet surgeon be revoked and that he should regard himself, for the time being, as *Minnesota*'s surgeon only. Later in the month, Whelan recommended that Gilchrist be transferred to USS *Wabash*; that Surgeon Thomas Dillard, who outranked Gilchrist and was the new fleet surgeon, be transferred from USS *Cumberland* to *Minnesota*; and that Surgeon Samuel Jackson, who was outranked by Dillard and Gilchrist, be transferred from *Wabash* to *Cumberland*. Such moves aligned the surgeons' rank with the rating or prestige of their assigned vessel and were needed, according to Whelan, "to maintain proper regard for the relative position of medical officers."[21]

Whelan's recommendations for fleet-surgeon appointments were probably not simplified by special requests. Acting Rear Admiral S.P. Lee, flag officer of the NABS, learned in December 1863 that his fleet surgeon, William Maxwell Wood, would soon be reassigned. Lee wanted his friend, Surgeon James C. Palmer, to take Wood's place and asked Assistant Secretary of the Navy Gustavus V. Fox whether that appointment could be made. Palmer had, as Lee knew, recently been named fleet surgeon of the WGBS. The extent to which Assistant Secretary Fox intervened is not known, but Palmer remained with the WGBS throughout the rest of the war. Lee, however, got his second choice, Surgeon John L. Fox, even though at least two surgeons, David Harlan and J. Dickinson Miller, were senior to him, were evidently healthy enough for sea service, and had not yet been a fleet surgeon. It is unclear if Whelan recommended Surgeon Fox; various factors could have prevented the assignment of Harlan or Miller as NABS fleet surgeon.[22]

A fleet surgeon exercised general supervision of a squadron's medical officers and was subordinate to the squadron commander, its flag officer. All communications from squadron medical officers to BUMED were channeled through the fleet surgeon, who received and approved all of their requisitions before forwarding them. He cooperated with the BUMED chief and with the flag officer, advised the latter on measures for maintaining health and caring for the sick and wounded, and kept a journal and notebook to be sent to the secretary of the navy. He also acted as the flagship's surgeon and was thus included in its allowed complement. In February 1865, Whelan said of Surgeon William Maxwell Wood, fleet surgeon of the NABS: "He is the surgeon of the flag ship, medical purveyor [supply officer] of the squadron, beside his extensive duties as medical supervisor of a fleet, and is allowed no clerical assistance." In 1863, Fleet Surgeon James C. Palmer of the WGBS, wrote Whelan that "writing and copying official letters and various other papers occupy so many hours, every day, as to leave hardly any time for action, and frequently more important duties." (Officers routinely made copies of at least outgoing correspondence.) Palmer asked for a clerk, a request endorsed by the WGBS's Commodore Henry H. Bell and by Whelan.[23]

On January 31, 1862, Surgeon George Clymer, fleet surgeon of the SABS, wrote from Port Royal, South Carolina, to summarize the state of his squadron as of the final quarter of 1861. He had medical officers on 30 different vessels and an officer ashore with a Marine battalion; thus, he had 31 groups of reports to compile and submit. He had 6 vessels without a medical officer; their medical care was provided by a storeship and the flagship. Since the beginning of the year, 8 more vessels, had arrived. The squadron, which had bombarded Port Royal on November 7, 1861, had an average of about 5,700 crewmen, with about 120 sick per day. Thus, when he wrote, Clymer had overall responsibility for the medical care of men on 44 vessels. In early 1860, in contrast, the Home Squadron, which was the navy's largest, had 13 vessels.[24]

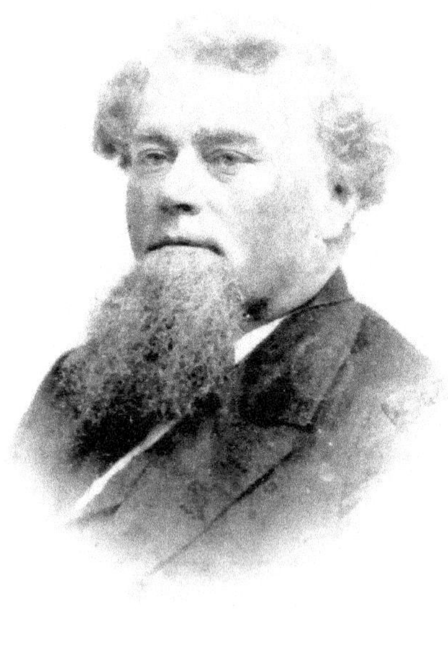

Surgeon William Maxwell Wood, who served as fleet surgeon for the WGBS and then for the NABS (NHHC, image NH 100178).

In at least one instance, involving the WGBS, the duties of Fleet Surgeon Jonathan M. Foltz were so "onerous and arduous" that an additional surgeon was assigned to the flagship, USS *Hartford*; this was in addition to two other medical officers already present. The same may have been true for the NABS, whose flagship, USS *Minnesota*, carried in early 1863 a fleet surgeon in addition to a full surgeon and two assistant surgeons. It is also possible that a fleet surgeon could be considered a supernumerary officer, perhaps as a member of the flag officer's staff.[25]

Shore Assignments

Most shore assignments for medical officers were to a navy yard—a facility for the docking, repair, and supply of naval vessel—or to an establishment considered within the yard's command and geographic limits, such as a naval hospital, rendezvous, or receiving ship. Among the navy's functional navy yards in early 1863 were those at or near Portsmouth (New Hampshire), Boston, New York, Philadelphia, Washington (DC), and Pensacola. Navy yards each had a high-ranking line officer as commandant. Medical officers could also be assigned to a naval station, which consisted of one or more facilities important enough to require a commandant of high rank. Wartime naval stations were located at Baltimore, where storage facilities and a receiving ship were situated, and near Norfolk, Virginia, where the station included a hospital and Marine guard. (Navy yards and naval stations could have numerous fairly widely dispersed elements that were not necessarily in the city or town after which the yard or station was named. The temporary hospital at the Norfolk station was on the outskirts of Norfolk, but the permanent hospital was closer to Gosport, on the opposite side of the Elizabeth River.) Medical officers assigned to a navy yard or naval station were responsible to both the commandant and BUMED.[26]

The man assigned as the medical officer of a navy yard was always a full surgeon, who may have had an assistant surgeon to help him. A full surgeon was usually placed in charge of medical personnel of a receiving ship, permanent hospital, or rendezvous, although such facilities often had assistant surgeons as well. A navy yard's surgeon was responsible for medical supplies issued to vessels fitting out at the yard, or received from vessels arriving there, and for providing medical care to naval and Marine Corps personnel attached to the yard. Most medical officers assigned to a station served in that station's hospital.[27]

One exception was Surgeon Robert T. Maccoun, assigned in mid–1863 to the naval station at Baltimore, which had no associated hospital.

Maccoun, as a "general agent" for BUMED, was in charge of medical supplies for naval vessels preparing for or returning from a cruise. He was to examine and forward requisitions from vessels to BUMED and see to the proper routing of supplies sent from the central supply facility (the medical laboratory in Brooklyn) and intended for vessels at Baltimore (including the receiving ship *Allegheny*) and Hampton Roads, Virginia, or for the Norfolk Naval Hospital. Whelan told Fleet Surgeon William Maxwell Wood of the NABS that surgical instruments needing repair could be sent to Maccoun at Baltimore, who was charged with attending "to all such matters," rather than to the medical laboratory. Maccoun was also to relieve Surgeon Daniel Egbert, *Allegheny*'s surgeon, when necessary.[28]

Before the war, it was not unusual for shore assignments to last at least three years, especially for senior surgeons. For example, Surgeon Isaac Brinkerhoff, whose naval service started in 1829, was posted to the naval rendezvous in Boston from June 1857 to June 1860, and Surgeon Edward Gilchrist, in the navy since 1832, was assigned to the Boston Naval Hospital (in Chelsea, Massachusetts) from April 1854 to February 1858. This remained true, to some extent, during the war. Surgeon Lewis B. Hunter, for example, entered the navy in 1828 and served at the naval rendezvous in Philadelphia from December 1861 to January 1865, and Surgeon M.G. Delaney, in the navy since 1833, was assigned to the Portsmouth (New Hampshire) Navy Yard from July 1861 to February 1865. (The name *Portsmouth* was sometimes applied to facilities associated with the Norfolk yard or station because of their proximity to Portsmouth, Virginia.) Surgeons who were placed on the retired list because of age, but were still able to work, often served much of the war at a shore facility.[29]

It appears that Whelan tried to alternate sea assignments—which could be exhausting and expose men to unhealthy climates—with shore postings, or at least with short breaks before a return to sea. However, the struggle to provide medical care on vessels during the war made it impossible to keep medical officers, especially assistant surgeons, on shore for prolonged periods between their assignments afloat. Breaks from sea duty would surely have been welcomed and found conducive to physical and mental health. They could also provide medical and other experiences that might not be available at sea. Respites were often given to provide assistant surgeons time to prepare for the promotion examination. The general lack of extended wartime shore assignments is shown by the eligibility of assistant surgeons for promotion within a relatively short time—which had to include at least two years at sea—after their entry into the navy. Seven men appointed as assistant surgeon in

May 1861 passed the promotion examination in October 1863, and 20 appointed assistant surgeons in July 1861 passed the examination in June 1864.[30]

About two-thirds of the 150 or so regular-navy assistant surgeons commissioned from May 1861 through 1864 served their first assignment at a shore facility. Postings to receiving ships or hospitals each accounted for about 25 percent of initial assignments, and duty at a navy yard accounted for about 16 percent. Those assignments, which typically lasted less than three months, could have had numerous benefits. The receiving ship *Ohio*, at Boston, was the initial wartime assignment for at least 20 assistant surgeons. On a receiving ship—a stationary vessel on which recruits were gathered for processing, indoctrination, and preliminary training—a new medical officer could start experiencing shipboard life, examine and treat relatively healthy sailors, and begin learning about the endless paperwork expected from medical officers. New skills could be learned at hospitals and navy yards. In some cases, assignment to shore duty probably lasted only as long as it took for a new officer's vessel to be completed or repaired.[31]

Acting assistant surgeons were most commonly assigned directly to a vessel. Exceptions included Acting Assistant Surgeons David V. Whitney and George H. Cooke, whose first assignments were to the Boston Naval Hospital and the Norfolk Naval Hospital, respectively.[32]

In some instances, medical officers posted to a squadron were given shore assignments. For example, Surgeon Benjamin F. Gibbs was assigned to the WGBS in September 1862 and immediately posted to the squadron's hospital being built at Pensacola. Since there was no established shore station in the area, and because he had, at times, to draw a ration—available, by law, to officers when on sea duty only—he asked whether he could be credited with sea service and receive sea pay. That request was granted, and subsequent medical officers initially assigned by the Navy Department to the Pensacola hospital had their orders modified to show them posted to the squadron, which entitled them to sea pay and sea-service credit while they worked ashore.[33]

Medical officers were sometimes assigned to provide care in army hospitals. In July 1863, Assistant Surgeon Isaac H. Hazelton of USS *Paul Jones* and Assistant Surgeon John T. Luck of USS *Ottawa*, were conveyed to Port Royal on an army hospital ship carrying army wounded and then to hospitals at Beaufort, South Carolina, to assist army surgeons. That service, approved by Rear Admiral John A. Dahlgren of the SABS, resulted in *Paul Jones* and *Ottawa* being without a medical officer.[34]

Courts

Whenever a naval officer of the medical, paymaster, or engineer corps was the subject of a court of inquiry or court-martial, the court was to consist, in part, of officers of that staff. Thus, medical officers sat in judgment of other medical officers. Courts could consume considerable time, during which their members were away from their regular duties.[35]

Secretary Welles in June 1864 received a complaint from a woman who claimed that she had met two intoxicated medical officers during a visit to the Norfolk Naval Hospital. One was "so drunk he could scarcely speak," and the other "was barely able to walk" from drunkenness. The next month, a court of inquiry was convened at the Norfolk Naval Station to ascertain the facts of the encounter. The court consisted of Commodore John W. Livingston, commandant of the station, as court president, Surgeons Lewis B. Hunter and William Maxwell Wood as court members, and Passed Assistant Surgeon John Paul Quinn as the judge advocate (prosecutor).[36]

The accused were Surgeons Solomon Sharp and William Johnson, Jr. No testimony suggested that either man was intoxicated at the time in question or had a drinking problem, but Fleet Surgeon John L. Fox of the NABS indicated that Sharp might appear drunk because of a speech impairment (caused by partial paralysis) in addition to "his fullness of habit [ruddiness] and carefulness of locomotion." Commodore Livingston confirmed that Sharp's florid complexion, speech difficulty, and unsteady gait might make him appear intoxicated. Fleet Surgeon Fox testified that Johnson, whom he had known since the latter's childhood, had two ophthalmic conditions that could make his eyes look bloodshot. Two days after first session, the court declared that there was nothing to sustain the allegations and that no further action was warranted.[37]

In April 1865, a court-martial convened aboard USS *Alabama* to try Acting Assistant Surgeon John F. Henry on multiple charges related to his allegedly being intoxicated in December 1864 while serving on USS *Delaware*. In addition to a line officer as court president and a captain's clerk as judge advocate, two of the six court members—Daniel D.T. Nestell and H.R. Watts—were acting assistant surgeons. (One of the court members, a line officer, was excused a few days into the trial because of his need to be with his vessel, which was ordered to another location.) After a trial of 10 days, Henry was acquitted of two charges but found guilty of two others: "scandalous conduct" (intoxication to the point of fighting, quarreling, and resisting the authority of another officer) and being "culpably inefficient to perform his duty." Henry was sentenced to forfeit any pay and subsistence due him and to be dismissed from the navy. The court also sentenced one of the witnesses to two months of imprisonment for his "contradictory evidence and prevarication."[38]

The urgent need for medical officers on vessels mandated that most assistant and acting assistant surgeons be assigned to duty afloat. Full surgeons were needed for sea duty as fleet surgeons and as medical officers on larger vessels, while older officers at that grade often served at shore facilities. The navy had too many vessels for each to be supplied with a medical officer or surgeon's steward. Shore assignments varied and could provide a welcome break from the taxing requirements of sea duty.

Chapter 7

Conducting Physical Examinations

Applicants for appointment as assistant surgeons were not the only subjects of physical examination by medical officers. Other examined persons included those enlisting in the navy or Marine Corps, prospective and actual students at the U.S. Naval Academy, and members of the navy or Marines who were ill or injured (or claimed to be) or were suspected to be physically incapable of performing their duties.

Recruits

Naval and Marine Corps rendezvous were operated in large Eastern port cites and along main waterways in the interior. The busiest rendezvous were in New York City, where at least five were open at the same time. Other facilities enlisting large numbers of men were in Brooklyn (not yet a borough of New York City), Boston, and Philadelphia. The remaining sites included Portland and Kittery, Maine; Burlington, Vermont; New Bedford, Massachusetts; Portsmouth, New Hampshire; Baltimore; Washington, D.C.; Erie, Pennsylvania; Cincinnati; Chicago; Cairo, Illinois; St. Louis; Louisville; and Memphis. Not all of these rendezvous were open simultaneously. In early 1863, the rendezvous in Portland lacked a medical officer, which necessitated sending recruits to Boston for examination.[1]

The medical officer present at rendezvous, especially the larger facilities, was generally a surgeon or passed assistant surgeon. Not only was a rendezvous a safe place to assign a surgeon who had been placed on the retired list because of age, older surgeons were experienced performing physical examinations and had a good idea of the physical and mental conditions that should disqualify a man from naval service. A man deemed suitable to join the navy by a line officer at the rendezvous was subjected to physical examination by the surgeon, who was guided by brief written instructions. The applicant was to remove all his clothes and demonstrate that he, and his limbs, could move freely. The surgeon would test the man's senses, perform a complete examination, and try to discover any predilection to convulsions or insanity. He would look for convincing evidence that the applicant had received a smallpox vaccination—a characteristic scar, for example—or had a previous case of the disease. (Before the war, evidence of vaccination or a previous case of smallpox would have obviated the need for vaccination upon arrival at the receiving ship. On December 31, 1861, however, BUMED chief Whelan ordered that *all* recruits be vaccinated promptly after boarding the receiving ship.) An applicant with physical defects could be allowed into the navy if the rendezvous commander and surgeon believed that the defects did not disqualify him from performing the duties of his rating. Those defects, however, had to be enumerated fully by the surgeon to prevent their being used later as the basis for a pension claim.[2]

Whelan acknowledged that guidelines for examining recruits were not very specific and relied on medical officers' judgment and experience. When a surgeon asked whether a venereal disease disqualified an applicant, Whelan replied that "judgment should be predicated on the condition of the man, rather than upon the name of the disease." Gonorrhea, if simple and recent, should not necessarily be a reason for rejection if the applicant was otherwise sound. The decision for a man with syphilis should "depend altogether upon the character of the disease, at the time, and the general condition of the individual."[3]

Careful physical examination, and documentation of the same, helped to ensure that the navy received recruits able to do their duty. Thoroughness on the part of rendezvous surgeons also helped to protect the navy against unjust pension claims, against losing salary advances and bounties to men who then claimed disability, and against the inconvenience and loss of time dealing with recruits who simply had a change of heart and sought a discharge. A frequent tactic of men who regretted enlisting was to assert that disqualifying defects were missed by the rendezvous surgeon, an action that might necessitate reexamination. Surgeon Gustavus R.B. Horner related a prewar story of a surgeon who had properly pronounced a recruit fit, had his judgment reversed after the recruit feigned lameness, and was fined by the secretary of the navy the amount that the man, who was discharged, had been advanced in pay.[4]

After a surgeon at the Norfolk Naval Hospital recommended the discharge of men who had recently been enlisted in New York, Whelan asked the medical officer of the rendezvous, Surgeon Charles Chase, to explain how the sailors' disabilities—extensive tooth decay in one and asthma in another—had been overlooked. Chase stated that because his careful examination had revealed nothing to justify the applicants' rejection, their problems must have arisen after he had seen them. Surgeon John J. Abernethy, also assigned to a New York rendezvous, gave a similar answer when questioned by Whelan. Among the more than 1,700 applicants he had passed during the previous six months, said Abernethy, "it would not be strange if some of them should prove after a trial of several months, owing to exposure, and change of life, and habits, unfit for the service." Whether Whelan found such arguments believable is impossible to say.[5]

An applicant judged fit at a rendezvous proceeded to a receiving ship, where he was examined and vaccinated by the vessel's surgeon. The vessel's officers took possession of two rendezvous-prepared lists that stated details about the recruit, including his physical description. The description was important in combatting fraudulent tactics, such as having a skilled man enlist as an able seaman—who was entitled to a relatively high salary advance—and substituting an unskilled and possibly unfit man to report to the receiving ship in his place. The skilled man could then enlist at multiple other rendezvous and keep collecting advances while the navy ended up with men who did not measure up to their expectations.[6]

Some medical officers, frustrated with unfit enlistees who were somehow approved by rendezvous surgeons, sought ways to alert their colleagues about "well-known invalids or malingerers." Surgeon Edward Shippen returned such applicants to rendezvous surgeons with an explanatory note and acknowledged that unfit men might appear healthy when attempting to enlist. "It is a pity," wrote Shippen to Whelan, "that we are not able to mark such men, for, if discharged, [they] will undoubtedly endeavor to repeat the same operation elsewhere." Surgeon Solomon Sharp, stationed at the Norfolk Naval Hospital, described one Henry P. Seaman, who had been previously discharged from the navy because of dementia. Seaman reenlisted, appeared three months later at the same hospital with essentially the same diagnosis, and became dangerous enough to be put in double irons. Sharp suggested applying a scarificator (a device used in wet cupping) to Seaman's left buttock to make two overlapping sets of incisions, perpendicular to each other, and then alerting rendezvous officers of the distinctive crosshatched scar. Scarificators were rarely used on the buttocks, so the mark was likely to draw a surgeon's attention. "The idea is not original with me," wrote Sharp, "but it can scarcely fall under the stigma of cruelty." Whelan agreed to warn rendezvous surgeons about

Seaman but rejected the idea of using a scarificator to mark any man who had been found unfit to serve.[7]

In May 1861, a newspaper correspondent described one of the New York rendezvous as being located on "one of the dirtiest streets in the city" amid "the double odor or old junk and loose morals." In August 1864, a man wishing to enlist described two of the city's rendezvous as seemingly "selected with special reference to inconvenience ... and too mean and dirty for business." The officers at one rendezvous were "pent up in a small hole, with a reeking crowd of all conditions and nations blocking the hall and stairway." Occupying the rest of the building were "shopkeepers, sharpers and hangers-on" on the lookout for recruits to swindle. Recruits were offered allowances for travel and housing, three-month advances on salary, and bounties that were made more attractive as enthusiasm for joining the navy waned later in the war. Various parties endeavored to fraudulently gain a share of those funds by acting as agents or brokers to facilitate recruitment, getting applicants drunk, bribing officials, and other measures. The degree, if any, to which medical officers were involved in this unscrupulous activity has not been determined.[8]

Assistant Surgeon Joseph O. Burnett was assigned in August 1864 to the naval rendezvous at Kittery, Maine, and to the ship *Vandalia* at the nearby Portsmouth, New Hampshire, Navy Yard. He testified in November 1864 to a court of inquiry that he had been offered bribes at

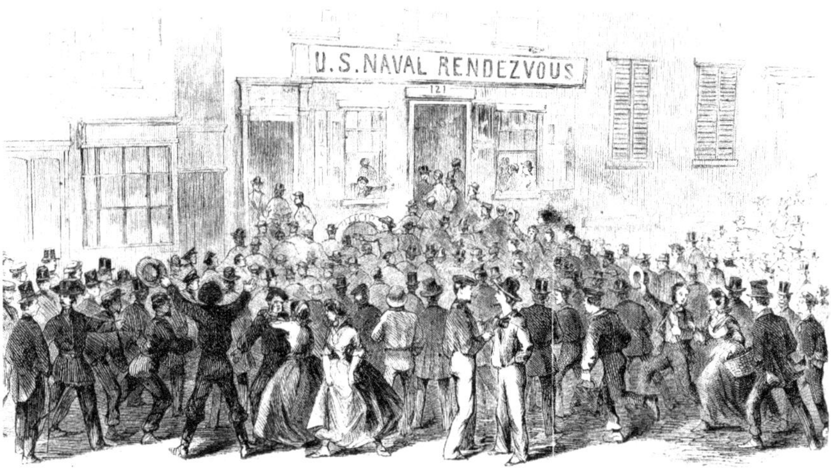

A rush of applicants eager to join the navy, with onlookers, at a naval rendezvous in New York City. Successful enlistment required passing a physical examination conducted by a naval medical officer (*Frank Leslie's Illustrated Newspaper*, May 25, 1861).

least 50 times to allow specific men into the navy; he claimed to have rejected all bribes. Among recruits on *Vandalia,* he said, were unfit men formerly discharged from the navy but allowed to reenlist at the Portsmouth rendezvous. Various naval recruits with supposedly disqualifying physical conditions testified that their enlistment was handled by a broker, who told them that the Kittery rendezvous surgeon had to be paid. One enlistee said that he had a hernia but did not so disclose to the surgeon, who did not look for one. Another claimed he was blind in one eye and saw poorly with the other but that his broker assured him he would be admitted "as the doctor was all right." Burnett testified that he always examined applicants thoroughly, after they had completely disrobed, as specified in naval regulations.[9]

After Surgeon William E. Taylor expressed concerns about some of the recruits arriving at his receiving ship, Whelan told him he had a duty to decline to accept any man he had reasonable doubts about. If a board of medical officers then found the recruit fit, Taylor would be exonerated from all responsibility for the man's condition. Even requiring more rigid examinations at rendezvous, admitted Whelan, might not help the situation, "especially at a time when the ingenuity of designing people [dishonest agents and brokers] is taxed to the uttermost to impose upon the service an indifferent class of men."[10]

Naval Academy

A medical officer was stationed at the U.S. Naval Academy—relocated from Annapolis to Newport, Rhode Island, for the duration of the war—to provide care for its students and staff. Admission to the academy required passing an examination administered by the institution's academic board and a physical examination by its surgeon and two other medical officers assigned by the Navy Department. Those physicians were to ensure that an applicant was "qualified to endure the arduous duties of an officer of the navy both at the time of his examination, and, probably, during the rest of his life, until age shall disable him."[11]

In 1863, proposed changes to the academy's regulations included minimum height requirements for the various ages of applicants, who had to be more than 14 and less than 18 years old. These ranged from 4 ft., 10 in. for a 14-year-old applicant to 5 ft., 4 in. for a nearly 18-year-old candidate. Whelan argued against strict application of the limits, especially for a 14-year-old, because short stature at that age did not rule out future development into "a man of fair proportions." Furthermore, "shape, activity, and stamina" were essential in naval officers and might well be more common in men measuring 5 ft., 3 in. than in men a foot taller. In place of the height requirements, argued Whelan, a paragraph should be added to the regulations stating that attention would be paid to applicants' stature, that no young man manifestly undersized for his age would be admitted, and that in instances of doubt about an applicant's physical condition, "any marked deviation from the usual standard of height will add materially to the consideration for rejection." Contrary to Whelan's urging, the medical board for examination of applicants added the height requirements in 1864, but Whelan's suggested paragraph was also included verbatim.[12]

Before the war, academy regulations required a physical inspection to allow a student to rise from a lower to a higher class "because of the rapid constitutional changes belonging to the transition state from youth to adolescence, or manhood." They also required a "physical examination of rigid character" at graduation but omitted details about who would conduct that examination. In 1864, Whelan—ignorant of existing academy regulations, wanting to clarify them, or suspecting that all were not followed—recommended that members of the academy's graduating class be examined by three medical officers, one of them being the academy's surgeon, before they assumed active duty in the navy. During a student's time at the academy, "disease, or defects, may be undergoing slow, but progressive development, not sufficient perhaps to arrest the attention of the medical officers of the academy, but which might, in the course of short exposure to climatic and atmospheric vicissitudes, prove serious impediments in the way of future usefulness." Whelan urged that the physical examination of Naval Academy graduates should assess "the external senses as sight, hearing &c as well as extend ... through physical and rational signs, into the general condition of the candidate for naval commission. Doing so would give the [Navy] Department the best assurance that the pupil it had fostered, and educated should repay in usefulness the care and kindness of his government." The wording of academy regulations was not altered in response to Whelan's suggestion, and it is unclear whether changes were made in the conduct of the physical examination performed at graduation.[13]

Surveys

Naval personnel were subject to a physical examination called a survey when they were suspected of being unfit for duty. A survey could be ordered as early as a recruit's reporting to a receiving ship, since that vessel's commander and surgeon were to examine all recruits upon arrival. If the commander thought a recruit unfit, he would report the fact to the station commander, who would order a survey by three officers. At least one of those officers had to be a medical officer, and if practicable, that medical officer should be senior to the rendezvous surgeon where the subject was enlisted. A finding of unfitness would be reported to the secretary of the navy for a decision. Outcomes might include a furlough to allow recovery, discharge from the navy, or admission to a hospital.[14]

The commander of a vessel in active service was to report any crewmember he thought to be unfit to the senior officer in command (usually the flag officer), who would order a survey by at least one medical officer, three if practicable. Information about possible unfitness could be relayed to a flag officer by his fleet surgeon, who was obligated to report any officers or men he deemed unfit. For such surveys, it was desirable to call upon medical officers not assigned to the subject's vessel, since it was likely that a surgeon who had already evaluated the subject had formed an opinion about his fitness. A finding of unfitness was to be sent to the secretary of the navy or the flag officer for a decision. A survey could also be conducted to determine eligibility for a pension. Copies of a certificate, made out by the commander and surgeon of the vessel on which the injury or illness occurred, were to be sent to the secretary of the navy and BUMED, with another copy given to the person surveyed.[15]

BUMED chief Whelan was especially concerned about his medical officers filling out survey reports that would prove satisfactory to the Pension Office, which was administered by the Department of the Interior. The relationship between that office and BUMED was close because the documentation that naval officers provided had a large part in pension decisions. In the first 10 months of 1863, Whelan reported, BUMED had 344 case referrals from the Pension Office and adjusted 185 cases.[16]

Surgeons on vessels were required to keep a journal of daily practice to record all cases of special interest, especially those that might involve a pension claim, and to note whether the disease of injury occurred in the line of duty. When, however, a certificate of disability—as might result from a survey—or of death was submitted, it was to state the facts or circumstances leading to the opinion that the disease or injury was a result of duty. The opinion alone, which medical officers had gotten into the habit of providing, was insufficient for the Pension Office.[17]

When Fleet Surgeon Lewis B. Hunter of the NABS forwarded in

February 1865 a death certificate completed by Acting Assistant Surgeon George Hopkins, Whelan observed that Hopkins did "not seem to comprehend fully the requirements of the Pension Office" in using the "line of duty" phrase without explanation. "As you know," Whelan chided Hunter—implying that the fleet surgeon should not have forwarded an inadequate certificate—the office needed the "facts upon which the opinion is based, rather than the opinion itself." Whelan continued, "Every casualty, or disease, occurring on board ship may be associated with the performance of ordinary duty, but the Commissioner [of Pensions] does not take so wide of view of the subject."[18]

Medical officers conducted rigorous physical examinations of men wishing to join the navy. Doing so helped protect the service from unfit personnel and prevent the payment of pensions to men with preexisting disabilities. Men who were already serving but whose fitness was questioned were also subject to examination, with a key factor in the resulting report—affecting the payment of a pension—being evidence about whether the disability, if found, arose during the performance of duty. Whelan routinely encouraged medical offices to use their best judgment about how to define disabling conditions.

CHAPTER 8

Medical Supplies

THE CORNERSTONE OF BUMED's supply system was the medical laboratory at the New York Naval Hospital. Whelan took justifiable pride in the laboratory's ability to cope with the navy's tremendous wartime growth.

The Medical Laboratory

Before the mid–1840s, the navy's medical supplies were obtained through contracts awarded to the lowest bidders. There were no effective regulatory agencies to ensure that medicines sold in the United States met a standard of purity and quality. It took an astute buyer to identify goods that were not misrepresented or diluted with cheaper constituents.[1]

Starting in 1845, the navy's medicines and medical supplies became exempt from the contract system. That development coincided with a realization by Surgeon William S.W. Ruschenberger, stationed at the New York Naval Hospital, in Brooklyn, that the quality of the hospital's medicines was indifferent. According to Ruschenberger's account, he got permission from Surgeon Thomas Harris, BUMED chief, to manufacture the hospital's medicines onsite, an activity that expanded to supplying the New York Navy Yard (also in Brooklyn), to vessels fitting out there, and eventually to the whole navy. By late 1850, Ruschenberger's hospital and laboratory duties had been assumed by Surgeon Benjamin F. Bache, who in 1853 was relieved of his hospital assignment and named director of the laboratory, which was made a post distinct from the hospital.[2]

November 1853 was said to mark the formal organization of the laboratory. One of Bache's assistants, from October 1853 to July 1857, was Passed Assistant Surgeon Edward R. Squibb, who resigned from the navy in late 1857 to enter the drug-manufacturing business. Bache served at the laboratory throughout the war, even though he was placed on the retired list in 1863 because of his age.[3]

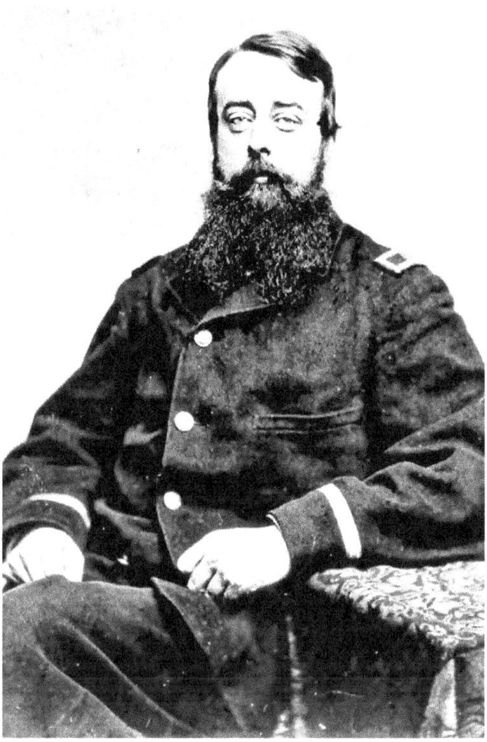

Surgeon Benjamin Franklin Bache, director of the USN's medical laboratory in Brooklyn. Bache attained the grade of surgeon in 1828, but the lace on his cuffs, which appears to reflect uniform regulations in effect early in the Civil War, is that of a surgeon with less than 12 years at that grade (Official U.S. Navy photograph in Sobocinski, "Dr. Bache").

Many medicinal items at the time were of vegetable origin and could be sold and used in relatively crude form—as dried roots, bark, or leaves, for example. Other items had to be processed into forms, such as a tinctures or extracts, before they could be used. Those forms could be purchased premade or prepared by apothecaries in their shops. Other medicines, called chemicals—acids, chloroform, and ether, for example—had to be manufactured from raw materials and could be bought premade or made onsite. Large amounts of crude ingredients and finished medicines were imported into the United States, arriving primarily at New York, Boston, Philadelphia, and Baltimore.[4]

The laboratory's officers used their best judgment, backed by meticulous visual and chemical examination, in purchasing articles in their crude state, out of which they manufactured finished medicines of uniform quality and strength. There was ample opportunity for finding materials of high quality in New York, where drug wholesalers and other suppliers of medical goods abounded. Nevertheless, avoiding poor-quality raw materials was a challenge, said Whelan, because the "adulteration of medicines has attained the refinement of a science; and the devices for eluding casual, or physical, inspection will keep pace with the increased value of medicines under the tariff, tax, etc." Because of widespread drug adulteration, civilian physicians could never be sure that patients were receiving the prescribed medication in the desired concentration. Naval officers, on the other hand, had "the great advantage of knowing precisely the strength of articles they prescribe; the profession generally will acknowledge this to be a signal benefit."[5]

Most of the navy's wartime medical supplies emanated from the laboratory. Surgical instruments, bedding, and certain other items were purchased by and repaired through the laboratory. The facility also examined articles offered under contract to other navy bureaus. According to Whelan, they included "soap, candles, oils, whiskey, coloring matter, and texture of cloth, paints, etc." The laboratory, observed Whelan, was "about the only institution known to the government where the officers perform all the clerical labor; and it is great: no clerks, or writers are allowed." He boasted in 1863 that the laboratory impressed the army's surgeon general, William A. Hammond, to the extent that he was using it as a model for army laboratories. The laboratory's staffing in 1864 was two medical officers and nine men and boys.[6]

Whelan routinely wrote Welles to ask the Treasury Department to allow the duty-free importation of drug shipments—evidently intended for the laboratory—which were stored in a bonded warehouse in New York. Although some such shipments contained crude drugs, such as opium, others contained quinine sulfate, whose manufacture was complex enough that only two American drug companies, both in Philadelphia, produced it. It is unclear whether the laboratory manufactured quinine in insufficient quantities or did not make it at all and found that the imported products compared favorably in price and quantity with Philadelphia-made quinine.[7]

Whelan's trust in the laboratory and the associated supply system was evident early in the war when he turned down an offer by Wyeth and Brother, of Philadelphia, to supply medicines to the navy. The process, he told Welles, made the navy "independent of any other means of obtaining medical supplies; it is ample, in organization and equipment, to meet all probable demands for anything of this description. It assures us most reliable medicines and at reduced and uniform prices." It is unclear whether Edward R. Squibb—his former assistant and, by then, a major supplier of the army—made a similar inquiry. Whelan had similar confidence in the laboratory's skill in purchasing surgical instruments and declined an offer from Snowden and Brother of Philadelphia to supply such implements. "The Messrs Snowden," acknowledged Whelan, "enjoy a well deserved reputation in their business, & would furnish articles of undoubted quality if required."[8]

One testimonial to the quality of the laboratory's work came in

1863 from Charles H. Nichols, MD, superintendent of the Government Hospital for the Insane near Washington City, whose patients included naval personnel with mental illness. Whelan allowed Nichols to purchase medicines and liquors at cost from the laboratory. "The medicines are prepared with such care and the bottles so closely stopped," wrote Nichols, "that tinctures [alcohol-based formulations] and other volatile preparations may safely be relied upon to keep for an indefinite length of time. We have recently opened bottles of tinctures put up at the Naval Laboratory in 1857 and found that nothing had been lost by evaporation, either in strength or quantity." Although the market was glutted with adulterated liquors, Nichols had found "the wines and brandies and other liquors selected by the Director of the Laboratory, pure and in every respect of the best quality." He was glad to pay the laboratory's prices, which were "quite moderate in comparison with those which have ruled in the market."[9]

The Supply Process

BUMED issued tables that showed amounts of supplies allowed for vessels of various types or complements. Medical officers were to replenish their supplies by indicating the needed amounts on a requisition form. In squadrons, the forms would be gathered and approved by the fleet surgeon, sent to BUMED for approval, and forwarded to the laboratory for filling. It is unclear whether similar tables existed for shore facilities. If they did, they likely included a wider variety of items and equipment and allowed for the compounding of prescriptions that were more complex than those conveniently prepared on a vessel. Officers at shore facilities that were part of a navy yard would presumably send their requisitions first to the yard's surgeon, who would send them to BUMED; otherwise, requisitions would be sent directly to BUMED. Requests for amounts exceeding those indicated on the allowance table, or for items not in the table, also went to BUMED for approval. Whelan was inclined to supply items in amounts that seemed reasonable and was usually reluctant to interfere with medical officers' judgments about what they needed to treat patients.[10]

Although the Bureau of Provisions and Clothing supplied vessels' regular rations, BUMED's supply tables included certain food items and other goods useful for sick patients—arrowroot and tapioca, for example—under the heading of "hospital stores." Whelan reported that hospital stores such as sugar, tea, coffee, rice, vinegar, and soap were obtained from government stores at contract prices, while fresh meats and other foods making up the daily diet of the sick were obtained from naval suppliers at contract prices. The extent to which such contract items were distributed through the laboratory is unknown.[11]

Whelan was also open to accepting recommendations for what should be carried, and in what amounts. Smaller vessels that did not have a dispensary—a space for the storage and preparation of medicines—were often equipped with a standard medicine chest intended for a complement of 80–100 men. In the summer of 1861, Whelan told Surgeon William S.W. Ruschenberger, serving at the Boston Navy Yard, that it would be acceptable to customize the supply of medicines to vessels' ability to store them rather than use prefilled chests. Whelan asked Surgeon Bache of Brooklyn's medical laboratory to visit USS *Unadilla*, a new gunboat fitting out at New York, to determine if its so-called dispensing locker was roomy enough that a medicine chest would not be needed. If so, Bache was to create a list of drugs and other supplies that *Unadilla* and the 22 other vessels of identical design could carry. To both Ruschenberger and Bache, Whelan suggested the expedient of using narrow strips of copper—rather than metal clasps, which cost about $18 a set—to hold bottles in place. The amount saved might be trivial for a single ship, but in light of the many vessels being fitted out, not just those of the *Unadilla* type, the total savings were worth considering. After all, Whelan needed to keep within his budgeted expenditures.[12]

Although most goods came from the laboratory, Whelan sometimes had them purchased elsewhere. Ale, whiskey, mattresses, and pillows, for example, were bought in Philadelphia in 1864 for delivery to depots or hospitals at Pensacola and New Orleans, which were used by the WGBS. Goods meant for a squadron were typically delivered by supply ships to individual vessels, to their flagship for distribution to individual squadron vessels, or to shore installations used by the squadron. During 1863, a supply ship left a northern port about every 15 days with goods meant for the WGBS or its Pensacola and New Orleans depots. Supply ships involved in that effort included *Bermuda*, *Circassian*, and *Union*, leaving from New York, Philadelphia, and Boston; all three vessels had a medical officer on board. Whelan used the same supply ships to transport medical personnel to and from squadrons and to carry patients who needed long-term care to northern naval hospitals. Surgeons on vessels in need of supplies between deliveries might be able to obtain what was wanted from other squadron vessels or from a shore hospital.[13]

Whelan and other naval officers seemed wary of shipping goods over land because of the enhanced danger of breakage or other loss.

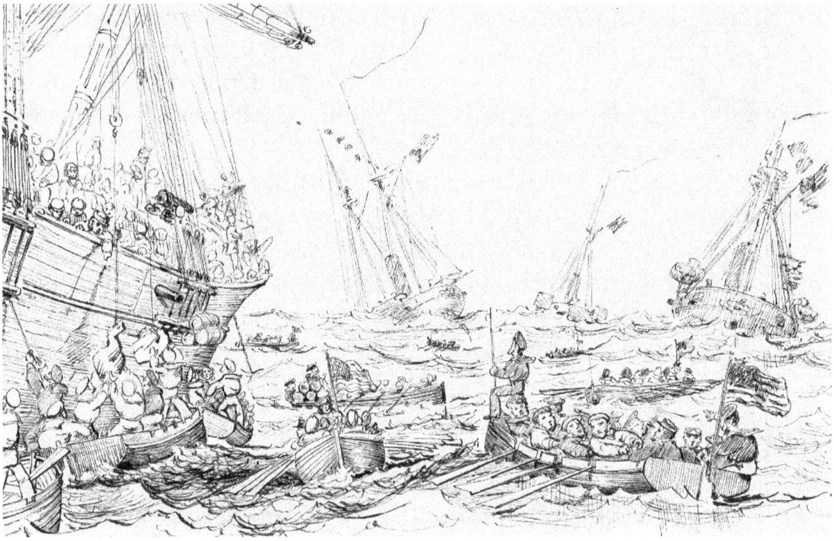

A supply steamer, possibly USS *Circassian*, lowering goods to boats for delivery to individual vessels of a squadron. Supply steamers could be called upon to transport patients to northern ports for hospitalization. Illustration by C. Ellery Steadman, an assistant surgeon during the war who served on *Circassian* (Civil War Photograph Collection, vol. 14, MOLLUS-MASS, USAHEC).

Whelan told the fleet surgeon of the Mississippi Squadron to exercise his judgment about whether it might be better to purchase supplies locally (in St. Louis) rather than use land transportation, with its additional cost and likely breakage. The fleet surgeon of the NABS wrote in mid–1863 that he would not entrust medical shipments to the military railroad between New Bern and Beaufort, North Carolina, "upon which our property disappears." When the fleet surgeon of the WGBS complained of receiving a box marked "muslin"—probably intended for bandages—that actually contained wrapping paper, Whelan replied that "it seems almost manifest that the box could not have left the laboratory in that condition; the contents must have been purloined somewhere, leaving the box to answer the invoice till the deficit was discovered." Shipments to Mare Island, California, were sent by the laboratory via steamer to Panama, where the U.S. consul and naval storekeeper arranged for their transport across the isthmus by rail and then by steamer to San Francisco.[14]

Vessels being equipped for a cruise obtained their medical supplies from the surgeon of the yard or station. Those returning from a cruise offloaded their supplies, which would be accounted for and transferred to the medical laboratory for inspection and possible repackaging and reissuance. The accounting practices used at depots that were not under the purview of a yard surgeon—for example, the depots at Cairo, Illinois (for the Mississippi Squadron), and at Pensacola and New Orleans—have not been determined.[15]

The supplying of naval hospitals presumably resembled that of vessels in terms of ordering and delivery. It was probably a simpler operation because the surgeon of a hospital had, at most, only a few other medical officers under his command, should have had a firmer grasp of the supplies needed, and could probably communicate more quickly, by letter or telegram, with Whelan.

Other Sources of Supplies

Whelan was generally disinclined to ask for outside assistance in providing medical supplies. In December 1862, he authorized Surgeon William Grier, at the naval hospital at Mound City, Illinois, not only to purchase goods locally when necessary, but also to call on the army's medical purveyor, who had helped in the past. Supplies could, however, be ordered quarterly, filled by the laboratory in Brooklyn, and shipped to Cairo.[16]

In August 1863, Whelan told Surgeon James C. Palmer, about to become fleet surgeon of the WGBS, that medical officers—presumably acting assistant surgeons—had gotten into the habit of requesting supplies from army medical storekeepers. (The practice may have been permitted by the outgoing fleet surgeon, Jonathan M. Foltz, who admired the amount and variety of army supplies.) Although the storekeepers complied "in a spirit of great liberality and kindness," they never indicated the price of the goods supplied. Consequently, the navy was "constantly incurring an indebtedness, the extent of which is only to be known, when we shall be called upon to pay." Since the medical storekeepers provided supplies in bulk, rather than break up packages, vessels ended up with amounts largely in excess of what they needed. Whelan thus urged Palmer to discourage the practice and have his officers requisition exactly what they needed through BUMED. Much of the problem, admitted Whelan, was that many medical officers, especially the volunteers, "are without experience and, I am sorry to say, without much apparent desire to familiarize themselves with their duties."[17]

The navy also received assistance, at times, from civilian relief agencies. The Western Sanitary Commission, for example, provided supplies for the navy's hospital ship *Red Rover*, and the U.S. Sanitary

Commission helped to procure officers and attendants for the Mississippi Squadron. In June 1864, Fleet Surgeon John L. Fox of the NABS asked Whelan about accepting aid from the U.S. Sanitary Commission. Whelan responded, "We have the means and facilities ... to furnish our people with everything needful; and if we can supply all our wants within ourselves. I should prefer to leave the Sanitary Commission to bestow its resources where they are so much more urgently required [to various sections of the army]." Whelan had been asked before about accepting assistance but was "at a loss to indicate at that time, how far, or in what way the Commission could assist us." Whelan left Fox to apply his own judgment about whether to accept "the proffers of assistance from the Sanitary Commission."[18]

Supply Problems

Complaints about the medical-supply operation centered around not initially having been issued the needed supplies or not receiving goods ordered by requisition. Surgeon Jonathan M. Foltz, fleet surgeon of the WGBS, complained that "not a vessel arrives [for service in the squadron] that does not immediately apply for such necessities as should have been sent with it." Acting Assistant Surgeon E. Boylston Jackson, assigned to USS *James L. Davis* of the EGBS, stated that his vessel was inadequately fitted out at the Philadelphia Navy Yard. Not only was he short of medicines, he was denied an amputation saw and was told by the yard's medical officer, Surgeon James M. Greene, that he could obtain a much better saw from the ship's carpenter. Jackson was willing to accept Greene's suggestion if it reflected the views of BUMED but thought it was "quite as reasonable to suppose the cook's knife would answer the place of an amputation knife as the former." Jackson claimed that medical officers of other vessels equipped at Philadelphia had similar or worse experiences. Assistant Surgeon Herman P. Babcock, assigned to USS *Agawam* of the NABS, said that supplies he had requisitioned had not been delivered and that red tape was getting in the way.[19]

Surgeon Greene also drew attention when prices he had paid when equipping a vessel at the Philadelphia yard greatly exceeded those for similar items provided by the medical laboratory. The difference, said Whelan was "evidence of the economy of the laboratory outfit, or its opposite under the purchase system." A possible reason for the high prices Greene had paid was that, as that officer explained, "almost every thing medical in Philadelphia has been exhausted by the army."[20]

Fleet Surgeon Foltz told Whelan of "the abundance, variety and quality of all supplies furnished the sick and wounded of the army," compared with the navy, in the hospitals at New Orleans. Whelan answered that the navy's medical supplies were as good in quality as the army's but might not compare in variety or amount. Furthermore, "the people of the whole country, through the sanitary organizations, are pouring their comforts and luxuries into the hands of the medical officers of the army until ... the excess of supplies of whatever kind greatly exceeds any probable demand." On the other hand, the navy had to depend on annual congressional appropriations to provide for its patients. Whelan, evidently weary of Foltz's frequent complaints, reminded him, "You have never been denied anything you have ever asked; on the contrary, you have almost uniformly left me to anticipate wants, which you could much better express."[21]

Indeed, Whelan believed that USS *Hartford*, flagship of the WGBS, on which Foltz served, was abundantly supplied because Foltz had described the vessel as "incumbered and crowded with fleet surgeon's stores, while some twenty boxes are stored in the sick bay." Surgeon George Clymer, fleet surgeon of the SABS, described the same situation on flagship *Wabash*. The vessel's space for its own medical supplies was full, but *Wabash* also carried supplies for the squadron, which were stored in the sickbay, "to the great encumbrance of the bay, and the great inconvenience of fulfilling requisitions for the squadron." Additional material recently delivered by a supply ship had to be transferred to the storeship *Courier* "until such disposition can be made of them as will afford access to their contents."[22]

The problem of being oversupplied most likely stemmed from medical officers—many of them with no previous naval experience—lacking confidence in regular deliveries from the medical laboratory and consequently ordering more than they would need until the next supply ship was supposed to arrive. Whelan preferred quarterly requisitions because larger orders intended to last longer strained the laboratory's ability to fill them while maintaining an adequate stock. Using the flagship to receive and distribute a squadron's medical supplies may have worked before the war when squadrons were much smaller, but the large number of vessels constituting a wartime blockading squadron made it difficult to find room on the flagship to store deliveries meant for that squadron.[23]

Whelan's idea of how the supply system should operate was sometimes incompatible with local conditions or with what other officers believed would work better. Surgeon Benjamin F. Gibbs, in charge at the Pensacola Naval Hospital, ordered not only for the hospital but also, at times, for the WGBS. He preferred annual or semiannual ordering—and showed no inclination to comply with Whelan's preference for quarterly requisitions—because, in the absence of clerical assistance, it took less of his time, and because it was better to have a surplus than a shortage of supplies. In the past, said Gibbs, shortages had resulted from supplies being damaged by sea water, from supply vessels being "exceedingly irregular" in arriving, and from rigidly enforced quarantine regulations (for yellow fever) preventing the timely docking of those supply ships. In mid–1863, supplies for vessels of the WGBS that were on blockade duty were drawn from USS *Pensacola* off of New Orleans, while supplies for WGBS ships on the lower Mississippi were drawn from the depot at or near the Pensacola Naval Hospital. This arrangement, in which the hospital's surgeon (Gibbs) was subordinate to a fleet surgeon (Foltz), was evidently necessitated, in part, by the dispersal of the squadron, and was probably improvised by Fleet Surgeon Foltz without Whelan's knowledge. Gibbs suggested establishing a post at New Orleans that would be the sole supply center for the WGBS.[24]

Whelan rarely, if ever, complained about lacking adequate funds to purchase, prepare, and ship medical supplies, yet he did alter requisitions that he thought called for excessive amounts. In July 1864, he called the attention of Fleet Surgeon James C. Palmer of the WGBS to the "enormous increase of price of whiskey, wines, &c" and asked him to moderate the prescribing of alcohol by the younger medical officers in the squadron. "Our appropriations are definite, & with the prices varying daily, unless we exercise great prudence in such expenditures, we shall have certain deficiencies in our funds." A year earlier, Whelan informed Fleet Surgeon Clymer of the SABS that the price of glass was increasing. Thus, he asked Clymer to "collect all the glass, or laboratory packings, for which you have no use and, after proper stowage in casks or barrels with sand or sawdust, return them" to the medical laboratory by supply steamer. Clymer was to tell his officers not to discard or destroy "property of this kind" that they were not using but to give it to him to ship back.

Medical supply problems were inevitable because of the amounts needed, the great dispersal of forces, irregularities in delivery, and distrust or ignorance of the supply system on the part of inexperienced medical officers. Although the medical laboratory in Brooklyn performed well in furnishing supplies, it sometimes became necessary for surgeons to procure items locally or establish new distribution models. BUMED chief Whelan's trust in the judgment of his senior officers allowed such improvisations to work.

Chapter 9

Surgeons at Sea

A MEDICAL OFFICER'S RESPONSIBILITIES on a vessel started well before sailing. Naval regulations set forth the duties of surgeons and assistant surgeons, but when a surgeon was not present—as was the case on so many ships—the assistant surgeon assumed the duties assigned by regulations to the higher-ranking officer. Many of the same responsibilities presumably fell on surgeons' stewards in charge, since they were the only medical providers on their vessels.[1]

Preparing to Sail

On joining his vessel, a surgeon was to assume charge of all medical supplies and take steps to bring amounts up to those allowed or needed. He had a storeroom, called the dispensary, for those supplies, although some articles—those that did not fit in the dispensary or were unlikely to be constantly needed—might be stowed elsewhere. Smaller vessels that did not have a dedicated space for medical supplies might be issued a medical chest. The dispensary would ideally be located adjacent to, or at least not far from, the sickbay, which was typically on the berth deck, the level that housed the officers and men.[2]

The surgeon would ensure that any men assigned to assist him knew their responsibilities. Those men would include a surgeon's steward, nurses (on larger vessels), and crewmembers who, during battle, were to help the sick and wounded to the appropriate location. He would instruct selected crewmembers on the use of tourniquets, which he would distribute when combat seemed imminent. (As Flag Officer David G. Farragut of the WGBS observed, "More men lose their lives by bleeding to death from want of early attention, than from the severity of the wounds.") On large vessels, the surgeon might see that some apparatus, perhaps "a cot with a spare sacking bottom" was prepared for the lowering of wounded men to a deck where they could be treated.[3]

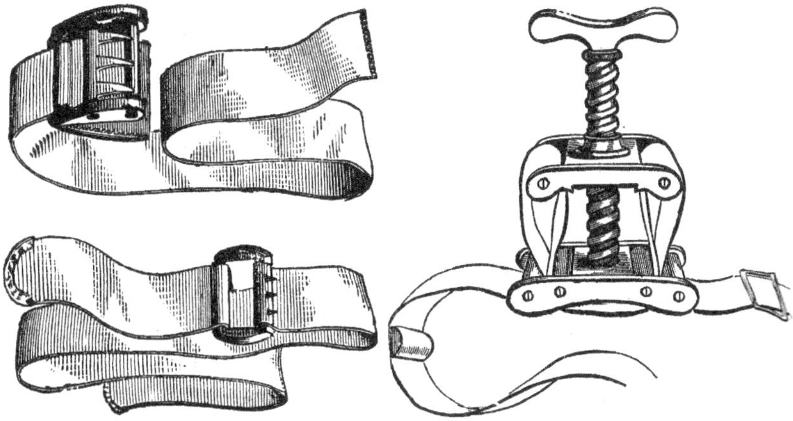

Field tourniquets, left, of the type distributed to selected crewmembers by a vessel's medical officer. A Petit or screw-type tourniquet, right, was likely included among a medical officer's surgical instruments (*American Armamentarium Chirurgicum* [New York: George Tiemann, 1889]).

The surgeon examined the crew to determine if there was a need for anyone to be vaccinated against smallpox and, if necessary, he administered vaccine before sailing. Other measures that would help ensure the crew's health—attending to cleanliness and the soundness of the food and water supplies, for example—were within the surgeon's purview.[4]

When off duty, a medical officer could retire to his stateroom. Plans for *Milwaukee*-class monitors show staterooms being about 6 by 7 feet; the height of quarters in the original *Monitor* was 8½ feet. Commissioned officers other than the captain typically dined together.[5]

Sickbay

Every morning, crewmembers needing or desiring medical attention presented themselves to the surgeon. That encounter might be at the dispensary, as was the case on USS *Circassian* and USS *Silver Lake*. Surgeons were challenged by the various motives of the patients they dealt with. Some men wished to be on the sick list—and excused from duty—when they did not belong on it, while others wished to stay off the sick list but wanted medicines. Still others wanted to be on the list but preferred to treat themselves or be attended by another medical officer, on another vessel, or on shore. Men with valid complaints but fit to work might be treated or given medication, while those unfit to work were placed on the sick list. One version of the sick list, given to the commander, enumerated the men and their medical problems, and a shorter version, the binnacle list, was left at the binnacle (the housing of the ship's compass) to inform officers about men excused from duty and who (before abolition of the spirit ration) the surgeon had determined should not get their daily gill of whiskey. Men placed on the sick list stayed in sickbay, also called the ship's hospital. There a patient might occupy a hanging cot rather than his usual hammock. On vessels that did not have a dedicated sickbay, patients would stay in their usual sleeping place or trade places with a healthy sailor so as to be somewhat out of the way. The surgeon generally visited sickbay in the evening and at other times when needed. His assistants, if available, prepared prescriptions, changed dressings, and performed other routine duties.[6]

Although physicians believed that patients needed quiet and plenty of fresh air, sickbays provided neither. Conditions were almost always crowded, ventilation was poor because hatches and ports were often closed while at sea, the temperature was uncomfortable because of proximity to the ship's galley or boilers, and noise was constant because of the normal operations of the ship and crew. Nor was sickbay, which was often above the water line, always a safe place to be. In February 1862, USS *Vermont* encountered a gale that broke through various ports and destroyed the dispensary, which was on the lower gun deck. *Vermont*'s surgeon reported that "the immense volume of water which entered broke adrift every movable article in the sickbay, making a complete wreck of the whole." Fortunately, the sick had been moved below and apparently escaped harm.[7]

Medical officers maintained a journal of practice, in which were recorded the names and details of sickbay patients, along with their medical problems, treatment, and statements about whether their illness or injury originated in the line of duty. Diagnoses, including injuries, were to be recorded using a standard nomenclature of diseases, in terms of Greek and Latin origin, which facilitated BUMED's compilation of statistics. Among the seemingly arcane paperwork were quarterly determinations of the average number of sick and their cost of care, for which fractions were reported not as decimals but with the denominator being the number of days in the quarter. Accounts of the treatment of men who were not admitted to sickbay were often omitted from official reports, so BUMED statistics resulting from hospitalization on vessels understate the actual number of men who were injured or ill.[8]

Smaller vessels frequently had little or no room for a sickbay and might not have enough medical personnel to provide skilled care. Patients who were too ill to receive adequate treatment or would need long-time care were often transferred to a larger squadron vessel to take advantage of better facilities or to await transfer to a shore facility, possibly via a supply or transport steamer. Fleet Surgeon George Clymer of the SABS reported that the flagship *Wabash*, a steam screw frigate, had become by February 1862 "the receptacle of the sick of the other vessels (which were constantly coming and going) here to await the opportunity of sending them North." At the time, *Wabash*'s sickbay was crowded not only with patients but with medical supplies. Surgeon Henry O. Mayo of USS *Powhatan*, also in the SABS, reported that he had neither the room nor medical manpower to treat other vessels' patients. *Powhatan*, he wrote, although a large ship with a complement of nearly 300, had only a single deck, most of which was occupied by officers' quarters and machinery. That situation left "very limited space on the berth deck forward for our own sick of whom we have a large number, diarrhea and dysentery being rife among us." Assistant Surgeon William L. Wheeler of the SABS's USS *Patapsco*, a *Passaic*-class ironclad with a complement of about 100, alluded to the short time that sick crewmembers remained aboard. "I cannot speak with certainty as to the rapidity with which patients convalesce on board of this vessel," he wrote, "for the reason that most of them have been sent away."[9]

Sending patients from blockading squadrons to Northern naval hospitals was not without complications. In 1862, naval patients carried to New York on the army transport *Atlantic* had to leave the vessel on their own upon reaching the dock because nobody on board was assigned to see that they arrived at their intended destination, the New York Naval Hospital. Whelan recommended that a naval commissioned or warrant officer be in charge of patients on transports to ensure the safe arrival of those men at the intended hospital. If that could not happen, then some arrangement to accomplish the same purpose should be made between the transport's captain (especially for a non–USN transport) and the squadron commander under whom the patients served. An alternative, wrote Whelan, would be to keep patients on squadron vessels, except in extreme cases, until regular naval supply steamers—most or all of which had a medical officer and were accustomed to carrying patients—could take them north. Within a few days of Whelan's recommendations, Secretary Welles issued a general order to put them into place. Naval commanders relinquishing patients to a transport were to take special care—including assigning a responsible person to accompany them, if necessary—to ensure the patients' prompt placement in the intended hospital. Unless the situation was urgent, the order continued, patients were to be sent north on naval supply ships only, or at least on other naval vessels.[10]

It is unclear how, or whether, northern hospitals were alerted to the impending arrival of patients from squadrons. The transfer of men from one vessel to another was certainly recorded, but it may not have been possible to relay the names and numbers of men being sent north before they arrived there. Since supply steamers serving the squadrons sailed, to the extent possible, on a regular schedule, their return dates were fairly predictable. Thus, hospitals at least knew that new patients might be coming.

Battle Stations

In preparation for battle, the surgeon and his assistants cleared unneeded articles from the area set aside for reception of the wounded and arranged surgical instruments, bandages, and other items that might be needed. The wounded were typically taken to the cockpit, a relatively shielded portion of the vessel, which was ideally below water level. That location was often the wardroom, which was surrounded by officers' staterooms. There, the officers' dining table was likely to serve as the operating platform. Lamps were hung, and assistants brought in pails, mops, and kegs of water. Sand was available to sprinkle on the deck, which was liable to become slippery with water and blood.[11]

Patients in sickbay were moved, if possible, to a safer part of the vessel. The exposure of sickbays to enemy fire, especially in wooden ships, was demonstrated repeatedly during the war. While passing the forts below New Orleans in April 1862, for example, USS *Hartford* was hit numerous times, with one shot damaging the sickbay and dispensary. In June 1862, *Hartford*, in trying to pass Vicksburg on the Mississippi River, was hit by a 10-inch projectile that passed through the forward shell room, smashed 20 empty shells, and rolled into the space and under the table where Fleet Surgeon Jonathan Foltz was performing an amputation. (It is unclear whether Foltz was in sickbay, the cockpit, or neither during this episode.) USS *Cumberland*, facing ironclad CSS *Virginia* in the March 1862 Battle of Hampton Roads, received a shot that did ghastly damage to its sickbay, where some of her wounded had been carried. Many men who survived that shot went down with *Cumberland* when she sank after being rammed by *Virginia*.[12]

The surgeon or his assistants removed or placed behind closed doors any supplies that might shatter and release caustic or inflammable substances if hit by an enemy shot. In the event of fire, medical

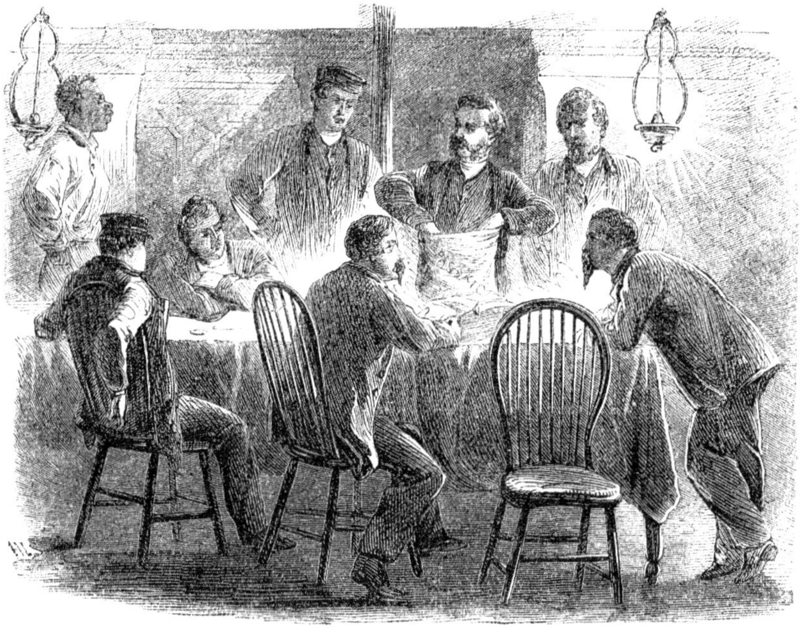

Officers receiving mail in the wardroom of USS *Passaic*, an ironclad monitor. The dining table, surrounded by officers' staterooms, was probably used as an operating platform for men wounded in battle. Edgar Holden, who served on *Passaic* as an assistant surgeon, described a syndrome he called "ironclad fever" and wrote wartime articles about life on the vessel (Holden, "First Cruise").

personnel were to be prepared to destroy any inflammable fluids or other medical stores that would increase the fire. Among such supplies would be the anesthetic ether, alcohol—if in the concentrated form used in pharmaceutical processes and as a preservative—and possibly whiskey and brandy. Ether, which is highly volatile and can ignite in the presence of open flames or heat sources, would probably not be kept near the cockpit, which was illuminated by lamps; chloroform would be the likely anesthetic.[13]

Once the wounded—who could include enemy personnel brought aboard—began arriving in the cockpit, they would be triaged, if necessary, so that those with nondangerous injuries were put aside and life-threating wounds were attended to first. Patients thought to be mortally wounded would ideally be put in a comfortable position and possibly be given an analgesic such as opium or morphine.[14]

In the tense and hectic atmosphere of battle, wrote Surgeon William S.W. Ruschenberger, "there is no substitute in the cockpit ... for coolness and sound professional knowledge.... On such an occasion a skillful surgeon is a blessing and a hope; but an ignorant one is a curse, an ally to the enemy." After the November 1861 Battle of Port Royal Sound, Whelan was gratified to read the reports of medical officers of the vessels involved. "Inasmuch as the incidents of actual warfare are novel to so many members of the corps," he wrote to Fleet Surgeon George Clymer of the SABS, "it is a subject of special congratulation that one and all proved so competent to meet the exigencies of a naval engagement." Whelan commented on the valuable lessons learned by officers who were new to combat: "The experience of that day will forcibly illustrate the difference between a capital operation [such as amputation] performed in the well prepared rooms of a [shore] hospital, and the same occurrence in the dimly lighted 'mainhold' of a frigate, or in the more restricted, and comfortless, quarters of the berth deck of smaller vessels."[15]

Expeditions

Vessels stationed close to shore and in the vicinity of enemy troops were sometimes called upon to participate in boat expeditions, which had various goals, such as capturing blockade runners, taking prisoners, or destroying salt works. The missions might include Marines and were sometimes conducted in cooperation with the army. The efforts could involve relatively few men, as in July 1864, when men in four boats from USS *Hartford* and USS *Brooklyn* boarded and burned a blockade runner that had run ashore near Fort Morgan, at the mouth of Mobile Bay. Assistant Surgeon William Commons of USS *Hartford* accompanied that foray, during which no Union casualties were sustained. Many other boat expeditions evidently did not include a medical officer. Official guidance regarding boat expeditions were sparse, mentioning only the need to carry "articles for the care of the sick and wounded," listed as tourniquets, bandages, lint, medicines, and surgical instruments. In 1846, Surgeon William S.W. Ruschenberger recommended that boat expeditions, which were "not infrequent," should be equipped with a portable box, with a shoulder strap, to carry surgical instruments and dressings.[16]

Early in 1862, five boats from the SABS and 2,500 soldiers of a Union army division headed toward Port Royal Ferry, South Carolina—on the Coosaw River, north of Beaufort—to capture and destroy enemy forts. Among the men in the boats, which carried howitzers, was Assistant Surgeon James J. Magee of USS *Wabash*. After the expedition,

Magee wrote a long report for Flag Officer George Clymer with his recommendations regarding medical supplies and personnel that should be included in boat expeditions (Appendix C). Whelan praised Magee for the zeal, intelligence, and energy displayed in his communication. The document is particularly informative in indicating the likely duties of an expedition's medical officer. Whelan might well have been impressed, for concepts that he valued highly—planning, efficiency, teamwork, and the relief of suffering—were emphasized in Magee's suggestions. It is unclear whether the navy took any of Magee's comments to heart.[17]

Surgeons' Exposure to Danger

Being staff rather than line officers did not protect naval surgeons from the hazards of shipboard life during war. About 50 Union naval medical officers died, at sea or ashore, between the bombardment of Fort Sumter in mid–April 1861 and the end of April 1865. Several deaths occurred among older or disabled officers on the retired list, and others occurred among nonelderly surgeons who had evidently been taken ill, were detached from duty, and died at home—or at least not at a naval facility. Many deaths occurred in naval hospitals, but how many were caused by illness or injury occurring at sea is unknown.[18]

The exact circumstances surrounding the deaths of medical officers serving on vessels are often unreported in available records. In some instances, death appears to have been unrelated to disease or combat. Acting Assistant Surgeon John M. Whitney drowned in Florida's St. Johns River in August 1864 while serving on USS *Norwich*, but what led to that incident is unclear. According to a man representing himself as the sole survivor of USS *Bainbridge*, that vessel encountered a gale on August 21, 1863, while sailing from New York to Port Royal and capsized; among the men who were missing and presumed dead were Acting Assistant Surgeon E.H. Allis and Surgeon's Steward S. Horace Smith. Assistant Surgeon Charles H. Pile, assigned to USS *Paul Jones*, died on December 23, 1862, at St. Simons, Georgia. Although a newspaper reported that he had succumbed to fever, Acting Assistant Surgeon Samuel P. Boyer recorded in his diary that Pile "died from the effects of chloroform, which he used to inhale at night, it being an old habit of his."[19]

In other cases, medical officers clearly died of disease. Assistant Surgeon Charles H. Covell died of dysentery aboard USS *Colorado* in August 1861, and Acting Assistant Surgeon Thomas McHenry, assigned to USS *Pursuit*, died during the night of August 19, 1863, of remittent fever at the marine hospital in Key West. Fleet Surgeon Edward Gilchrist of the EGBS reported that McHenry had been ill and was prescribing for himself but did not appear on death's door that morning.[20]

Combat took its toll on medical officers. On May 22, 1863, USS *Penobscot* took enemy fire near Fort Fisher, North Carolina, with one shot killing Assistant Surgeon Edward A. Pierson and seriously wounding Surgeon's Steward Julius C. Force. On January 31, 1863, off of Charleston, a shot from a Confederate ironclad penetrated a boiler of USS *Mercedita* and caused other serious damage. Assistant Surgeon Jacob H. Gotwald was scalded by steam while tending to a wounded man and died on February 2.[21]

During the January 15, 1865, assault on Fort Fisher, North Carolina, Assistant Surgeon William Longshaw, Jr., was one of a landing party of 241 men from USS *Minnesota*. While tending to a wounded man near the enemy works, Longshaw was "shot in the head and instantly killed."[22]

Assistant Surgeon Henry A. Danker died on August 5, 1864, when his vessel, USS *Tecumseh*, struck a torpedo (mine) and sank during the Battle of Mobile Bay. A torpedo was also responsible for the death of Assistant Surgeon Samuel H. Peltz, who was aboard USS *Patapsco* when she sank after striking the device in Charleston Bay on January 15, 1865.[23]

A small number of medical officers—exactly how many is unclear—were taken prisoner by Confederate forces. After USS *Water Witch* was captured on June 3, 1864, south of Savannah, her medical officer, Acting Assistant Surgeon W.H. Pierson was transported to the Confederate naval hospital in Savannah, where he cared for Union wounded. Citing the practice, which he believed was in effect, of releasing captured medical officers, Pierson appealed on July 6 to Stephen R. Mallory, the Confederate secretary of the navy, to be returned to Union lines. Ten days later, Pierson learned that he was to be treated as other prisoners of war, and he was sent to Camp Oglethorpe, near Macon, Georgia, where he arrived on July 17. (Agreements and practices regarding the release and parole of prisoners changed frequently during the war.) He was later moved to Charleston, and he was released to Union officials on September 3, 1864, after a total confinement of three months.[24]

On May 6, 1864, USS *Granite City* was captured at Calcasieu Pass, Louisiana. Assistant Surgeon Edmund C. Ver Meulen was reportedly among the crew taken prisoner, but details about his captivity are elusive. By November 1864, he was available to the U.S. Navy Department for a new assignment.[25]

Assistant Surgeon Thomas N. Penrose became a prisoner when

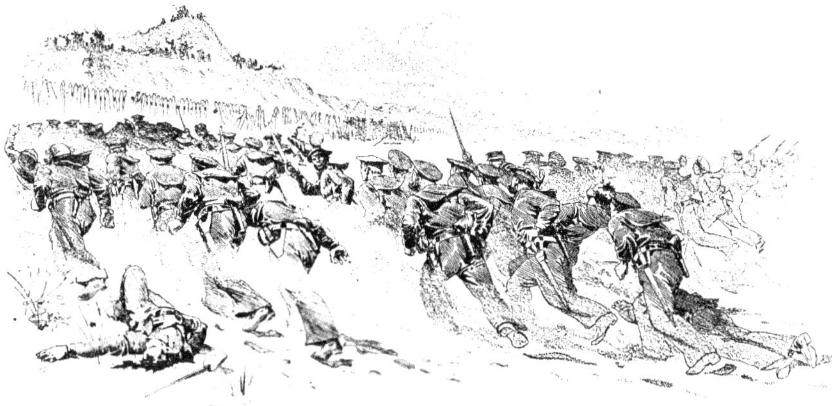

Assault by Union sailors and Marines on Fort Fisher, North Carolina, on January 15, 1865. Assistant Surgeon William Longshaw, Jr., USN, part of the landing party from USS *Minnesota*, was killed while tending to a wounded man (Selfridge, "Navy at Fort Fisher").

his ship, USS *Harriet Lane*, was captured on January 1, 1863, in Galveston Bay, Texas. Penrose was paroled and arrived at New Orleans on or before February 26.[26]

On January 21, 1863, USS *Morning Light* was captured close to Sabine Pass, near the Texas–Louisiana border. The ship's medical officer, Acting Assistant Surgeon John W. Sherfy, was taken prisoner. Soon after his capture, Sherfy received a Confederate offer to be sent to the Federal fleet under a flag of truce, but he declined because he felt a duty to care for his fellow prisoners. He and others were moved from Sabine City, Texas, to Houston, and then to Camp Groce, near Hempstead, Texas, about 50 miles northwest of Houston, where he spent about six months. There followed a three-week march of close to 300 miles, during which Sherfy accompanied enlisted prisoners, to Camp Instruction, about 10 miles from Shreveport, Louisiana; along the way, the men rested for two days at Camp Ford, near Tyler, Texas. At Camp Instruction, Confederate surgeons assumed responsibility for the treatment of sick prisoners, so Sherfy asked to be sent to the Federal lines; the request was granted. He left Camp Instruction in February 1864 and entered Union-controlled territory in early March 1864, about 14 months after his capture.[27]

Sherfy wrote, in addition to a formal report to Secretary Welles, a detailed account of his captivity and the suffering of his fellow prisoners to BUMED chief Whelan (Appendix D). The latter document, wrote Whelan showed "evidences of interest, zeal and the genuine heroism of our profession," and prompted him to congratulate himself and the Navy Department "that our unfortunate prisoners in Texas fell under the charge of an officer who displayed at once the disposition, and the ability to render them such signal assistance." In the account, Sherfy apologized for his routine reports being late and deviating from the exact form required by regulations, so Whelan saw in Sherfy qualities that he repeatedly regretted were absent from many acting assistant surgeons—attention to detail and a manifest devotion to duty.[28]

On September 8, 1863, USS *Clifton* was captured at Sabine Pass, not far from where *Morning Light* surrendered earlier in the year. The vessel's medical officer, Acting Assistant Surgeon Daniel D.T. Nestell, was taken prisoner and endured an ordeal similar, though shorter, to that of Sherfy. For about three months, Nestell and Sherfy were both at Camp Groce, although there were apparently confined separately and did not care for the same patients. In December, Nestell and other prisoners were marched to Camp Ford, where Nestell's request to be released was granted. He left Camp Ford on January 31, 1864, swore in writing not to divulge any information that would affect the interests of the Confederacy, entered the Union lines, and after a number of stops, arrived at New York on February 29.[29]

On February 14, 1863, USS *Queen of the West*, a ram of the Mississippi Marine Brigade, was captured on the Red River in Louisiana, and its medical officer, Assistant Surgeon David S. Booth, was taken prisoner. Booth was an army officer, and *Queen of the West*, although commanded by Colonel Charles Rivers Ellet of the army, was operating under the direction of Acting Rear Admiral David D. Porter, flag officer of the Mississippi Squadron. Booth was released outright or paroled and arrived by February 26, 1863, at New Orleans, where he reported to Rear Admiral David. G. Farragut.[30]

Surgeons assigned to vessels had varied responsibilities connected with the prevention and treatment of medical problems. Those duties could extend to boat expeditions and, in case of capture, to the care of fellow prisoners. Service afloat exposed medical officers to the same dangers faced by the rest of the crew, and their valor and devotion to duty were sources of pride for BUMED chief Whelan.

Chapter 10

General Health Concerns

The medical department, simply by virtue of the number and varied background of officers on its rolls, could probably not have operated under a strictly uniform model of medical care. For the most part, the department did not dictate how its officers should perform the clinical aspect of their duty—maintaining health and managing wounds or illnesses. One notable exception was the requirement that all recruits be vaccinated against smallpox shortly after joining a receiving ship. Vaccine, procured from the medical laboratory in Brooklyn, was also a component of the medical supplies issued to vessels of all sizes. The prevention of disease was a goal common to all medical officers, and BUMED chief Whelan was eager for reports and suggestions on the topic.[1]

Whelan seemed averse to interfering with officers' freedom to exercise their best judgment. Nevertheless, allopathic practices—rather than those of various medical sectarians—were the norm in the navy, a circumstance that seems to have had Whelan's blessing. The favoring of allopaths is apparent by the presence of items in the medical supply table that sectarians generally abhorred (e.g., mercury-containing compounds, bloodletting instruments) and the absence of some plant-based remedies that sectarians promoted (e.g., *Lobelia inflata* [Indian tobacco], *Eupatorium perfoliatum* [boneset]). Furthermore, the process for examining candidates for admission to the medical corps evidently favored graduates of allopathic schools, and sectarians complained that they were excluded from practicing medicine in the army and navy.[2]

Acting Assistant Surgeon Samuel P. Boyer, a recent graduate of the University of Pennsylvania in Philadelphia, commented that the eclectic school, a group of sectarian practitioners, would object to bloodletting, calomel, and tartar emetic, "whereas we allopaths, like sensible physicians, use all three remedies." Calomel (mild chloride of mercury) had many uses and was often prescribed as a laxative or to regulate the actions of the liver. It also had serious adverse effects, including necrosis of the gums and jaw. Tartar emetic (antimony and potassium tartrate), also capable of producing adverse effects, was often prescribed to induce vomiting. (Physicians commonly sought to clear the gastrointestinal tract of supposedly irritating matter—not just overt poisons—by inducing vomiting or defecation.) Although sectarians had historically cited the treatments mentioned by Boyer as examples of allopaths' harsh or "heroic" methods, the use of those methods by allopaths had declined in the decades before the Civil War.[3]

In 1863, Surgeon General William A. Hammond ordered calomel and tartar emetic removed from the army's standard supply table because he was convinced that the agents, as currently used, were causing more harm than good.[4] Whelan sent a copy of Hammond's order to Fleet Surgeon Ninian Pinkney of the Mississippi Squadron and commented,

> I do not propose to imitate the example of the Surgeon General; but if his course be wise, its results will ultimately inure to our department, as well as to that for which the order was specifically designed. We have in the navy, as there is in the army, a large number of inexperienced officers whose ideas of the practice of medicine consist mainly, if not exclusively, in the administration of drugs, whose traditional value is a constant source of disappointment. It would be a great gain to inculcate upon this class of officers, the importance of hygienic measures as a means not only of preventing but of curing disease; if successful, it would supersede routine practice by intelligent observation, and thoughtful diagnosis; tending to the true advancement of the profession.[5]

Despite the absence of formal treatment protocols, certain modes of therapy seem to have been fairly common. Thus, when a sailor suffering from diarrhea was transferred to the naval hospital at Memphis, the medical officer last caring for him thought it sufficient to report that the patient had received "the usual treatment." That treatment probably consisted of opium to check the diarrhea, possibly preceded by a laxative—perhaps castor oil or a mercury compound—to expel any irritating material, and an astringent to control bowel inflammation. Another example, often advocated in respectable publications of the time, is the use of "alkaline treatment"—an oral solution of potassium bicarbonate, for example—as part of the management of rheumatism. Assistant Surgeon Charles Carter recorded prescribing alkaline treatment with no other details, such as the actual medicine used, as if it would be understood by other physicians. Other common treatments included opiates for pain or cough, quinine for malaria, and colchicum for rheumatism.[6]

Quinine and mercury, neither of which was benign, were prescribed commonly and—according to some observers—indiscriminately, interchangeably, and often for no apparent reason. Acting Assistant Surgeon R.O. Mason prescribed quinine, which was widely considered the treatment of choice for malaria, for a patient with bronchitis. That might seem an odd use for quinine, but there was support in the literature for doing so. Surgeon Edward Shippen prescribed calomel, which was often used as laxative or to regulate the liver, for a patient with pneumonia—another seemingly unusual choice of therapy but one that was consistent with recommendations in a major medical textbook.[7]

Many patients had multiple medical problems, and the lack of detailed records makes it impossible to determine whether recorded treatments were for undisclosed conditions or were otherwise reasonable. In addition, surgeons often applied the preventive measure of administering purgatives to "keep the bowels open." That intervention—one supposed benefit of which was to remove or prevent the accumulation of toxins—was common enough that medical officers frequently saw no reason to explain in their reports why it was used. Such omissions, especially when the agents used had many possible indications, complicate the evaluation of how various conditions were treated and whether prescribing proclivities show medical officers, as a group, as being guided by any particular clinical doctrine. In any event, it is easy to understand how physicians could be seen as ignorant or cavalier in their prescribing of drugs, especially those with meaningful adverse effects, and why advocates of gentler therapies had their followers.[8]

Whelan tried to provide medical officers with current medical information. The table of allowances for vessels included Wood and Bache's *Dispensatory of the United States*—a comprehensive and well-referenced book describing medicines, including those used by sectarians, and their uses—as well as a formulary that contained recipes for prescriptions. By early 1861, the *Dispensatory* was out of print, and Whelan was awaiting a new edition to distribute. The formulary usually issued, by Ellis, was also out of print, so Whelan substituted Griffith's formulary instead.[9] BUMED also supplied a copy of the quarterly *American Journal of the Medical Sciences* to medical officers of the permanent, but not the volunteer, navy.[10]

Whelan evidently perused the medical literature and was willing to try new treatments. Thus, after he read an article advocating the use of picked oakum as a cheap and effective dressing for pus-producing wounds, he sent copies to medical officers and instructed navy-yard surgeons to substitute it for patent lint when filling requisitions. (Oakum, used for caulking seams or joints in ships, was made by shredding or unraveling used fragments of tarred rope.)[11]

When Fleet Surgeon Charles D. Maxwell of the Pacific Squadron asked for an "electro magnetic battery" (probably for treating nerve injuries), Whelan replied that he would gladly send one if he knew "which of the many, rather pretentious apparatus" Maxwell preferred. Treatment with electricity was unconventional and sometimes considered quackery but had its advocates. Whelan admitted using a recently introduced device by a Boston maker and was "satisfied its results would not compensate the cost of transportation."[12]

Medicinal Alcohol

One issue, that of medicinal alcohol, demonstrated Whelan's need to balance the desires of many medical and line officers against his need to uphold the law and the authority of Secretary Welles. At the beginning of the war, sailors' daily ration included four ounces (a gill) of distilled spirits, usually whiskey, which was supplied by the Bureau of Provisions and Clothing, rather than by BUMED, and stored in the vessel's spirit room. The spirit ration was traditionally thought useful in combatting fatigue and in fortifying men exposed to harsh conditions; it was not issued to officers, midshipmen, or seamen younger than 21 years. Many medical and line officers favored continuing the spirit ration, but Congress, which was influenced by the temperance movement, abolished it as of September 1, 1862. The Navy Department, in seeking to improve the navy's efficiency, supported the legislation. The law did not apply to nondistilled beverages such as ale, beer, or wine, which were allowed on naval vessels as private stores only, subject to the approval of the commanding officer. Thus, officers often enjoyed wine with their meals. The only distilled spirits allowed on vessels were those used for medical purposes under the control of medical officers. Secretary Welles issued general orders to inform naval personnel of the legislation and how it would be implemented.[13]

There was good reason to believe that liquor was not conducive to good naval discipline and health. In April 1862, a few months before the spirit ration was abolished, Commander Percival Drayton of the SABS, senior officer at Fernandina, Florida, complained about trading schooners operating under permits granted by the Treasury Department. Such vessels delivered legitimate supplies, as was intended, but also "carried on a most disgraceful trade in almost poisonous liquors, retailed at most exorbitant prices to the sailors," which resulted in "considerable mischief ... both ashore and afloat." The "more or less floating grogshops" readily sold bottles of spirits for $2 each when they were worth, in Drayton's estimation, only 10¢. A month later, Drayton complained again, this time that liquor, brought by a sutler aboard supply ship *Massachusetts,* was finding its way into the hands of sailors and soldiers. Since selling liquor was so profitable, it was displacing, among the sutler's wares, items that might actually contribute to the comfort of officers or crews. Drayton believed that "nothing but the greatest care in keeping the men from excesses of any kind will enable us to retain the vessels this summer in a healthy condition."[14]

Before abolition of the spirit ration, the alcoholic beverages in medical allowance tables included ale, brandy, port, and sherry; whiskey that was needed medicinally was obtained from the spirit room. After the ration was abolished, the tables allowed ale, whiskey, port, and sherry. Distilled alcohol was also a constituent of various tinctures in the allowance tables. (In tinctures, the alcohol acted as a solvent for the active constituents of medicinal substances.)[15]

Alcoholic beverages were prescribed for many indications but probably most commonly as stimulants for patients suffering from physical or mental shock, prostration, or debility. Alcohol was considered a stimulant because its early effects were to quicken the pulse, induce flushing, and elevate mood, but its depressant properties were also well recognized. Whiskey was often used or suggested as a vehicle for quinine administration. Quinine was usually effective for treating malaria and could easily be given as a pill. The drug was thought by many to also be useful in preventing the disease, but giving it for that purpose to men who were not ill was sometimes difficult because of quinine's extreme bitterness. Mixing quinine with whiskey supposedly made the medicine easier to ingest, and adding the drug to barrels of whiskey allowed the simultaneous administration of quinine and the spirit ration.[16]

Shortly before the abandonment of the spirit ration, Commodore Charles Wilkes, Flag Officer of the James River Flotilla feared that "stoppage of the whisky ration will have a disastrous effect upon the crews," which were exposed to the night air on the river. Although he was advised to give his men quinine in the spirit ration, he declined because thought he lacked the authority to ruin the ration for men who were not sick by turning it into "a nauseating dose." After the ration was abolished, NABS Fleet Surgeon William Maxwell Wood recommended administering prophylactic quinine "in strong coffee which is a much better medium than whisky."[17]

When medical officers asked about obtaining more alcohol than was indicated on the allowance lists, Whelan admitted that the limits were modest and were "not to be overly construed." Since whiskey could no longer be obtained from the spirit room, some increased use of medicinal spirits was to be expected. However, said, Whelan, the small

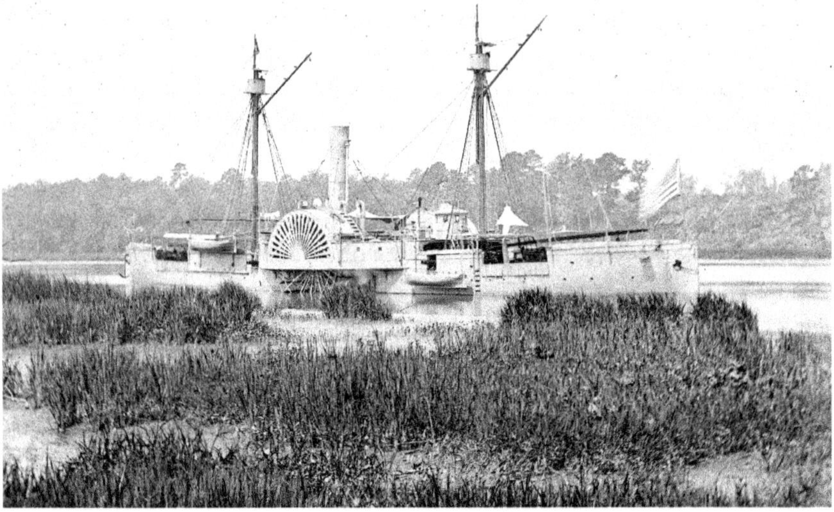

USS *Mendota* on the James River. Swampy areas around the river were conducive to the breeding of mosquitoes that transmitted the malaria parasite. The river's water was deemed unfit to drink because it contained decaying animal and vegetable material, was polluted by vessels, and received drainage from huge encampments of soldiers accompanied by cattle and horses (Library of Congress, control no. 2018666839).

official allowance also reflected the fact that "the [medical] profession differs so widely about the use of spirits, as to divest it of the character of an established necessity of practice." Additional high-quality medicinal whiskey could be requisitioned through the medical laboratory in Brooklyn, Whelan told one surgeon, but if he wanted the "inferior and cheaper article [previously used for the spirit ration] than [what] we supply" for medical use, he could obtain it from the Bureau of Provisions and Clothing.[18]

Whelan emphasized the obligation of the medical bureau to adhere to the ration-abolishing law, the passage of which the Navy Department favored because "of the amount of intemperance prevailing in the Navy." He added, "If our department can be made, in any manner, subservient to the craving consequent upon long indulgence, the object of the statute would be frustrated, and large expense imposed upon us. Medical officers must be looked to, to aid the reform, which Congress has initiated." Indeed, because the Bureau of Provisions and Clothing was no longer supplying spirit-room whiskey, any liquor used by medical officers had to be paid for by BUMED.[19]

Much of the opinion behind liberal use of whiskey was expressed by surgeons of long experience. After Fleet Surgeon John L. Fox of the NABS, asked for large amounts of whiskey—both for fortifying crews in harsh condition and for administering prophylactic quinine—Whelan cited numerous examples of stressed sailors doing well without the whiskey and doubted that the liquor enhanced the actions of quinine. Fleet Surgeon George Clymer of the SABS described "a regulated allowance of whiskey" as "indispensable for health, and efficiency, and, indeed, to save many [men] from breaking down entirely."[20]

Clymer's letter elicited a memorandum from Whelan, in which the bureau chief disagreed "with diffidence" with the opinion of "so judicious and intelligent an officer." Whelan admitted that whiskey given to exhausted men "proves a momentary comfort," but asserted that the effect was short-lived and necessitated repeated doses. "Whiskey," stated Whelan, "is a simple stimulant, and nothing more." Simple hygienic measures, he said, would be more judicious. They included having the men bathe in the ocean and giving them strong coffee or tea, possibly with ice. "Oatmeal, mixed with water," wrote Whelan, "is familiar to sea-going men and engineers as a means of assuaging thirst." Furthermore, decks should be kept as dry as possible so that "the sailor in profuse perspiration from hard work should have a place to rest himself where he will not be exposed to rheumatism or cold." Frequent changes of clothing would also make sailors more comfortable. If a restorative agent was indicated, Whelan wrote to Surgeon James Suddards, "the tinctures upon our list, as ginger and capsicum [cayenne pepper], diluted, would perhaps answer all the objects for which whiskey, and brandy, is used."[21]

Young physicians, thought Whelan, also bore some responsibility for the demand for whiskey. He acknowledged that liquors "constitute an easy offhand prescription, to be sure," yet he urged a fleet surgeon to "impose some caution upon the younger members for our department" about choosing that route of therapy. "Prudence, in the use of spiritous liquors, in our department," he wrote to Fleet Surgeon Gustavus R.B. Horner of the EGBS, "is enjoined, especially upon the younger and less experienced officers of our branch of the service."[22]

What Whelan considered overuse of alcohol was not confined to naval vessels. In July 1863, he told Surgeon Solomon Sharp, who was ordering supplies for the naval hospital at Norfolk, that he was approving his requisition. By agreeing to furnish articles in the requisition that were absent from the allowance table, Whelan demonstrated his willingness to allow Sharp to prescribe as he wished. Whelan was surprised, however, by the "very large demand for liquors, wines, and tinctures, simply for the reason that it affords such a striking contrast to the practice to other hospitals, with a larger number of patients, and doubtless, with as great a variety of disease." Since the spirit ration was not issued to patients in shore hospitals, Sharp could not blame the removal of spirit-room whiskey as necessitating large orders for spiritous liquors. Whelan had no intention of creating "impediments to the proper discharge of duty on the part of medical officers"—and did not order Sharp to markedly reduce the use of medicinal alcohol—but he clearly implied that he would keep an eye on alcohol usage at Norfolk and wanted to see it drop.[23]

Hygienic Measures

Whelan's hope that medical officers would pay more attention to hygienic measures was just one example of the value he placed on providing men with a healthful living environment and wholesome sustenance. In March 1864, for example, he recommended various improvements to receiving ships. Once a permanent position for the stationary vessels was determined, their nonessential articles could be removed and replaced with an apparatus to heat the ship with steam or warm air. An additional deck and "apertures for light" might be added to create a "quite habitable" space. He recommended gas lighting, which would consume less oxygen and be less odorous and smoky than oil lamps or candles. Fresh water could be taken aboard through a large pipe and directed wherever necessary or convenient. Making his proposed changes would help relieve the crowded conditions of receiving ships, which had resulted in many men being sent to hospitals with diseases that were "ascribed to the absence of comforts, and the defective means of heating during inclement seasons." Furthermore, the alterations would ease new recruits' introduction to ship life and "afford more cheerful and healthful temporary homes for the crews of ships undergoing repairs."[24]

Although BUMED was not responsible for buying and providing regular provisions, Whelan had much to say about what sailors were given to eat and how it was prepared. In December 1864, he made three suggestions, none of which appear to have been implemented during his life. First, steam-powered vessels should be equipped with a contrivance to allow steam to accomplish all the galley's boiling, which constituted "so large a portion of ships' cooking." That would not only reduce the need for wood fuel, it would allow much cooking even in "heavy boisterous weather" when fires could not be made and sailors most needed the comfort of hot food and beverages.[25]

Second, the use of a recently promoted form of boned and preserved beef and pork should be investigated. If its advertising was truthful, the meat was more nutritious than the unboned salt-packed meat that the navy was then currently using. Furthermore, the new product would occupy much less space. Whelan recommended obtaining samples of the meat and examining it after some period of storage.[26]

Third, Whelan urged carrying barrels of flour on vessels and adding ovens so that freshly baked bread could replace ship's bread, the dense and rock-hard biscuit also known as hardtack. He called ship's bread "an expensive form of a not over palatable necessary" that was often declared unfit for consumption because of moldering or weevil infestation. "Every one who has lived on ship board," he added, "cannot fail to have remarked the peculiar odor emanating from the best cared for bread room." Barrels of flour would take up less room than barrels of hardtack, and fresh bread, because of its superior nutritional value, could be issued in lesser amounts. Overall, he argued, implementing his suggestions would also save money.[27]

The navy ration, and the extent to which it was issued and consumed, concerned surgeons not only because sailors needed adequate nutrition to perform their duties, but because it was commonly believed that a diet lacking in fresh food—especially fruits and vegetables, but also meat—would likely lead to scurvy (*scorbutus*, in medical terminology). In December 1861, scurvy, now known to result from vitamin C deficiency, was reported on vessels of the SABS and attributed to an insufficient supply of fresh provisions, which had arrived just three times in three months. Whelan recommended to Secretary Welles that deliveries to blockading vessels be made more frequently with more abundant supplies. Whelan mentioned the need for vegetables but also recommended antiscorbutic measures he had noted in the medical literature: beer or ale should be substituted for wine, and fresh bread substituted for hardtack. To the SABS's fleet surgeon, George Clymer, Whelan suggested providing men with more potatoes—as another surgeon had recommended during the Mexican War—and lime juice, both of which he was sending to the SABS. He repeated his suggestions about beer, ale, and fresh bread while mentioning additional recommendations from the literature, such as maintaining dryness and proper ventilation on ships and issuing flannel clothing.[28]

Assistant Surgeon J.C. Spear reported in July 1862 that scurvy was appearing on James River vessels, that fresh provisions were not arriving regularly, and that crews did not like portions of the regular ration. Canned beef and mixed desiccated vegetables (sardonically called "desecrated vegetables") were often rejected by the men, such that "but a small part of the ration is used for food." Spear praised canned tomatoes as retaining their freshness and having antiscorbutic effects. Surgeon William Maxwell Wood, dispatched to observe and report on sanitary conditions on the river, recommended increasing the frequency of delivery of fresh provisions. "Even though the material effect of this change in ration might not be certain," wrote Wood, "the moral effect upon men engaged in this depressing service of having the food they prefer would be of a sanitary character."[29]

Whelan was quick to take issue with an 1863 article in the *American Medical Times* in which a USN passed assistant surgeon suggested that the navy ration lacked antiscorbutic content. Not only had the article's author resigned from the USN in the mid–1850s, noted Whelan, the current ration, and the way it was distributed, made his concern inapplicable. In fact, preserved items in the current ration—such as dried fruit, pickles, and desiccated vegetables—may have contained some vitamin C, and fresh produce could be substituted from time to time for items in the ration. Perhaps the problems reported in 1861 and 1862 had largely been addressed, for Whelan pointed out that supply steamers left the North on a regular schedule with "large quantities of fresh provisions." The periodical's editors acknowledged in print that the article had been written by the named author more than 10 years earlier, was sent to them by an army surgeon, and was meant to illustrate the causes and prevention of scurvy rather than to critique the current ration.[30]

Surgeon Wood, in observing conditions on the James River, noted that the river water was turbid, objectionable, and liable to cause diarrhea if ingested. He wrote that steam vessels could produce plenty of drinking water if equipped with easily available fresh-water condensers. Whelan repeated that recommendation to Secretary Welles and explained why the river water was unsafe. Not only were many naval and other vessels scattered on the river's surface, encampments of 90,000 to 100,000 men, accompanied by horses and cattle, were along its banks. The resulting drainage into the river, along with decomposing animal and vegetable matter already in the river, would certainly make the water unhealthful to drink. Many steamers did produce their own water during the war, but the influence of Whelan's recommendation is unknown.[31]

Special Concerns About Ironclads

Complaints about life on early ironclad vessels were numerous and usually centered on their poor ventilation and excessive heat, conditions that were antithetical to most physicians' concept of a healthful living environment. Medical officers also mentioned that drinking water produced by condensers and stored in iron tanks had reddish sediment, with one surgeon reporting that the amount of iron in his vessel's drinking water was "so great, as to render it at times as dark as coffee." Interior lighting was so poor as to cause eyestrain—men did not want to make the vessel interior warmer by burning candles—and there was a general indisposition to walk the iron decks for exercise. There was little or nothing that medical officers could do to correct defects in ship design and engineering other than bring them to the attention of Whelan and, through him, Secretary Welles. However, knowing about the problems themselves could prompt consideration about how to respond to them medically. Whelan, in fact, appreciated being informed of health concerns, a characteristic that did not go unnoticed. After he thanked Fleet Surgeon George Clymer of the SABS for forwarding reports from medical officers about health on ironclads, Clymer quickly sent those officers "a copy of the Bureau's gratifying appreciation of their reports, and recognition of their labors."[32]

The reports forwarded in mid–1863 by Clymer were from officers serving on *Passaic*-class monitors: USS *Catskill*, *Patapsco*, and *Nahant*. They indicated that men were suffering from the vessels' extreme temperatures, which in July measured 92°F–102°F on the berth deck (where sailors tried to sleep), 130°F–135°F in the fireroom, and at least 140°F in the galley. One officer wrote that galley temperatures were too high to be measured with an ordinary thermometer.[33]

The ventilation system took air from the turret, which was filled with gunpowder smoke during battle, routed it via blowers primarily to the furnace rather than to living spaces, and returned it to the turret, where the blowers recycled it. That portion of air reaching the living spaces, reported Assistant Surgeon W.L. Wheeler of *Patapsco*, first traveled beneath the berth deck and "through the ship's stowage, and bilge, coming in contact with everything contained therein, and finally escapes to us heavy with sickly odors—one of the most prominent being that of bilge water." (Water naturally collected in the bilge, the lowest part of the vessel, and contained "every variety of filth and vermin." In steamers, oil and grease were added to the mix. Physicians of the time believed that plenty of fresh air was needed for good health and that crowded quarters and rank air engendered disease.) One of Wheeler's fellow officers found the stench of air entering his room so objectionable that he kept his ventilation grating closed. *Patapsco*'s captain improved matters by ordering the bilge washed out daily, but even that action left some living areas "very disagreeable." Ventilation might improve in port when various hatches were opened, but at sea, the openings had to be closed, and the only way to breathe fresh air was to go up to the turret, which was impractical for most of the crew.[34]

Clymer informed Whelan that the SABS's flag officer, Rear Admiral Samuel F. Du Pont, asked that some sort of disinfecting liquid be issued to the squadron's ironclads. (In the terminology of the time, a disinfectant was an agent used to counteract an unhealthful atmosphere or neutralize decomposing matter that might accumulate on walls and floors.) The original recommendation came from Commander John L. Worden of USS *Montauk*, another of the SABS's *Passaic*-class monitors, who feared that, despite efforts to maintain cleanliness and dryness, men would likely "suffer much discomfort, and, perhaps, some impairment of health, from the effluvia from their holds, unless a corrective of these noxious effluvia be furnished to them." Whelan said that some agent could certainly be supplied but opined that unless ironclads were built to allow frequent changes of air and easier, more thorough cleaning of the vessels, "the use of disinfectants of whatever pretentions would be of small avail."[35]

Whelan suggested that when ironclads were in port, their crews could be transferred to other vessels or to barracks on shore. Even if brief, time away from the vessels would help to "break up the chain of adverse influences, which must in continuous residence in such vessels, for a protracted period, result in rendering the crew sickly, and inefficient." Assistant Surgeon Wheeler thought having "a consort to each monitor, to sleep in" was an admirable idea, but the extent to which it was carried out has not been determined.[36]

The conditions on ironclads resulted in men suffering from heat exhaustion, sluggishness, loss of strength, and "want of recuperative power." Reports about such effects might, thought one medical officer, "seem extravagant to those who have never lived in a monitor under closed hatches, at sea, in the summertime." Another stated, "there are many influences at work undermining the constitutions of those of long residence in a vessel of this class that must be experienced in order to be perfectly understood." Assistant Surgeon C. Ellery Stedman reported that illness and weakness aboard *Nahant* seemed to affect the vessel's best men, "some of them being remarkable as specimens of manly strength and symmetry." Every crewmember, suggested Stedman, ought to be rotated out and relieved by a healthy replacement "if the government wants their services during the coming winter, tho many will never be the men they were." Stedman observed that the youngest members of the crew endured the conditions the best, and he recommended that "no man that has seen more than 23 years ought to be sent on board a monitor." Assistant Surgeon Edgar Holden, who served on USS *Passaic*, described a condition that he called "iron-clad fever," in which initial symptoms resembled those of typhus, progressed to severe headache, and then led to aphonia (inability to speak.) Aphonia, reported Holden, usually signaled a fatal outcome.[37]

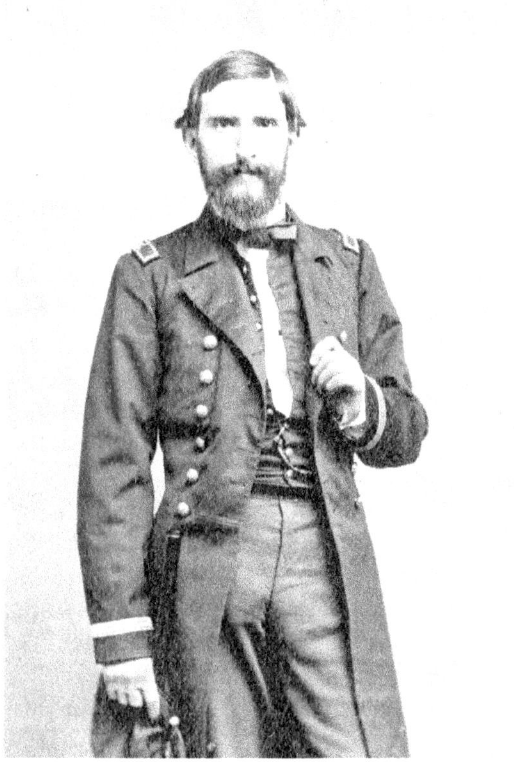

Assistant Surgeon C. Ellery Stedman, who described health conditions on ironclads and drew scenes of Civil War naval life. Although Stedman resigned from the navy in 1865 as an assistant surgeon, the lace on his sleeves reflects mid-war uniform specifications for a passed assistant surgeon (Civil War Photograph Collection, vol. 14, MOLLUS-MASS, USAHEC).

The *Passaic*-class vessels were supposed to represent an improvement over USS *Monitor*, yet their troubles largely echoed those reported on *Monitor* more than a year earlier. In May 1862, Lieutenant William N. Jeffers, commanding *Monitor*, reported that "if the hatches were all closed (as they must be at sea) in this warm weather the crew would be unable to live for forty-eight hours shut up. Quite one-third of the crew are now suffering from debility." Several men working in the galley, wrote Jeffers, had "already literally wilted down by the intense heat of its position against the rear end of the boiler." Heat was also a problem on USS *Chickasaw*, a *Milwaukee*-class monitor. According to an October 1864 report by that vessel's commander, Lieutenant G.H. Perkins, ventilation was poor, with "the heat in the midship portion of the vessel being so intense as to prevent living below."[38]

The maladies attributed to service on ironclads apparently abated late in the war when improvements were made in the vessels' ventilation.

In late 1865, BUMED chief Phineas J. Horwitz characterized the ventilation in early ironclads as having been "based on a wrong principle, that of forcing fresh air through the hold, instead of pumping out the foul air and allowing fresh air to rush in from all the openings above." Early vessels were forced to close hatches and thus diminish the entry of fresh air "when at anchor, with a sea just sufficient to wash the deck." That situation was remedied, wrote Horwitz, by adding "iron tubes, some three or four feet in height ... that could be trimmed to the wind, and thus send a steady stream of cool, fresh air below." Modern physician–historians have suggested that causes of ironclad fever may have included carbon monoxide intoxication, toxic agents in drinking water, a bacterial organism in the vessels' ductwork, or viral encephalopathy.[39] Another possibility is that some material used in constructing the vessels—perhaps in treating the metal—acted as a toxin in the closed and overheated interior of early ironclads.[40]

BUMED reported in late 1865 that statistics on sickness did not support the notion that ironclads were less healthy than wooden vessels. Many medical officers who served on ironclads would have disagreed. "It amounts to no more or less than an axiom," wrote Assistant Surgeon Wheeler of *Patapsco*, "that the residents of monitors must suffer more ... than those of well-ventilated vessels." Many men, he reported, "constantly complain of headaches, are evidently not well, and yet there is no particular symptom to indicate any particular disease." Wheeler made a vital point—one not acknowledged in the 1865 BUMED report—about illness on ironclads: "The sick report does not show the number of men who received treatment, as two thirds of them are not excused from duty." Indeed, sickness reports from vessels included only those men admitted to sickbay as unable to work; many other men were treated without their missing work.[41]

BUMED encouraged allopathic practice, but surgeons were still free to exercise reasonable medical judgment as long as it did not incur large expenses or violate the spirit or letter of the law. Dealing with medicinal alcohol and the abolition of the spirit ration tested that balance. Whelan appreciated the value of hygienic measures in preventing and controlling disease and was grateful when surgeons displayed the same attitude. Medical officers could do little about the health problems thought to be particular to ironclads except to bring them to the attention of the Navy Department.

Chapter 11

Illness and Injury

Details about the number of men who became sick or were injured during the war, and how long their disability lasted, are vital in understanding the importance of health in the navy. Such information helps in appreciating the extent of suffering, how the loss of manpower affected the navy's fighting strength, and the need for BUMED to appoint an adequate number of medical caregivers and furnish the necessary supplies. Annual and postwar reports from BUMED summarized the navy's health in terms of numbers of patients treated. While the statistics are illuminating in some respects, they are far from complete, and their interpretation requires some caution.

General Limitations of BUMED Statistics

In its annual compilations, BUMED classified sickness reports according to their sources—hospitals, receiving ships, navy yards, and vessels at sea—which differed in the susceptibility of their potential patients to various maladies and in the criteria for admission and treatment in a care facility. The primary occupants of receiving ships, for example, had recently been deemed fit to serve in the navy, so those ships' medical officers were relatively unlikely to treat seriously ill patients. Furthermore, a sailor on a receiving ship might be ill enough to be excused from duty—and thus reported among sickness statistics—but not sick enough to be sent to a hospital. Patients with the most serious or long-lasting conditions tended to end up in hospitals, which as expected, had the highest mortality rate among the four sources of sickness reports.

To be included in a sickness report, a man had to be disabled enough to be excused from duty. Men with minor complaints could be treated by medical officers, but if judged able to work, they were not admitted to a ship's sickbay; such cases did not appear in BUMED's published reports. Furthermore, surgeons' stewards in charge did not routinely submit sickness reports, and such reports from medical officers were often tardy, if submitted at all. In 1864, Fleet Surgeon James C. Palmer of the WGBS took steps that, if followed faithfully and applied to other squadrons, might have enhanced the completeness of sickness reports sent to BUMED. According to his orders, medical officers temporarily attending patients on vessels having no such officers would keep a journal of practice aboard those vessels. A vessel's journal would be under the charge of its surgeon's steward, if there was one, or by such crewmember assigned by the vessel's commander. The medical officer in temporary attendance on the last day of each quarter or year was responsible for completing the required BUMED reports. Regardless of how effective Palmer's efforts were, annual BUMED reports included the caveat that summary sickness statistics for squadrons did not incorporate reports from vessels to which a medical officer was not assigned.[1]

BUMED supplied medical officers with a list of 176 medical terms to be used, when possible, as diagnoses. The diagnoses were divided into 12 categories that, for the most part, pertained to the site of the ailment (e.g., digestive system, respiratory system), although some described the type of medical problem (e.g., fever, injury). Squadron medical officers—or the BUMED office itself—found the standard list inadequate and added diagnoses so that the total number on compilations of wartime reports numbered about 200. The intent behind standard terms was to simplify BUMED's tabulation of data, but their use did not eliminate possible confusion.

Concepts of disease applied by physicians of the Civil War era differed from those used today, with the result that certain terms, although familiar to practitioners of both eras, might not carry the same connotations. *Febris intermittens*, for example, translates easily to "intermittent fever" but describes a fever pattern—alternating elevated and normal temperatures—rather than a specific disease. Most intermittent fever probably resulted from malaria, a disease caused by mosquito-transmitted protozoan parasites, but there were other possible causes. To Civil War physicians ignorant of infectious microorganisms, *malaria* (bad air) referred to the environment that apparently gave rise to intermittent fever but not to the ailment itself. *Influenza*, as used in the mid–19th century, meant a severe form of *catarrhus* (catarrh, or inflammation of the mucous membranes of the air passages) occurring in epidemics, a definition in line with modern usage but lacking the implication of infection by influenza virus. Today, most Americans with uncomplicated catarrh would probably say instead that they had a cold.

A patient's medical record usually indicated a single diagnosis as his reason for hospital or sickbay admission, even if he had multiple medical problems. Thus, problems that were present but not the reason for admission were underreported, and deaths might be attributed to the admission diagnosis when a coexisting or later-developing condition was actually the culprit. Medical officers examining the same patient might arrive at different diagnoses, call the same disorder by different names, or disagree about what problem accounted for the patient's admission. Regardless of how the diagnosis nomenclature was intended to be used, the presence of medical officers—especially new acting assistant surgeons—unfamiliar with or having little concern for that nomenclature practically ensured inconsistency and errors in how the terms were applied.

In 1867, BUMED published detailed wartime diagnosis-specific prevalence and mortality data for squadrons only, and not—even though figures were certainly available—for hospitals, navy yards, or receiving ships. The same patient could be counted in reports from more than one type of facility for the same illness. Thus, a man treated in a vessel's sickbay and transferred to a shore hospital would account for two admissions, and his discharge from the sickbay would not necessarily imply that he had recovered sufficiently to resume his shipboard duties. The relative frequency of diagnoses probably differed between squadrons and hospitals because crewmen with common complaints—intermittent fever and catarrh, for example—could usually return to duty within a few days, and transferring them to a hospital ashore made little sense. Hospitals tended to receive patients with the more dangerous or longer-lasting disorders and those who did not respond adequately to shipboard treatment. BUMED's summaries of illness do not show average lengths of stay in medical facilities and thus do not allow precise determination of the effects of specific illnesses on naval manpower.

Although reported sickness statistics are informative, they fall short of providing a complete picture of how illness affected the navy's fighting efficiency. In mid–1863, for example, SABS Fleet Surgeon George Clymer wrote to BUMED chief Whelan about how exhaustion and illness were affecting his squadron's manpower. The squadron, on blockade duty and patrolling in and around Charleston Harbor, comprised about 7,000 men, but this, said Clymer, was about 1,000 less than its intended complement.[2]

When the squadron's flagship, USS *Wabash*, arrived from Port Royal at its station off of Charleston, she was 60 men short of her full complement of 630. Within a week, 163 *Wabash* crewmembers were transferred to other squadron vessels "to take the place of used up men." Fifty other men, reported Clymer, were out every night, all

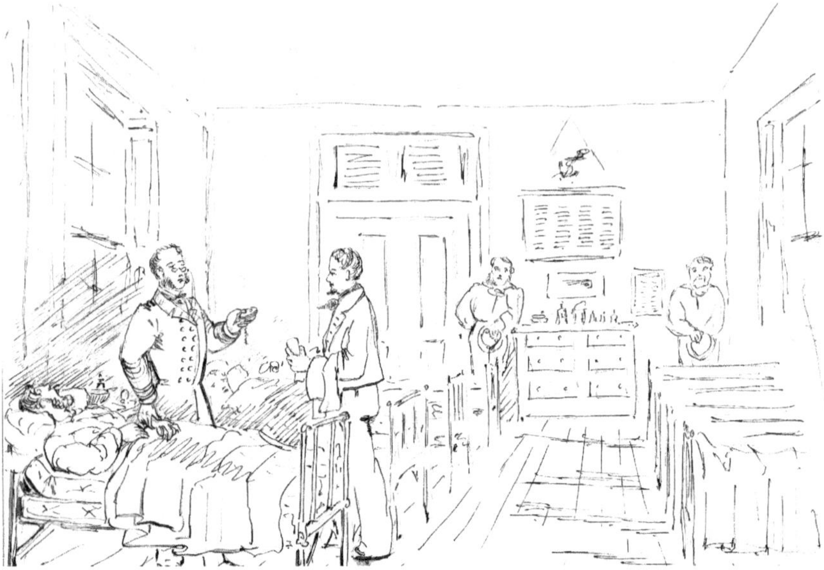

A medical officer and assistant, probably a surgeon's steward, attending to a hospital patient. BUMED preferred to have land-based hospitals receive patients with conditions that would not resolve quickly or were difficult to treat in a vessel's sickbay. Illustration by C. Ellery Stedman (Civil War Photograph Collection, vol. 14, MOLLUS-MASS, USAHEC).

night—largely on picket duty in boats—exposed to drenching rains and unable to perform other duties during the day. *Wabash*'s daily sick list contained about 30 men. Of her remaining 327 men, 50 were Marines and 54 were coal-heavers, which left 223 sailors "for whatever duty."[3]

Rear Admiral John A. Dahlgren, the SABS flag officer, concurred with Clymer about the severity of duty. Blockade duty was trying, and service on the squadron's ironclads, which were "either in action or in situations so exposed as to require constant readiness for action" made for a taxing existence "not easily understood except by personal experience."[4]

Many of the "used up" men mentioned by Clymer were probably on ironclads and suffering from the effects of poor ventilation—the vessels' hatches were kept closed when near Charleston—and from other unhealthful conditions. It is unclear exactly what diagnoses were used when such men were admitted to sickbay; one may have been *adynamia,* which referred loss of strength or vigor. Assistant Surgeon C. Ellery Stedman, of the SABS monitor USS *Nahant,* then at Port Royal, reported that so many men were ill or sent to other ships—to receive medical care or to fill in for those vessels' sick—that there were "too few men in the Engineer's Department to work [*Nahant*] to her station in

Wassaw Sound; so that we are delayed till a number of men can be sent aboard to take the place of the disabled." Many crewmembers on the SABS's ironclads, especially those manning the engines or boilers, felt poorly but were either not ill enough to be admitted to sickbay or were unwilling to be removed from duty because they wanted desperately to participate in action against Charleston's defenses. Some exhausted men may have been surveyed and deemed unfit for continued duty without being on the sick list at the time. The SABS's condition when Clymer wrote is simply not apparent from examining its compiled sickness statistics, and the same general limitation applies to the other sources of sickness reports.[5]

By their very nature, compiled sickness data do not indicate exactly *who* was stricken. The war effort was probably more influenced when the victim of illness or injury was an officer of great responsibility rather than a seaman. Flag Officer David G. Farragut of the WGBS reported in June 1862 that his own illness prompted him to yield to the judgment of other officers regarding an attack on Vicksburg. Rear Admiral John A. Dahlgren took command of the SABS in 1863 because the officer originally intended for that role, Rear Admiral Andrew H. Foote, died of a kidney ailment. Dahlgren then lost the services of four successive fleet captains (chiefs of staff) in about two months—the first sent home sick, the second killed in action, the third crippled by a leg broken in combat, and the fourth captured. Between the third and fourth losses, Dahlgren wrote to Secretary Welles that the misfortunes had seriously compromised him in the "transaction of public business."[6]

Overall Death and Sickness Rates

In the latter half of the war, the average annual death rate for all naval personnel was about 4 percent. A large proportion of those deaths, perhaps a fourth, were not accounted for in sickness reports and may have occurred in men who were on active duty but not attended by naval medical officers, in men who were on leave or furlough, or in men who were on the retired list and living essentially civilian lives. In contrast, the 1860 U.S. census showed that death during the year ending June 1, 1860, occurred in 0.72 percent of men who were 20–40 years old, a range probably encompassing most naval personnel. (Census officials were certain that deaths were underreported but could not speculate to what extent.) It is probable that the true wartime risk of death was higher, to a substantial but unknown degree, for men in the USN than for average American men with the same age distribution.[7]

Among patients included in medical officers' sickness reports for 1861–65 from all types of facilities, 1.70 percent died during the reported admission. The death rate was 0.57 percent (82 of 14,464 admissions) in navy yards' sick quarters, 1.06 percent (110 of 10,350) in receiving ships' sick quarters, 1.34 percent (2,837 of 211,677) in vessels' sickbays, and 4.88 percent (1,525 of 31,246) in shore hospitals. In the latter half of the war, a member of the navy was, on average, put on the sick list about 1.6 times a year.[8]

It is difficult to determine with precision the proportion of deaths that were caused by sickness versus combat. One major concern is that statistics for injuries do not specify whether they occurred in combat. Some drownings and fatal gunshot wounds, for example, may have been accidental. However, BUMED did report in December 1865 that 1,406 navy men (presumably including Marines) had been killed during the rebellion, with 1,638 wounded and 176 missing. BUMED reports for 1861–65 show 4,554 deaths occurring in hospitals, navy yards, receiving ships, and squadrons combined. Dividing the first death figure by the second—with the caveat that the numbers may not have been derived from identical data sets—suggests that about 31 percent of deaths resulted from combat, with the remainder (69%) caused by illness. That result is consistent with the general consensus that about two-third of deaths in the Civil War armed forces were caused by disease.[9]

Commonly Reported Diagnoses

During the second half of the war, BUMED reported that the three categories accounting for the most diagnoses in squadrons were, in descending order, diseases characterized by fever (febrile diseases), diseases of the digestive system, and diseases of the respiratory system. Because the prevalence and severity of individual diseases within a single category could vary widely, it is less helpful to know the frequently reported categories than the specific diagnoses; the latter can be determined by pooling data from the individual squadrons.[10]

Among sickbay cases in 1861–65, the most frequently reported admission diagnosis by far was intermittent fever, whose 22,111 cases accounted for 15.4 percent of the 144,038 total cases tabulated (Appendix E). Second through fifth most common were acute diarrhea, catarrh, remittent fever, and acute bronchitis, which accounted for 10.7 percent, 6.3 percent, 6.0 percent, and 3.4 percent of total cases, respectively. Although those five diagnoses together constituted 41.8 percent of admission diagnoses and probably led to great suffering and loss of manpower, their cases, when pooled, ended in only 319 deaths, for a 0.5 percent mortality rate.[11]

The five diagnoses whose cases ended in the most deaths were, in descending order, drowning (570 deaths), gunshot wound (448), remittent fever (202), typhoid fever (146), and yellow fever (132); when pooled, those deaths were 59.2 percent of 2,532 total reported squadron deaths. Three diagnoses shared the distinction of being among the 20 most common and being associated with at least 100 deaths: remittent fever, chronic diarrhea, and gunshot wound.[12]

Large differences existed among squadrons in the overall frequency of illness, the frequency of specific diagnoses, and overall mortality. For example, men of the SABS averaged being on the sick list 1.15 times a year, whereas those of the Mississippi Squadron averaged 2.44 times a year. From October 1, 1861, to June 30, 1865, the SABS, with an average complement of 6,436 men, reported intermittent fever 1,552 times (0.24 times/man), but during the shorter period of October 1, 1862, to June 30, 1865, the Mississippi Squadron, with an average complement of 5,408, reported intermittent fever 10,352 times (1.91 times/man). Among sickbay admissions during the war, 1.3 percent ended in death in the SABS, and 2.6 percent ended in death in the Mississippi Squadron.[13]

A comprehensive review of the ailments that afflicted the USN and how they were managed would be impractical here. Nevertheless, and despite the limitations of sickness summaries, it is worthwhile to comment briefly about some of the ailments that were the most common or worrisome or are otherwise of interest. Some of the more common treatments are mentioned here, but they could vary widely and depended on practitioners' preferences, individual attributes of the cases, and what medical supplies were available.

Fevers

Intermittent fever—characterized by alternating periods and elevated and normal (or near normal) body temperature—was probably most commonly caused by malaria (the disease) and was the navy's most common diagnosis in squadrons, accounting for 15.35 percent of sickbay admissions. Medical officers knew that intermittent fever was likely to be problematic in swampy areas during warm weather and often ascribed the disease to the bad air (*malaria* or miasma) resulting from decomposing vegetable and animal material in stagnant water. Such conditions favor the breeding of mosquitoes, among them *Anopheles*, which carries the infectious agent for malaria, a protozoan parasite of the genus *Plasmodium*. Mosquitoes, while certainly considered a nuisance, were not recognized at the time as transmitting the disease. Naval surgeons routinely advised, when there was a choice in the matter, having vessels anchor or operate where there was a constant breeze or away from marshes.[14]

With an overall associated death rate in squadrons of 0.20 percent, intermittent fever was rarely fatal, yet the disease was capable of reducing manpower considerably. During 1863, intermittent fever was reported as the sickbay admission diagnosis 1.07 times for every man in the Mississippi Squadron. That value is probably much lower than the actual rate, because cases on the many vessels without a medical officer were usually not reported, while the denominator used in computing the rate (the average squadron complement) presumably did not depend on the presence of a medical officer. With an average sickbay stay of, say, three or four days, the illness, if equally prevalent throughout the year, might not have a great effect on a vessel's efficiency. Intermittent fever, however, occurred most commonly in late summer and through the fall, so vessels might have a large percentage of their crews ill during those months.[15]

The preferred treatment for malaria was often quinine sulfate, although a solution of potassium arsenite, commonly called Fowler's solution, was also popular. Men admitted to sickbay with malaria were often well enough to return to duty within a few days, but they were also likely to return with recurrences of the disease. Quinine, sometimes mixed with whiskey, could be given to prevent malaria; the dosages in such instances were smaller than those used to treat the disease.[16]

Remittent fever, a condition in which the body temperature fluctuates but does not return to normal, was the 4th-most-common admission diagnosis in squadrons. Continued fever, in which the temperature is elevated with minimal fluctuation, was the 20th-most-common. Clinical thermometers were used only rarely during the Civil War, so temperature was estimated by touch, and it is likely that some fevers were mischaracterized. Also, microbiologic and other laboratories did not yet exist to help medical officers make diagnoses. Some patients said to have remittent or continued fever may have suffered from malaria, mild typhoid fever, or another disease. In squadrons, the reported mortality rate associated with an admission diagnosis of remittent fever was 2.34 percent, while that associated with continued fever was 0.52 percent. Treatment of remittent and continued fever resembled that of intermittent fever, with quinine being used frequently. One army clinician described two types of remittent fever, one that improved when treated with quinine and potassium arsenite and one that got worse with those drugs and was better treated with bleeding and large doses of calomel.[17]

Typhoid fever, caused by ingestion of food or drink contaminated with the bacterium *Salmonella typhi*, was stated as the admission diagnosis only 752 times in squadrons during the war—compared with 22,111 times for intermittent fever—yet was associated with a frightful mortality rate of 19.41 percent. Typhoid fever was sometimes difficult to distinguish from malaria, and the two diseases may have existed simultaneously in some patients. Among the treatments for typhoid fever was quinine, any benefit from which was probably the result of its activity against coexisting malaria.[18]

Yellow fever was similar, in squadrons, to typhoid fever in reported prevalence and associated death rate. Yellow fever, caused by a virus transmitted by the *Aedes aegypti* mosquito, was one of the war's most feared diseases because of the suffering of its victims, its propensity to decimate local populations, and the disruption caused by efforts to isolate people suffering from or exposed to the illness. During the war, the virus was common in areas with tropical climates, such as the West Indies. It was thought that persons with the disease or coming from areas with outbreaks could spread it to others, although transmission actually occurred after an infected person was bitten by a local *A. aegypti* mosquito, which transmitted the virus by biting someone else. The insects' part in disease transmission was not appreciated at the time.[19]

Ports required quarantines for vessels carrying persons with yellow fever or coming from areas with the disease. When yellow fever broke out at Key West, the USN endeavored to keep its vessels away from that locale. Vessels that were or had been carrying infected persons were sent north, because cooler climates were thought to be less hospitable to the disease. Cooler surroundings were indeed less favorable to the breeding of *A. aegypti*, although sanitary measures could go a long way in controlling the disease. That was proven when Major General Benjamin Butler, commanding the Union occupying force in New Orleans in 1862, enforced a yellow-fever quarantine and ordered that the city's streets be cleaned to reduce the miasmic conditions that favored disease. Those measures reduced the *A. aegypti* population, and continuation of the sanitation rules helped to protect New Orleans from major outbreaks of yellow fever throughout the rest of the war.[20]

Yellow fever could incapacitate crews quickly and make their vessels almost useless, as was demonstrated when the disease struck the EGBS in the summer of 1864. In early August, 38 of 53 men on USS *Chambers* were on the sick list, presumably with yellow fever. The fever affected so many men on USS *Roebuck* that at one time, only five men and one officer, out of a complement of about 69, were available for duty.

Between mid–May and mid–August, 7 ships—out of 28 in the squadron, excluding tenders—were sent north to escape the fever and place the crew in a more favorable climate. In describing the outbreak, Secretary Welles called yellow fever "so much and so justly dreaded" but reported that sending vessels north "has been in its effects salutary." He also claimed that despite the EGBS's reduction in strength, there was "no serious interruption" in maintaining the blockade.[21]

Among just five EGBS vessels—USS *Nita, Dale, Wanderer, Eugenie,* and *Chambers*—there were well over 30 deaths during that summer from yellow fever. Additional deaths undoubtedly occurred on other ships of the squadron. BUMED reported after the war, however, that the EGBS had only 64 sickbay admissions for yellow fever, with 10 associated deaths, for all of 1864. Part of the discrepancy can reasonably be attributed to the absence or illness of medical officers on the stricken ships, and thus the nonsubmission of sickness reports. The magnitude of the difference, however, casts doubt on the accuracy of the BUMED disease compilations in general.[22]

Treatment of yellow fever varied among practitioners and might include bleeding or administration of mercury-containing compounds or quinine. No particular strategy seemed especially popular or effective. One experienced physician characterized yellow fever as a self-limiting disease that should be managed rather than treated. "All that is to be done," he maintained, "is to keep the patient alive for a certain time, and he will get well."[23]

After *Roebuck*, one of the EGBS vessels struck by yellow fever, arrived at Portsmouth, New Hampshire, she underwent a number of so-called disinfection processes to rid her structure and atmosphere of odorous or injurious constituents. They included treating parts of the ship with copperas (hydrated ferrous sulfate) dissolved in water, fumigation by dipping a red-hot bolt (a solid cast-iron artillery projectile) in tar, and leaving open containers of copperas and chloride of lime (calcium hypochlorite) about the ship.[24]

Surgeons may sometimes have entered yellow fever or another disease as the admission diagnosis when the patient actually had dengue, or breakbone fever. Dengue, which was not included in BUMED's standard nomenclature, was added separately as a diagnosis 150 times—55 times in the NABS and 95 times in the WGBS—with all such entries reported for 1863. Other cases of dengue, however, were mentioned in correspondence concerning the WGBS vessel USS *Brooklyn* in July 1862, when she was serving on the Mississippi River. Still other cases were mentioned as occurring in October 1864 in Mobile Bay. Those cases were apparently omitted or classified under a different diagnosis in sickness reports submitted to BUMED. Unlike yellow fever, which was often fatal, no deaths were associated with an admission diagnosis of dengue.[25]

Dengue is caused by a virus transmitted by mosquitoes. During the war, dengue and yellow fever occurred in similar locales, and the presence of dengue was commonly thought to precede the arrival of yellow fever. Dengue caused fever and severe pains in the back, limbs, and joints. Because its prognosis was almost always favorable, the most important treatment was pain control, usually with opium.[26]

Medical officers worried about smallpox (*variola*) because of the suffering of its victims, its ability to spread, and the disruption it caused to normal operations. Transmission of the disease occurs primarily through inhalation of the variola virus contained in droplets sneezed or coughed by infected persons; such transmission typically requires fairly prolonged face-to-face contact. Transmission can also result from contact with bedding or clothing contaminated by the fluid from sores of an infected person. All of those conditions were likely to exist on ships. Wartime methods of preventing spread of the disease included isolating patients in special wards, hospitals, or hospital ships and burning the bedding and clothing of patient and caregivers.

Vaccination against smallpox was routine in the navy and was apparently fairly effective. The material used for vaccination, called "vaccine virus" or "vaccine matter," could consist of fluid from the lesions of cows or humans with cowpox or from humans with smallpox. Scabs from people who had formed lesions after vaccination could also be used after being mixed with water. Whelan reported that BUMED procured scabs through an arrangement with a city institution in New York. Vaccination was not foolproof and could result in unusual lesions or unexpected illness. That phenomenon, termed "spurious vaccination," was commonly attributed to impure vaccine.[27]

Smallpox was stated as the sickbay admission diagnosis 300 times during the war and was associated with 35 deaths. A related diagnosis, varioloid or *varioloides*, was a mild form of smallpox occurring in persons who had been vaccinated or had a previous case of smallpox. Varioloid was the sickbay admission diagnosis 198 times and was associated with 4 deaths.[28]

Treatment of variola and varioloid was nonspecific and might consist of purging with laxatives, attempting to reduce the fever with exposure to cool air or sponging with cool water, and application of a topical formulation, such as mercurial ointment.[29]

Among the other diagnoses classified as fevers were measles and erysipelas (a skin infection usually caused today by streptococcus), which were sickbay admission diagnoses 624 and 523 times, respectively. Measles and erysipelas were associated with death in 17 and 15 cases, respectively.[30]

Diarrhea and Dysentery

When combined, acute diarrhea, chronic diarrhea, and acute dysentery were reported in squadrons nearly as often as intermittent fever. The terms *diarrhea* and *dysentery* were sometimes used interchangeably, with some physicians using the latter to denote diarrhea accompanied by pain, mucus, or blood. Patients with acute cases of diarrhea—meaning those of sudden onset and of short duration—nearly always recovered, with a death rate of 0.33 percent, but an admission diagnosis of chronic diarrhea was more ominous, with a death rate of 5.68 percent. The diagnoses of acute and chronic dysentery had mortality rates of 1.50 percent and 4.04 percent, respectively. Fortunately, chronic dysentery was an uncommon admission diagnosis in squadrons, accounting for only about 400 cases during the war. The chronic forms of diarrhea and dysentery were often associated with weight loss and weakness.[31]

Among the causes of diarrhea and dysentery were microbial contamination of food or drink and a poor diet. Ingestion of river water was sometimes cited as causing diarrhea and led to recommendations to use drinking water distilled from condensers on steamers. Another cause could be unhealthy rations or overindulgence in fresh fruit or vegetables, as might occur during or after foraging excursions on shore. Diarrhea could also be a symptom of other illnesses, such as malaria, typhoid and yellow fever, and influenza, but in such instances, those diseases, rather than diarrhea, were probably more likely to be designated as the admission diagnosis.[32]

Diarrhea was often thought to result from bowel inflammation or irritation, so laxatives, such as calomel or castor oil, might be given first to rid the gut of offending matter. An astringent, such as tannic acid, might follow to reduce the gut's production of mucus or blood. That might be accompanied by an opium formulation to check the diarrhea itself.[33]

Diseases of the Respiratory Tract

Among the respiratory tract diagnoses that were of concern because of their frequency or death rate were catarrh, acute bronchitis, pneumonia, and pulmonary tuberculosis. There was probably a fair amount of overlap between the very common diagnoses of catarrh and acute bronchitis, with catarrh being a more benign illness in terms of mortality (0.02 percent for catarrh, 0.42 percent for acute bronchitis). Treatment for either might include an expectorant, such as syrup of squill, to loosen secretions, and an opium formulation to suppress cough.[34]

Pneumonia, which was associated with a death rate of 7.73 percent, could follow catarrh or bronchitis and might also be a consequence of other diseases, such as measles and smallpox. Fortunately, pneumonia was relatively infrequent, accounting for only 1.13 percent of more than 144,000 sickbay admissions. Commonly recommended treatments for pneumonia included bleeding (to reduce the workload of the lungs), opium to reduce coughing and its associated pain, and administration of calomel and tartar emetic.[35]

Phthisis pulmonalis, or pulmonary tuberculosis, had about the same death rate (7.31%) as pneumonia when designated as the sickbay admission diagnosis. Its occurrence was somewhat less frequent than that of pneumonia, accounting for 0.80 percent for admissions. Patients with pulmonary tuberculosis were often advised to exercise and adjust their diet. Medicine might be prescribed for cough, but there seemed to be no drug therapy commonly believed to have much effect on the course of the disease.[36]

Rheumatism

Acute and chronic rheumatism ranked 6th and 8th in frequency among squadron admission diagnoses, respectively, and together constituted about 6 percent of those admissions. Many—perhaps most—cases of acute and chronic rheumatism were manifestations of rheumatic fever, which can result from a streptococcal infection such as strep throat or scarlet fever. Many cases of tonsillitis, the 18th most common sickbay admission diagnosis, were probably strep throat. *Scarlatina* (scarlet fever) appeared only 27 times during the war as a sickbay admission diagnosis. Rheumatism could also be a reactive arthritis, an inflammatory response to diseases such as gonorrhea, syphilis, scurvy, malaria, and dysentery. Rheumatism was characterized by inflammation of one or more large joints—the internal organs, including the heart, might also be affected—accompanied by fever and general debility. Patients with serious cases of rheumatism could be essentially immobile and helpless because moving about was so painful. It is no surprise, then, that a man with rheumatism might not be able to perform his duty.[37]

Oral therapy for rheumatism might include potassium iodide, "alkaline treatment" with potassium or sodium bicarbonate, or a preparation of colchicum—the active ingredient of which, colchicine, is still used for gout. Various liniments could also be applied topically.[38]

Scurvy

Scurvy, caused by vitamin C deficiency—a fact not known at the time—was a constant worry of medical officers, who routinely recommended that crews be provided with fresh provisions, especially fruits and vegetables, to prevent the disease; the same types of foods constituted its treatment. The disease was reported 521 times as a sickbay admission diagnosis (0.36 percent of such diagnoses), with three associated deaths. It was probably present in many other sailors who were not ill enough to be excused from duty. Scurvy can cause weakness, gum disease, skin hemorrhages, and poor wound healing. It can also interfere with the treatment of injuries or other diseases.[39]

Sexually Transmitted Diseases

Gonorrhea and primary syphilis were the 16th and 18th most common sickbay admission diagnoses, respectively, with each accounting for about 2,100 admissions (1.5 percent of admissions each). Secondary syphilis was somewhat less common as an admission diagnosis, appearing about 1,300 times and accounting for slightly under 1 percent of all admission diagnoses. No deaths occurred during admissions attributed to gonorrhea or syphilis. Venereal disease was probably present in many men who were not admitted to sickbay.[40]

Gonorrhea might be treated with urethral injections of a silver nitrate or zinc solution or with an oral formulation of cubebs (derived from berries) or copaiba (a plant resin), the latter two for their supposed anti-inflammatory effects. Calomel might be given initially to open the bowels and in later stages of the disease. Stricture, or narrowing, of the urethra was a complication of gonorrhea and might necessitate the use of an instrument (catheter or bougie) to dilate the constriction. Such devices were normally supplied to medical officers as were syringes for urethral injections. Stricture of the urethra, which could arise from injury or diseases other than gonorrhea, was indicated as the sickbay admission diagnosis 352 times during the war, with two associated deaths.[41]

Treatment for the chancres of syphilis might include application of silver nitrate or a mercurial ointment, and oral treatment frequently included calomel or some other mercurial drug.[42]

Dental Disease

Among the diagnoses in BUMED's nomenclature were *odontalgia* (toothache) and *caries*. The latter term referred to softening and disintegration of bone tissue and was not limited to tooth decay. Odontalgia and caries were sickbay admission diagnosis 324 and 23 times, respectively, with no associated deaths for either disorder.[43]

Naval surgeons were supplied with dental instruments, which consisted of (according to one commentator) only one pair each of straight and curved forceps. Extracting teeth was probably the most common dental procedure performed. Acting Assistant Surgeon Samuel P. Boyer described treating two sailors who were "cursing and damning" teeth that they wanted removed. Boyer extracted the teeth, with the result that the satisfied sailors "left me rejoicing."[44]

The USN appears to have appointed no men during the war to specifically provide dental care, although the topic was discussed in 1853. Surgeon Thomas Harris, who preceded William Whelan as BUMED chief, had no doubt that men at sea would benefit from the availability of an experienced dentist and considered having one per squadron as ample. Discussions involving Harris and Secretary of the Navy John P. Kennedy centered not on appointing dentists but on whether the education of naval surgeons produced, or could be made to produce, practitioners able to provide a higher degree of dental care. Harris stated that the medical education of men appointed as naval surgeons included the "physiology and pathology of the teeth" and "the practice of such operations on the same, as may be considered essential to the health and comfort of the officers and men on ship board." That, thought Harris, was sufficient, and additional instruction "to embrace any thing like a complete and practical knowledge of the nicer manipulations of dentistry" was "altogether impracticable without a neglect of other, and much more important branches" of the medical profession. Harris described dentistry, which was traditionally learned through apprenticeship, as "an art separate and distinct from the profession of Medicine, and one requiring a manual dexterity, which can only be acquired by long and extensive practice." Furthermore, providing the instruments and other supplies needed for a high level of dental practice would entail much expense.[45]

As for appointing dentists—rather than expecting surgeons to acquire dental skills—Harris believed that no colleges in the United States or Europe were devoted to the teaching of dentistry. In this he was incorrect, as the Baltimore College of Dental Surgery was established in 1840, but his overall point—that formal dental education was scarce—was correct. By 1865, only four dental schools existed in the United States. Any further consideration of appointing dentists was put off until after the war.[46]

BUMED appears not to have gathered much data on the frequency of dental complaints during the Civil War. Given that many such problems would probably not disable a man from duty, the squadron statistics on odontalgia and caries are likely to be poor indicators of the navy's dental health.

Seasickness

Seasickness, or *nausea marina*, did not appear in the BUMED's standard nomenclature of disease or compiled sickness statistics. It could, however, incapacitate men and interfere with naval operations.

USS *Minnesota*, flagship of the Atlantic Blockading Squadron, left Boston in May 1861 but needed a passed assistant surgeon. Flag Officer Silas H. Stringham informed Secretary Welles that the fleet surgeon (Thomas Dillard) "has always been sick at sea for the past ten years, and I fear it may be [the] case now." Stringham needed an experienced medical officer because his assistant surgeon had never been to sea before.[47]

In June 1863, USS *Marion* left New York in search of commerce raider CSS *Tacony*. *Marion* encountered violent weather and sustained serious damage. One factor that convinced *Marion*'s commander, Lieutenant E. Orville Matthews, to return to New York was that "all the midshipmen and acting lieutenants (midshipmen of first class)" were seasick.[48]

Medical officers had no good way to treat seasickness. "It is worse than useless to swallow drugs," opined one surgeon. Suggestion for managing the ailment included getting plenty of fresh air, viewing the horizon or distant land rather than the ship's spars and rigging, and consuming moderate amounts of food when possible. Eating strongly flavored articles, such as smoked herring or ginger cakes—again, in moderation—was sometimes helpful in preventing seasickness and during the recovery phase.[49]

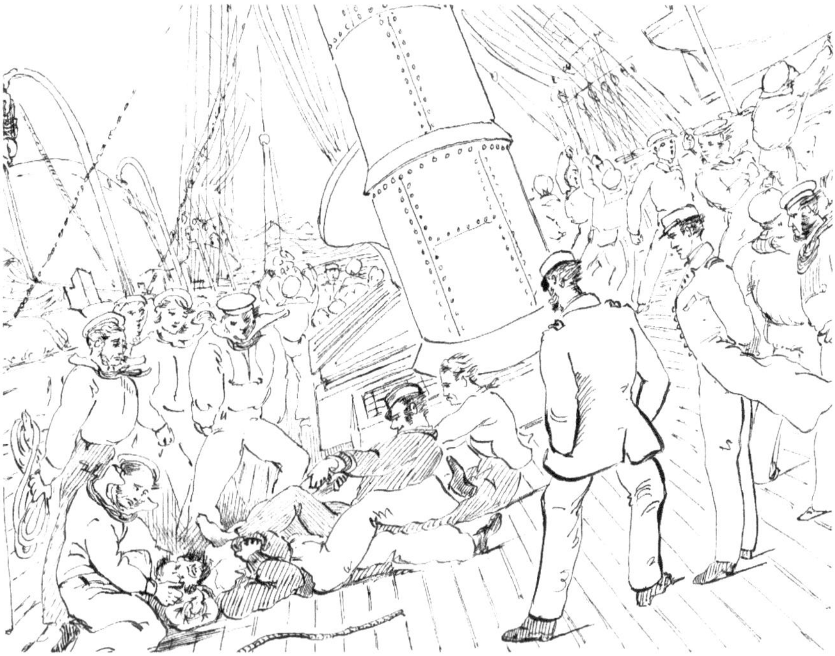

A medical officer (seated, in dark jacket and trousers) and assistants treating a sailor with a dislocated shoulder during a gale. Partial and complete dislocations were fairly common in squadrons but were not reported to be associated with any deaths. Many such injuries may have gone unreported if the victims were able to resume duty, as might occur with a dislocated finger. Illustration by C. Ellery Stedman (Civil War Photograph Collection, vol. 14, MOLLUS-MASS, USAHEC).

Injuries

The injury most commonly reported as a sickbay admission diagnosis was contusion, or bruise. Typically caused by impact with a blunt object, contusions were commonly associated with normal shipboard activity but would have to be fairly serious to disable a man enough to miss duty. Contusions also occurred during battle. If a contusion was accompanied by broken skin, the injury was called a contused wound. Contusions and contused wounds were the 7th- and 11th-most-common diagnoses for sickbays, accounting for 3,660 and 2,737 admissions, and 12 and 16 deaths, respectively, for mortality rates of 0.33 percent and 0.58 percent.[50]

Vulnus sclopecticum or *vulnus sclopetarium* (gunshot wound) was the 19th-most-common sickbay diagnosis, with 1,970 admission and 448 deaths (mortality rate, 22.74 percent). In addition to injuries from handheld or shoulder-fired weapons, the diagnosis also included wounds from the projectiles of naval or shore artillery.[51]

The diagnosis of *submersio*—probably intended to mean drowning—was classified as an injury and accounted for 570 sickbay admissions, with all such patients dying. In light of the 100 percent death rate, it seems likely that most or all of the victims were dead when recovered—if recovered at all—were presumed to have drowned, and were entered on the sick list so that their fate could be accounted for in BUMED's bookkeeping. If any men were resuscitated after nearly drowning, they must have been classified under a diagnosis other than *submersio*. Men lost when their ship was sunk, were swept overboard, or were otherwise lost at sea were presumably counted as drowning victims.[52]

Injuries varied so widely in their nature and seriousness that it is impractical to describe their general treatment, although arresting heavy bleeding was certainly a top priority. Surgeons would have been expected to reset bones, apply splints, remove foreign objects, and give medicine, such as opium, to help control pain. Extensive damage to a limb might necessitate amputation. Surgical removal of a limb was performed when its risks, including inevitable postoperative infection, were thought to be more survivable than those of leaving the shattered limb in place. Major surgery was almost always performed with chloroform or ether as a general anesthetic.[53]

BUMED's statistics on disease and mortality, especially those based on squadron reports, must be interpreted with caution but probably still give a good indication of the most common and dangerous diagnoses faced by medical officers. The majority of sickness appears to have been of infectious origin, although some ailments, such as scurvy and certain cases of diarrhea, were related to diet. Statistics for injuries do not allow easy differentiation between those related to shipboard accidents and combat. Gunshot wounds had a fairly high mortality rate, while all reported cases of drowning were fatal.

Chapter 12

Hospital Ships

The Union's Civil War navy did not have any vessels that were intended, before their construction, for the main purpose of caring for or transporting sick and wounded men. To be sure, multiple ships performed those functions, usually for relatively short periods of time and not necessarily as their primary mission.

Many USN vessels had a sickbay to care for their own men, and it was not unusual for smaller vessels that did not have a medical officer or space for a sickbay to transfer patients to a vessel that was better equipped to treat them. Because blockading squadrons operated off of territory that was largely under Confederate control, shore-based naval hospitals might not be within easy reach. Perhaps the most common solution for such a situation, at least for men who were not critically ill but needed long-term care, was to transport them to a large naval hospital via a supply ship that had finished its deliveries and was returning north. According to an 1863 schedule, USS *New Berne*, a supply ship for the NABS, left New York every month on the 1st and 15th and arrived at its farthest point, Old Inlet, North Carolina, on the 6th and 20th. The return trip, leaving Old Inlet on the 6th and 20th of the month, was faster, arriving at New York on the 9th and 23rd. *New Berne*'s medical staffing consisted of Acting Assistant Surgeon John E. Cobb, possibly assisted by a surgeon's steward. Supply ships that transported patients were seldom, if ever, called hospital ships.[1]

A warship might be called upon to transport patients. After the August 1864 Battle of Mobile Bay, for instance, USN gunboat *Metacomet* carried about 60 seriously wounded men, including Confederate Flag Officer Franklin Buchanan, to the USN hospital at Pensacola, a trip that took five or six hours. That task probably did not qualify *Metacomet*, in the minds of most medical officers, as a hospital ship.[2]

Vessels called hospital ships were most commonly used when a shore-based hospital was not conveniently close and when sending patients north seemed problematic. Timely conveyance to the North might be too unpredictable, for example, or patients might be either too ill to tolerate sea travel or likely to recovery too quickly to justify a trip to and from a faraway hospital. In such situations—and in keeping with long-standing naval practice—a large vessel, often a storeship, anchored in a Union-controlled port and received patients while it continued some of its normal activities. A surgeon took charge of a hospital ship's medical accommodations. A line officer was in overall command, however, because hospital ships had personnel devoted to functions other than patient care, and an officer with the authority to command them—which medical officers lacked—was needed.[3]

USS *Ben Morgan*

The USN's April 1861 abandonment of the Norfolk Navy Yard left the Norfolk Naval Hospital intact and available for Confederate use and deprived the USN of a hospital in that region. Thus, Surgeon Thomas Dillard, fleet surgeon of the Atlantic Blockading Squadron suggested in October 1861 to Flag Officer Louis M. Goldsborough "the necessity of establishing a hospital, on shore, for the sick of the squadron; or, if it be deemed more expedient, a hospital ship, permanently moored near Fortress Monroe." Should the latter be preferred, wrote Dillard, "the vessel selected should be solely appropriated to the use, and accommodation, of the sick. A store-ship would be unsuitable for such a purpose, evidently so, from the crowded condition of such a vessel with stores, and the consequent confusion and noise, in transferring provisions &c, to, and from it."[4]

The need for hospital accommodations led to the selection of USS *Ben Morgan* (sometimes called *Benjamin Morgan*) to be fitted up to receive patients. *Ben Morgan* had formerly been named *Mediator*, a sailing ship launched in 1826 and purchased by the USN in May 1861. By early November 1861, newspapers were reporting that *Ben Morgan* was at Fortress Monroe being prepared for hospital duty.[5]

Ben Morgan, evidently moored at Hampton Roads, began admitting patients no later than December 1861. The vessel's medical officer was Assistant Surgeon James H. Macomber, who appears to have been transferred from storeship USS *Brandywine* of the NABS, which itself may have cared for patients from other squadron vessels. In fact, hospital tickets suggest that Macomber transferred some of his *Brandywine* patients to his own care on *Ben Morgan*. In May 1862, Union forces regained control of the Norfolk facilities, with the U.S. Army initially occupying the naval hospital there. In June 1862, the USN began sending patients to a temporary hospital, which was under Macomber's supervision and located near Fort Norfolk, across the Elizabeth River from the Norfolk Naval Hospital. At about that time, admissions to *Ben Morgan* ceased. Among the patients treated on *Ben Morgan* were sailors wounded during the March 1862 Battle of Hampton Roads. *Ben Morgan*, when no longer needed or deemed suitable as a hospital ship, was used as an ordnance vessel and storeship.[6]

Flag Officer Goldsborough, for one, never seemed at ease calling *Ben Morgan* a hospital ship and shared Surgeon Dillard's concern about such a vessel having nonmedical functions. While it was receiving patients, he called it a storeship at least once and referred to its hospital space as "the store ship's between-decks." It was also used, while at Hampton Roads, as a coal ship. Surgeon William Maxwell Wood, who became NABS fleet surgeon in January 1862, commented in 1863 from near Newport News, Virginia, that the vessel "never was, in my opinion, a fit recipient of sick, except under the pressing necessities, which caused her to be used as such, at the time we had no access to hospital facilities, and no control of territory in this neighborhood." In 1862, Wood referred to *Ben Morgan* as "the wretched hospital ship."[7]

Hospital Ships for the SABS

The Union capture of Port Royal, South Carolina, in November 1861 provided a convenient base of operations for the SABS, but the squadron had no hospital ashore and needed a means of providing for its sick and wounded men. Flagship *Wabash* took on the role of hospital and supply ship while awaiting the arrival from Boston of USS *Vermont*, which anchored at Port Royal on April 12, 1862, after being seriously damaged in a gale and requiring the assistance of other vessels. The original intended role at Port Royal of *Vermont*, whose construction began in 1818 as a ship of the line, was to be a receiving ship, but its huge size qualified it for other purposes.[8]

Vermont began admitting SABS patients no later than April 30, 1862, and continued to do so until about August 1864 under the supervision of Surgeons James Eversfield (until November 1863) and William Lowber (November 1863 through July 1864). During that time, *Vermont* also acted as a storeship, as a hub of logistical activities, and even as a jail for misbehaving men from other squadron vessels. In October 1863, BUMED chief Whelan reported that "storeship Vermont, stationed at Port Royal, S.C., affords imperfect accommodations for the sick, &c., of the small vessels employed in that quarter; the space allowed for this purpose is too small to make it of special benefit to the medical department, though it is confessedly a great convenience on many occasions." At about the same time, Fleet Surgeon William Johnson opined that *Vermont*, "being employed as a storeship as well as for the reception of sick men, is manifestly unfit for the accommodation of sick officers."[9]

In late July 1864, Secretary Welles ordered *Vermont* to New York for service as a receiving ship. Taking over most of *Vermont*'s role at Port Royal, starting in late May 1864, was USS *New Hampshire*. That vessel, also originally intended as a ship of the line, had an average ship's company of 977 during the second quarter of 1864. Its complement dropped to 500 during the next quarter, during which *New Hampshire* had a smallpox outbreak that necessitated moving its smallpox patients to USS *Valparaiso* and the well crewmembers to quarters on shore. (Patients from a smallpox outbreak earlier in 1864 had been placed on USS *Mohawk*.) *New Hampshire*'s hospital admitted 457 patients from late May through September 1864 and had an average hospital census of 66 for the third quarter of 1864. Patients appear to have been admitted through the end of the war, first under the charge of Surgeon William Lowber (until late October 1864) and then Surgeon Henry C. Nelson. In November 1864, Whelan called *New Hampshire*'s accommodations "entirely inadequate" for the SABS's needs.[10]

Also assisting at Port Royal—during at least the second and third quarters of 1864—was USS *Home*, with Acting Assistant Surgeon W.W. Howard in charge of its hospital. *Home*, with a crew of about 50, admitted 162 patients during those six months, with an average hospital census of approximately 22. From about October 1864 through March 1865, *Home* served as a hospital ship off of Charleston, South Carolina, admitting 90 patients during those months and having an average patient census of about 17. USS *Supply*, with Acting Assistant Surgeon Reuben Smith, admitted at least one patient at Port Royal during that period, in mid–July 1864. The need for vessels at Port Royal to take on patients was drastically reduced by the opening of a shore hospital on Saint Helena Island in late 1864.[11]

Other Hospital Ships in the Blockading Squadrons

Multiple other hospital ships have been identified, but details about their activities are elusive. Among them are USS *Tallahatchie* of the WGBS, which in April 1865 cared for men injured by torpedoes in or near Mobile Bay; USS *Wanderer*, of the EGBS, which operated near Key

West; and USS *Fort Jackson* of the NABS, which received men wounded during the December 1864 and January 1865 attacks on Fort Fisher, North Carolina. The NABS also used at least one vessel, USS *Louisiana*, at Beaufort, North Carolina, as a hospital ship. Flag Officer William W. McKean of the EGBS expressed in May 1862 his intention of turning frigate USS *St. Lawrence* into a storeship and hospital ship, but whether that happened is unclear.[12]

USS *Red Rover*

One vessel for which the term *hospital ship* seems much more appropriate was USS *Red Rover*, which served on the Mississippi River. *Red Rover*, a river steamboat, had been purchased in November 1861 by the Confederate States to serve as a barracks ship for the floating battery *New Orleans*. When Island Number 10 was taken by Union forces in April 1862, *Red Rover*, although damaged, fell into their hands.[13]

Flag Officer Andrew H. Foote of the Union's Western Gunboat Flotilla, had directed that some suitable vessel be fitted out at St. Louis as a hospital ship. *Red Rover* fit the bill, and her modifications were put in charge of an army assistant quartermaster, Captain George D. Wise. At that time, the flotilla was under army control, although its vessels were commanded and manned by naval personnel.[14]

By mid–June 1862, *Red Rover* was at Cairo, Illinois, ready to receive patients. On board were supplies sufficient for 200 men for three months, including "delicacies for the sick" and 300 tons of ice. Wise gushed about the vessel's furnishings, which included "bathrooms, laundry, elevator for the sick from the lower to the upper deck, amputating room, nine different water-closets, gauze blinds to the windows to keep the cinders and smoke from annoying the sick, two separate kitchens for sick and well, a regular corps of nurses, and two water-closets for every deck." Many of the supplies were contributed by the Western Sanitary Commission, a civilian relief agency that took a particular interest in assisting with the furnishing of hospital vessels. There were other hospital ships on the Mississippi—*R.C. Wood, D.A. January, City of Memphis*, and *City of Nashville*, for example—that belonged to the army or were chartered by the Commission.[15]

Red Rover's first two medical officers were George H. Bixby and George Hopkins, who were referred to the Commission from Boston by James M. Barnard. Bixby had served on the Commission-chartered hospital ship *Empress* during the Shiloh Campaign in April 1862 and was offered command of *Red Rover*'s medical department. On June 3, 1862,

Bixby accepted the appointment—offered on June 1 by Captain Charles H. Davis, who had replaced Foote as the flotilla's flag officer—as "assistant surgeon in the U.S. gunboat service [Western Gunboat Flotilla]." Bixby's appointment was probably an acting one, which Davis was allowed to grant with the approval of the secretary of the navy. Bixby was formally appointed as an acting assistant surgeon on November 7, 1862.[16]

A list of *Red Rover*'s crew, evidently prepared a few days before Bixby's June appointment, shows 35 men, headed by the vessel's captain, Albert McDaniels. The "doctor's department" consisted of 11 men—many, if not all, of whom were engaged by the Commission—including a druggist, two wardens, and eight male nurses. Two women were employed as matron and laundress. During much of *Red Rover*'s Civil War service, some portion of the nursing care was provided by the Sisters of the Holy Cross, and at least five African American women served as nurses under the Sisters' supervision. As the first female nurses to serve on a USN vessel, those women have been called the forerunners of the U.S. Navy Nurse Corps.[17]

Flag Officer Davis issued regulations to ensure efficient use of *Red Rover*. "It will be understood," he ruled, "that only those patients are to be sent to the hospital boat who it is to be expected to be sick for some time, and whose cases may require more quiet and better attention and accommodation than can be provided on board the vessels to whom they belong. Slight disorders and accidents will be treated by the surgeon under whose care they may happen to fall." Davis wanted the conditions "distinctly understood and uniformly adhered to."[18]

Red Rover's missions included caring for and transporting men who had been injured by an explosion on USS *Mound City* and in combat with ironclad ram CSS *Arkansas*. Many of *Red Rover*'s trips were for the purpose of transferring patients to hospitals at Memphis or farther north to Cairo or Mound City. At one point, *Red Rover* and the naval hospital at Mound City were full, and the ordnance vessel *Judge Torrence* had to be converted to a hospital ship for temporary service. *Red Rover* was a godsend to the many small Union vessels patrolling the Mississippi River and its tributaries.[19] Flag Officer Davis made that clear when he thanked the army quartermaster, Captain Wise, for the "judgment and humanity" he had displayed in converting the former barracks vessel into a hospital ship:

> No one but those who have witnessed it can comprehend the suffering to which our sick have been exposed by the absence of proper accommodations on board gunboats and by the necessity for frequent and sometimes hasty change of place. The wounded and the patients suffering from fever

> occupy, under the direction of the surgeon, those parts of the ship which are the most quiet and best ventilated. When the ship was cleared for action, as often happened when lying near Fort Pillow, it was necessary to take down their cots and hammocks more than quickly into out-of-way and uncomfortable places. This must always have been attended with pain and distress, if not positive injury. The arrival of the *Red Rover* will put a stop to all this, promote the efficiency of the squadron by procuring comfort and the means of restoration for the sick. All the conveniences and appliances of a hospital are fully provided, and to these are added the neatness and order essential to so large an establishment.[20]

Davis also expressed his thanks to Acting Assistant Surgeon Bixby after the *Mound City* explosion: "It is a source of deepest gratification to me to know that these poor wounded men are in the hands of so able, attentive, and humane a physician as yourself. I have witnessed your devotion to them with profound gratitude, and I am sure you must enjoy the highest of all rewards—the consciousness of having done your duty," Respect for Bixby was widespread. In 1863, James M. Barnard—who had urged Bixby to volunteer his services in the West and by then was an official of the U.S. Sanitary Commission—proudly referred to Bixby as "one of my boys."[21]

In the fall of 1862, control of the Western Gunboat Flotilla was transferred from the army to the navy—with *Red Rover* formally becoming a vessel of the USN—and the flotilla was thereafter known as the Mississippi Squadron. At about that time, an Illinois court having jurisdiction over *Red Rover* as a prize of war sold her to the Navy Department for about $9,300. The change in command seemed to have no effect on *Red Rover*'s activities. After the fall of Vicksburg in July 1863, Flag Officer David D. Porter divided the Mississippi River into districts, each with its own divisional officer and patrolled by its assigned vessels. *Red Rover* was not restricted to one zone or another but cruised up and down the river, from Cairo to New Orleans, picking up patients from and delivering medical and other supplies to squadron vessels.[22]

Shortly before the Mississippi Squadron came under USN control, Assistant Quartermaster Wise told Bixby that he (Bixby) would be as much in command of *Red Rover* as of a shore hospital and that he would need a pilot but not a captain. Although orders for *Red Rover*'s movements were often directed to Bixby, a line officer was the vessel's captain. There were, after all, many nonmedical crewmembers, who were outside of Bixby's command authority.[23]

Not all of the vessel's tasks were related to patient care. In one instance, *Red Rover* and *Judge Torrence* were directed to guard the

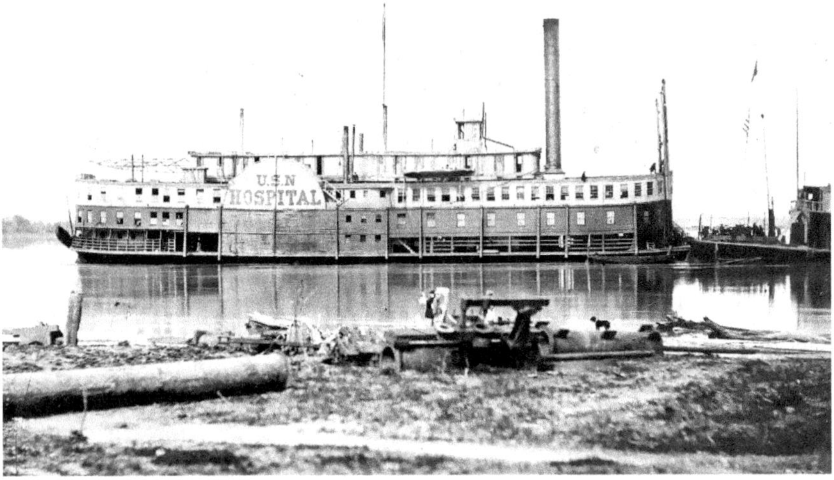

Naval hospital ship *Red Rover*, which served on the Mississippi River. The vessel's chief medical officer was Acting Assistant Surgeon George H. Bixby (NHHC, image NH 60501).

mouth of the White River while other squadron vessels went up the Arkansas River to attack Fort Hindman. In the aftermath of that battle, *Red Rover*, while about a mile below Napoleon, Arkansas, was hit twice by Confederate fire and returned fire with musketry. In June 1863, during the Vicksburg Campaign, Flag Officer Porter ordered *Red Rover* to be prepared to fire shells—her armament consisted of a 32-pounder—in the vicinity of Young's Point, Louisiana.[24]

Photographs of *Red Rover* show "U.S.N. Hospital" painted prominently on her sides. Although army and naval officers may have understood that the customs of war prohibited firing on facilities clearly marked as hospitals, no formal agreement on that point existed between Union and Confederate forces. General orders issued to the U.S. Army in April 1863 stated that hospitals were customarily designated by a flag (usually yellow) and that an "honorable belligerent allows himself to be guided by flags or signals of protection as much as the contingencies and necessities of the fight will permit." The orders added that deceiving the enemy by flags of protection was "an act of bad faith" and might justify refusal to respect such flags. Orders addressing the protection of hospital ships were issued in the USN's General Orders no. 551 of June 1900. They stated that hospital ships should have specified markings and were to be "respected and exempt from capture," provided that they were not used for any military purpose and did not "in any way hamper the movements of the combatants." Confederate forces were not bound by the U.S. Army's 1863 orders, and some of *Red Rover*'s activities, such as guarding the mouth of the White River and using her gun in an attacking manner—it that was ever done—might have been considered as invalidating any protection that her signage claimed.[25]

Bixby served on *Red Rover* through the end of the war. Whether Flag Officer Davis also granted *Red Rover*'s other physician, George Hopkins, the same title he had given Bixby is unclear, but Hopkins received his formal appointment as acting assistant surgeon on the same day in November 1862 as Bixby. During that month, a medical board that included Bixby deemed Hopkins unfit for duty because of his suffering from chronic dysentery "contracted from exposure to the influence of the climate and aggravated by great and constant exertion in the discharge of his duty for some months past." Hopkins was consequently granted a month's leave to recover in a more healthful climate. He continued to serve with the Mississippi Squadron until late December 1863, when he was detached and ordered to duty on USS *Tacony* of the NABS. Surgeon Ninian Pinkney was appointed in December 1862 as fleet surgeon of the Mississippi Squadron and made his headquarters on *Red Rover*. When administrative responsibilities made Pinkney unavailable to assist in patient care, Bixby probably had one other medical officer to assist him.[26]

Red Rover's last trip of the war was in December 1864, by which time she had admitted nearly 1,700 patients, with 157 deaths. There has been disagreement about which vessel should properly be called the USN's first hospital ship, with many favoring *Red Rover*. Much seems to depend on how the term is defined, with at least one author suggesting that the distinction belongs to USS *Intrepid* for her service in the First Barbary War (1801–5). Although *Red Rover*'s USN service was not exclusively medical, she was certainly the first USN vessel to be so well equipped, in furnishings and personnel, to provide patients with care and transportation.[27]

The Mississippi Squadron also used a number of hospital barges, about which little has been recorded. One was being prepared to receive patients in December 1862 while *Red Rover* was being repaired, and one called *Rebecca* was active in mid–1863. In September 1864, Lieutenant Commander Le Roy Fitch, commanding the 10th District of the Mississippi Squadron (the Cumberland and upper Ohio rivers) asked Flag Officer Porter for a barge for use as a hospital boat during the fall and winter. Not only did Fitch's vessels have little room for sick men, ice on the Ohio would make transporting patients to Cairo or Memphis difficult. Porter sent a barge to Fitch at Smithland, Kentucky, to be fitted up

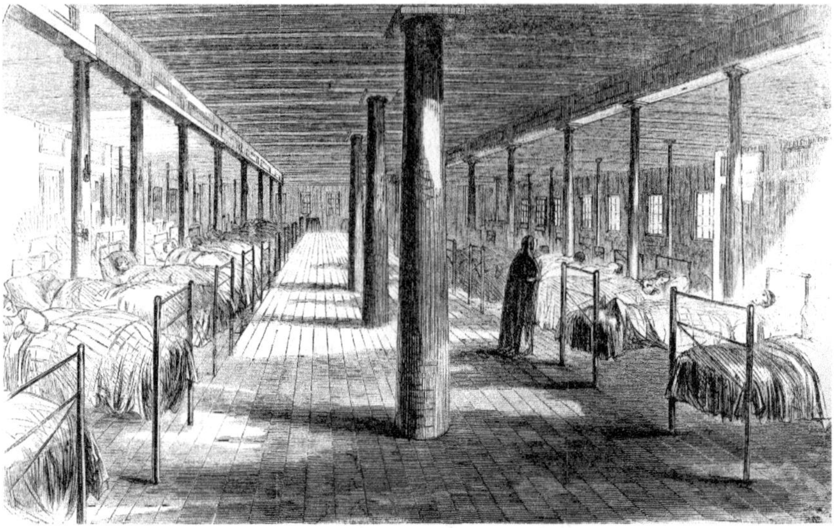

Interior of hospital ship *Red Rover.* The standing figure is a member of the Sisters of the Holy Cross, who provided nursing services for the vessel (*Harper's Weekly,* May 9, 1863).

by Fitch's carpenters. The vessel, known as hospital barge *Fitch,* admitted 58 patients in 1864 and 179 in 1865.[28]

One response to the lack of shore-based hospitals near areas patrolled by naval vessels was the employment of makeshift hospital ships that were typically crowded, uncomfortable, and busy with other tasks. *Red Rover,* which operated on the Mississippi River, was notable exception.

Chapter 13

Temporary Hospital Accommodations

After the USN lost control of the Pensacola and Norfolk Naval Hospitals during the first four months of 1861, it became apparent that the Boston, New York, and Philadelphia Naval Hospitals were, by themselves, insufficient for the service's rapidly growing needs. Not only did those facilities lack the space to provide for all of the seriously sick and wounded, they were not all located conveniently for blockading squadrons that patrolled the Atlantic and Gulf coasts and for the vessels on the Mississippi River and its tributaries.

Hospital ships provided some relief but could not compare with shore hospitals in having enough supplies, equipment, and personnel to provide high-quality care and comfort. Strategies for addressing the problem included constructing temporary buildings on the grounds of existing hospitals or at new locations. The navy also turned to other government agencies for assistance. Thus, naval patients were accepted at some army hospitals, at some marine hospitals—which were established to care for sick and injured civilian seamen (not for U.S. Marines) and were operated by the Treasury Department—and at the Government Hospital for the Insane in the District of Columbia, operated by the Interior Department.

Portland, Maine

In spring 1862, BUMED chief Whelan mentioned the possibility of admitting patients to the marine hospital at Portland, Maine. The building had an estimated capacity for 100–150 USN patients and was evidently available if desired. Whelan recommended paying whatever the Treasury Department saw fit to charge, up to that hospital's cost of $2.50 to $3.00 per patient per week, and noted that BUMED would have to provide its own medical attendance for naval patients. Whelan thought that the only drawback to using the marine hospital was its remoteness "from the usual sphere of our naval vessels." It appears that the Navy Department decided against using the Portland facility.[1]

Chelsea, Massachusetts

Overcrowding at the Boston Naval Hospital in Chelsea, Massachusetts, caused Whelan to suggest in March 1862 sending naval patients to the Boston Marine Hospital, also in Chelsea, a few hundred yards away from the naval hospital. The naval hospital had room for only 65–70 patients, whereas an additional 125–150 could be accommodated at the marine hospital, whose administrators were willing to help. Whelan proposed paying about 40¢ per patient per day, which was in line with the cost of patient support at the naval hospital.[2]

The marine hospital reportedly received patients directly from naval vessels, by transfer from the Boston Naval Hospital, and from the sick quarters at the Portsmouth, New Hampshire, Navy Yard. From June 1862 through April 1865, 648 naval and Marine Corps patients were admitted to the Boston Marine Hospital. Whelan reported that at one time in 1864 the marine hospital was treating 100 naval patients. An addition to the naval hospital, ready for occupancy in June 1865, removed the necessity for further naval use of the marine hospital.[3]

District of Columbia

During summer 1861, Whelan received permission to hospitalize sick and wounded naval patients in a section of the Government Hospital for the Insane in the District of Columbia, across the Anacostia River from Washington City. At first, the accommodations, which were separate from those for army and naval patients with mental illness, amounted to about 50 beds. A cottage on the hospital grounds was later made available to the navy as a quarantine hospital. The total number of beds at both sites for naval use was about 70. Whelan consistently pointed out that use of the facilities was granted through the courtesy of the Interior Department and was a great inconvenience to the facility.[4]

The preparation and charge of the so-called "general and quarantine naval hospitals" at the Government Hospital for the Insane were assigned to Surgeon Ninian Pinkney in June 1861. Pinkney served there through most of 1862 and was succeeded by Surgeon Francis M. Gunnell, whose assignment there lasted through most of 1865. Admissions numbered 215 in 1862, 317 in 1863, 367 in 1864, and 310 in 1865. The average patient census is unknown, but Gunnell reported 39 patients being present during one day in late 1863.[5]

In late 1863, Whelan requested an appropriation of $25,000 for the building of a naval hospital in Washington City. Not only did he wish to stop imposing on the Government Hospital for the Insane, the growing importance of Washington as a naval center necessitated a new facility. Congress approved the funds, but preparations for building did not begin until after BUMED assumed responsibility (from the Bureau of Yards and Docks) for the project in mid–1864. The property for the hospital, bounded by Pennsylvania Avenue SE and E Street SE on the north and south, and by Ninth and Tenth streets SE on the west and east, was already owned by the government. Architect Ammi B. Young was appointed to oversee the construction.[6]

Various unavoidable delays and substantial increases in the cost of labor and materials delayed the completion of the hospital and necessitated additional appropriations. The new facility opened on October 1, 1866, and was reported to have a capacity of 100 patients.[7]

Norfolk, Virginia

After the Norfolk Naval Hospital, near Gosport, was reclaimed by Union forces in May 1862, the building was initially occupied by the army for hospitalization of its sick and wounded. Over the next few months, army and navy officials discussed the return of the hospital to the navy, but while the transition was being arranged, a temporary naval shore hospital was needed. In late June 1862, Flag Officer Louis M. Goldsborough of the NABS obtained permission from Secretary Welles to occupy a building near Fort Norfolk for use as a temporary hospital. The fort was on the outskirts of the town of Norfolk and less than a mile away and across the Elizabeth River from the permanent Norfolk Naval Hospital.[8]

The building used for the temporary hospital was a plain, two-story, brick structure that had been used as a machine shop before the war. It had been occupied by Confederate forces, who removed the machinery, and then by Union troops as a barracks. When the medical department took possession, the structure's windows had been destroyed and most of the walls were unplastered. Part of the ground floor had been used as a stable and was "littered with an accumulation of manure," and the upper floor was "a mass of varied filth." Under the direction of Fleet Surgeon William Maxwell Wood, substantial repairs and improvements were made. Wood reported the building's capacity as 75 patients comfortably, or 100 by crowding.[9]

Assistant Surgeon James H. Macomber, formerly of USS *Brandywine,* was assigned charge of the temporary hospital, which began receiving patients from hospital ship *Ben Morgan* on or about June 21, 1862. Surgeon Solomon Sharp was at the Norfolk Naval Station by that date and was later assigned as surgeon of the station, but because no decision had been made about what exactly constituted the station, Sharp's responsibility for the temporary hospital was nebulous. Although it is unclear how many patients the temporary hospital was able to accommodate, Goldsborough and Wood believed that it could be made comfortable "for all patients likely to require hospital treatment" with the resources on hand, which included medical personnel formerly serving on *Ben Morgan.*[10]

A previous tenant, who represented the building's owner and was charged with its safety, claimed rent of $1,000 per month, but once he realized the extent of improvement and the fact that the government's occupation of the building had protected it, he no longer saw fit to demand rent. When the navy vacated the building around the end of August 1862, army authorities quickly took possession for use as quarters for runaway slaves.[11]

North Carolina

The hospitals in North Carolina that served the NABS were of at least two sorts: those controlled by the army, to which naval patients could be admitted, and temporary facilities set up by the navy. Use of a marine hospital was considered, but the extent to which it admitted naval patients in unknown. The burden of North Carolina hospitals was eased somewhat by the availability of the permanent Norfolk Naval Hospital, which transitioned from army to navy control during the summer of 1862.

In late September or early October 1862, Fleet Surgeon William Maxwell Wood arranged with army officials to have the army's Hammond General Hospital at Beaufort, North Carolina, admit patients from the portion of the NABS that was blockading Wilmington. The hospital, occupying a building formerly used as a hotel, was about two hours by rail from New Bern, could accommodate about 200 patients, and was staffed by "a corps of Sisters of Mercy." Whelan approved of the agreement and informed Wood that if no understanding had already been reached about compensation, the navy would pay 35¢ per day per patient, the same rate paid at Norfolk Naval Hospital while the army controlled that facility. Notwithstanding the availability of beds at Hammond General Hospital, Wood considered whatever hospital vessel was anchored at Beaufort—USS *Louisiana* during his tenure as fleet surgeon of the NABS—to be that city's naval hospital.[12]

Wood made a similar agreement for the acceptance of naval patients at the Treasury Department's marine hospital on Ocracoke Island (a barrier island) at Ocracoke Inlet. The army occupied the hospital, which had a capacity of about 90 beds and was 8–10 hours by ship from New Bern. The Ocracoke hospital—sometimes called the Portsmouth hospital because of its proximity to the island and town of Portsmouth, North Carolina—was across Ocracoke Inlet from Ocracoke Island, and Wood thought it and would be suitable for men who had suffered from malarious conditions while serving on North Carolina's rivers. (*Portsmouth* could also apply to naval facilities near Norfolk, Virginia, and near Portsmouth, New Hampshire.) How many naval patients were treated at the Ocracoke hospital is unknown.[13]

Wood reported that the vessels patrolling the sounds of North Carolina—the waters between the barrier islands and the mainland—and the associated rivers were "totally unfitted for the accommodation and treatment of diseases even of a few days duration." He thus approved of medical officers, who were already assigned to vessels, establishing temporary hospitals in convenient buildings on shore, where patients could be more conveniently treated without expending more medical manpower or supplies. Temporary hospitals included those at Washington (on the Pamlico River), Plymouth (on the Roanoke River), and New Bern (at the confluence of the Neuse and Trent rivers). Little has been recorded about the hospital at Washington, although it appears to have been admirably managed by the navy's Assistant Surgeon Michael Bradley.[14]

The Plymouth hospital—established by late August 1862 "in the best house in town"—was, according to Wood, originally intended for the joint use of the army and navy. It was managed by USN Acting Assistant Surgeon George R. Mann, who became ill and was replaced temporarily in September 1862 by Acting Assistant Surgeon George W. Gale. Because he was the only medical officer in the area, Gale reported that month that he was attending to both army and naval patients and was prescribing for 120 sick men. He described Plymouth as "a very unhealthy place for a hospital." The following month, Wood reported that the army had taken charge of the Plymouth hospital but was accommodating naval patients. By July 1863, the army had ceased using the hospital and left it for the sole use of the navy.[15]

The unhealthy environs of Plymouth entered into Wood's opinion about where to establish a single hospital—if such was the desire of the Navy Department—that would care for the personnel of all vessels in the sounds and associated rivers. In October 1862, he specifically recommended against having that hospital at New Bern for two reasons: first, its distance from Plymouth (about 240 miles), where the amount of illness was the greatest, and second, the likelihood of stormy weather further prolonging the transport of patients from Plymouth. If a single hospital were deemed appropriate for the sounds, Wood recommended placing it at Edenton, on Albemarle Sound, about 20 miles from Plymouth as the crow flies.[16]

Although New Bern was not, at the time, chosen as a site for the sole hospital serving the sounds, a small temporary naval facility was in operation there by mid–October 1862. Wood visited that hospital in July 1863 and found it "in great neglect and confusion, more however from the want of experience of the medical and other officers than from an intentional disregard for duty." The wards were filthy, the cellar was full of rubbish, and the grounds were overgrown with rank weeds. Wood took numerous steps to improve matters and suggested that a medical officer of the regular navy be assigned to take charge. Acting Assistant Surgeon George W. Wilson had been in charge but was away on other duty and had temporarily been replaced by Acting Assistant Surgeon Loren R. Boyce. According to Surgeon John L. Fox, who followed Wood as fleet surgeon of the NABS, the temporary naval hospital at New Bern was never intended to accommodate the sick of more than one or two vessels.[17]

In August 1863, after learning that the naval force in the sounds would be reduced, Wood closed the Washington and Plymouth hospitals and directed that sick and wounded men in the sounds be sent to the temporary naval hospital at New Bern. A year later, Fox proposed notifying medical officers in the sounds that the naval New Bern facility was intended for men with acute rather than chronic ailments and should not contain more than 12 patients. Men with chronic conditions requiring hospitalization or who were subject to discharge, suggested Fox, should be sent to a northern naval hospital, to the army's Hammond General Hospital at Beaufort, or—pending arrangements with the army's regional medical director—to the army hospital at New Bern. Use of an army hospital was to be a temporary measure until transfer to a northern naval hospital was possible. Without such restrictions on admissions to the navy's New Bern hospital, the medical officer there would have been overtaxed. Acting Assistant Surgeon Lucian H. Kendall, in charge of the hospital in March 1864, was also responsible for treating his own vessel's men plus patients from the navy yard, government schooners, and two other squadron vessels that lacked a medical officer.[18]

During the fall of 1864, the appearance of yellow fever at New Bern prompted the closure of the naval hospital there and the transfer of its patients to army hospitals at New Bern or Beaufort, North Carolina. Assistant Surgeon Herman P. Babcock of USS *Agawam* reported in March 1865 that he had visited the army's Foster Hospital at New Bern, at which some naval patients were present, but was hesitant to ask permission to continue admitting naval patients there because its space was needed for sick and wounded soldiers. He repeated the familiar complaint that most of the hospitalized naval patients "had disqualifying diseases on entering the service & should not have been shipped." A naval hospital for the sounds was needed, but the former temporary naval facility at New Bern was unfit for the purpose, and Babcock thought Roanoke Island would be a more suitable location. No naval vessels were available to transport patients to the Norfolk Naval Hospital, and the Dismal Swamp Canal was not an option for moving patients to Norfolk. Using the canal, which connected Albemarle Sound and the Chesapeake Bay, required two changes of boats—which, in any case, did not have suitable accommodations—and entailed constant delays. The only transports outside the sounds belonged to the army and went directly to New York. *Agawam*'s captain, Commander A.C. Rhind, thought that using the marine-hospital building on Ocracoke Island might be an option. How the situation was resolved is unclear.[19]

BUMED annual reports show 128 and 122 patients being admitted to the naval New Bern hospital in 1863 and 1864, respectively.[20]

Port Royal, South Carolina

In October 1863, Rear Admiral John A. Dahlgren, flag officer of the SABS, ordered Fleet Surgeon William Johnson to determine whether hospital accommodations could be found ashore in the vicinity of Port Royal for naval officers. The hospital ship *Vermont*, anchored at Port Royal, seemed unfit for sick officers, and Dahlgren believed that sending them north often removed them for a longer time than seemed necessary and had an "injurious effect upon the morale of the squadron." Johnson found that all suitable buildings at Beaufort, South Carolina, were already occupied by the Federal army, but he received an offer to have naval officers admitted to a Beaufort hospital established for army officers. Patients there paid 75¢ a day "for their board and enjoyment of the luxuries & delicacies so highly prized by the sick, that are obtained from the hospital fund and the Sanitary Commission." (In the army, the hospital fund was the cash value of rations that patients would ordinarily be entitled to but were presumably not using while hospitalized. That value was credited to the hospital and often used to purchase comfort items.) Should the army's offer be accepted, naval patients would be expected to pay the same daily charge.[21]

Johnson reported his findings to Dahlgren, suggested accepting the army's offer, and expressed his belief that the current system of sending sick enlisted men to a hospital ship would suffice for the time being. Johnson also suggested having sick officers subjected to medical surveys to determine whether they were candidates for short-term hospitalization—in which case the army hospital in Beaufort could be used—or needed more extended care and should be sent north. Dahlgren agreed, subject to the approval of BUMED. Johnson then asked Whelan for approval and a decision about what portion, if any, of the per diem payment would be assumed by BUMED. Whelan's response has not been found, but a similar arrangement was already in operation at New Bern, North Carolina.[22]

In August 1864, Dahlgren described the hospital ships at Port Royal as "the only legitimate [naval] establishments, provided for the reception of officers and men" of the SABS. Officers, he reported, were permitted to be hospitalized at Beaufort upon application, presumably at the aforementioned army hospital, and to be treated there by a naval medical officer; Dahlgren characterized treatment at Beaufort as "an indulgence."[23]

Despite Surgeon Johnson's view that hospital ships at Port Royal were adequate for the SABS's enlisted men, the Navy Department ordered in January 1864 that a site near Port Royal be selected for a hospital "for the sick, and wounded of the naval forces employed at that station." The new hospital was evidently intended to accommodate both officers and men and thus make it unnecessary to send any naval personnel to the army hospital at Beaufort. Whelan estimated that about 200 patients would be hospitalized at a new hospital per quarter, a number that was unlikely to decrease in the near future. Johnson, with Assistant Surgeons Adoniram B. Judson and Josiah H. Culver, carefully examined sites in the area and recommended the "lower portion of St. Helena Island, or Land's End, as the most favorable site, combining beauty of position, healthfulness, elevation, good supply of water, ready accessibility of shade trees, &c."[24]

Obtaining the land required the cooperation of tax commissioners of the Treasury Department because property in that area, having been forfeited to the United States in response to nonpayment of direct taxes, was subject to sale. President Lincoln subsequently had certain property reserved for "war, military, naval, revenue, and police purposes," including the land that Johnson had identified.[25]

Surgeon Johnson also submitted a plan for the hospital and believed that structures could be erected on the spot. The shortage of skilled workmen and the perceived difficulty in obtaining building materials, however, prompted him to recommended engaging a northern firm to prepare the building, transport it to the site, and put it up. Whelan thus hired George H. Davies of East Cambridge, Massachusetts, to proceed to Port Royal with men and materials to start construction at the Saint Helena site. After their arrival, work was delayed in mid–July 1864 because army authorities refused to grant the navy possession of the property. That complication may have necessitated a change in the hospital's location—which Whelan hoped would be "of no material consequence"—and by late August, Johnson reported that construction of the hospital on Saint Helena would probably be completed early. Whelan did not consider it important to furnish a ceiling for the officers' rooms, as the structure was already supposed to be "perfectly tight, and weather proof" and unnecessary expenses were to be avoided. He authorized Johnson's suggestion to have Dahlgren assign medical officers of the squadron for hospital duty; the alternative would have been for assignments to originate at the Navy Department.[26]

On November 4, 1864, Whelan reported the Saint Helena Island hospital as a "sufficiently modern building" that was almost ready for use, was based on plans furnished by medical officers of the SABS, and would be able to accommodate 150–175 patients. For 1864, admissions numbered 86 or 349 at the Port Royal (Saint Helena Island) hospital—different parts of the same BUMED report provided divergent numbers—and 31 at the Beaufort, South Carolina, hospital (probably the naval portion of the army hospital for officers). In 1865, 267 patients were admitted to the Port Royal hospital, with no figures reported for the hospital in Beaufort, South Carolina, which should have stopped admitting naval officers when the Port Royal hospital opened. The Port Royal hospital was closed on February 20, 1866.[27]

Key West and Egmont Key, Florida

In December 1861, the navy obtained permission from the Treasury Department to admit patients to the marine hospital at Key West.

Whelan believed the arrangement to be a good one because the naval vessels in the area—which would shortly constitute the EGBS—generally lacked appropriate accommodations for the sick. He also thought that, in the absence of an epidemic, the number of naval patients admitted would be too small to interfere with the hospital's usual care of merchant seamen. At that time, Whelan believed that a civilian physician employed by the Treasury Department was in charge of the hospital, but he learned in March 1862 that the facility was actually under command of an army medical officer. That officer, Assistant Surgeon William F. Cornick, had been at Key West since January 1861 but was about to be reassigned, so someone else—the Treasury Department preferred a civilian—was needed to take charge of the hospital.[28]

Whelan quickly recommended Acting Assistant Surgeon David T. Lewis to the Treasury Department, which offered Lewis the appointment on April 13, 1862. Whelan favored Lewis—who had entered the volunteer navy in September 1861 and was serving near Key West on USS *Ethan Allen*—because of his "long hospital experience, and habits of industry, and correct deportment." Exactly how Lewis qualified as a civilian is unclear. Whelan expected him to submit the usual paperwork associated with a naval hospital, but perhaps relieving him of the sea duty normally assigned to acting assistant surgeons effectively made him a civilian. Whelan told one correspondent that he presumed that Lewis was at liberty to resign his naval appointment. Lewis had not accepted the appointment by early June but eventually did and was admitting patients to the hospital by late July 1862.[29]

An outbreak of yellow fever starting in late July 1862 at Key West prompted Fleet Surgeon Gustavus R.B. Horner of the EGBS to recommend that hospital accommodations be prepared at Pensacola for the reception of patients with yellow fever or other malignant diseases. Confederate forces had captured the USN's Pensacola Navy Yard and nearby hospital in January 1861 and destroyed the yard and hospital when they evacuated in May 1862. (Pensacola was actually in the region for which the WGBS was responsible.) Thus, Horner realized that it would take some days to erect suitable temporary buildings. Flag Officer James L. Lardner, however, thought that housing patients with yellow fever anywhere near army troops at Pensacola was out of the question. The situation was managed by sending the affected patients north for hospital care and disinfecting their vessel at a northern station.[30]

Lewis died of yellow fever on September 3, 1862, at Key West. His hospital duties were assumed, at first, primarily by Fleet Surgeon Horner, with assistance from Assistant Surgeon William K. Van

Reypen. By early 1863, Acting Assistant Surgeon George J. Sweet began assisting Horner, and by summer 1863, Sweet appears to have assumed charge.[31]

Another outbreak of yellow fever during 1864 prompted Flag Officer Theodorus Bailey to establish coaling and hospital facilities distant from Key West, which he considered "the center of the disease." He thus ordered an officer to construct a wharf and hospital at Tampa Bay; the site chosen was Egmont Key, at the mouth of the bay. The hospital was intended to accommodate 30 patients.[32]

It is unclear how many naval patients were admitted to the Key West and Egmont Key Hospitals. Information gathered from hospital tickets indicates an average of 20 patients admitted monthly at Key West from October 1861 through May 1865, with peaks of 46 in September 1862, 37 in October 1864, and 39 in March 1865. The 1862 and 1864 peaks correspond to epidemics of yellow fever.[33]

Pensacola

The USN's Pensacola Navy Yard and surrounding buildings, including the naval hospital, were seized by Southern troops in January 1861 and set on fire on May 9, 1862, when Confederate forces abandoned the facilities. The area was quickly reoccupied by Union forces, but the total destruction of the hospital prompted questions from USN medical officers about when a hospital near Pensacola might be made available for use of the WGBS. (The navy yard and hospital were often referred to as being at Warrington, a town that adjoined the yard and was several miles from Pensacola.) In late May 1862, Whelan remarked that rebuilding the hospital was too new a topic to have received consideration, and he predicted that the uncertainty about the state of affairs around Pensacola would probably prevent any immediate restoration of the facilities in the area. By late October 1862, a temporary hospital was being built on the grounds of the navy yard—rather than on the site of the destroyed hospital, which was about a half mile west of the yard—and put in charge of Surgeon Benjamin F. Gibbs. The yard's chapel served as the nucleus of the temporary structures.[34]

In mid–1863, the temporary hospital was reported to have a capacity of 66 patients, with an average occupancy of 39 patients for February–May 1863. At that time, staffing consisted of one surgeon, two assistant surgeons, one surgeon's steward, three male nurses, one cook (a male contraband), and six attendants (one female and five male contrabands). What the workers were paid is unknown, but Whelan pointed out that the pay for male and female contrabands was not to exceed $10 and $6 per month, respectively.[35]

In June 1863, WGBS Fleet Surgeon Jonathan M. Foltz, anticipating USN attacks on Mobile and Galveston, recommended expanding the hospital's capacity by 200 beds, and the building of "large additions" appear to have started by late 1863. In March 1864, Fleet Surgeon James C. Palmer visited the hospital, took lodging in its partially completed wing, and reported his observations to Whelan. "The hospital is a mere shed," he began, "two stories high, and raised about two feet, upon brick piers." The walls were constructed of newly sawn pine, which had already shrunk enough that "daylight streams through innumerable crevices." Ventilation was defective, and the walls were too thin to prevent the interior from becoming intolerably warm during summer. Palmer identified numerous other faults but was encouraged that Flag Officer Farragut supported his suggestions for improving the facility. Palmer hoped for a creditable result, although he anticipated that a permanent hospital would be erected after the war—as was the case—on the site of the destroyed one, "whose foundations, with many indestructible materials, are ready to be brought into use." In late 1864, Whelan reported that, although much remained to be done, enough progress had been made to accommodate the invalids of the WGBS as well as casualties from the Battle of Mobile Bay.[36]

The temporary Pensacola hospital admitted 48 patients in 1862, 453 in 1863, 824 in 1864, and 738 in 1865. It was demolished in 1875, and a "medium-sized pavilion" was built on the grounds of the old naval hospital.[37]

Pilot Town and New Orleans, Louisiana

In preparation for the bombardment of Forts Jackson and Saint Philip and the eventual capture of New Orleans, Flag Officer David G. Farragut of the WGBS, took possession of the abandoned village of Pilot Town, on the Southwest Pass of the Mississippi River. There, a large building, formerly a hotel or boarding house, and at least one other nearby structure were chosen by early April 1862 to serve as a naval hospital. Farragut assigned Surgeon Philip S. Wales of USS *Colorado* to take charge. According to a newspaper correspondent, Wales began work "without a single carpenter, nurse or steward" and was expected to have the hospital ready for 150 patients.[38]

By early June 1862, after the capture of New Orleans, Wales was being helped by Assistant Surgeons Charles H. Burbank of USS *Santee*,

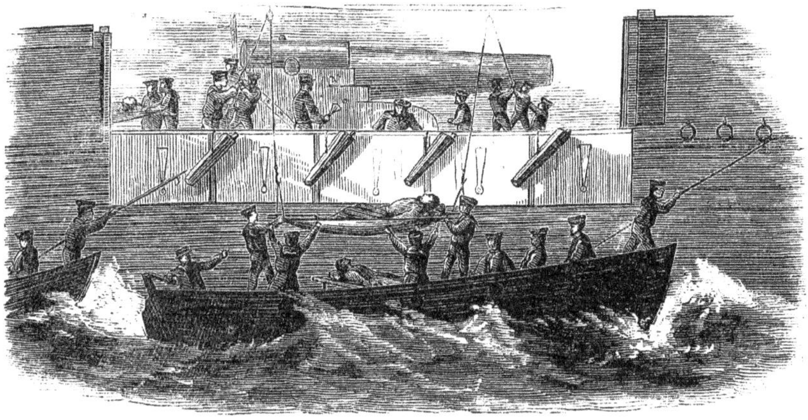

Wounded men from various vessels being transferred to USS *Metacomet* after the Battle of Mobile Bay on August 5, 1864. *Metacomet* transported about 60 men, including Confederate Flag Officer Franklin Buchanan, to the temporary USN hospital at Pensacola (*Harper's Weekly*, October 29, 1864).

John O. Burt of *Colorado*, and John J. Clark, who had recently arrived for duty with the WGBS. At that time, the hospital was reportedly treating 53 patients. On about July 20, 1862, Wales was relieved by Surgeon Charles H. Wheelwright, but Wheelwright quickly became ill and died at the Pilot Town hospital on July 30. Burbank, who then took charge, reported that the hospital was transferred to Pensacola around mid–September 1862. Burbank was probably referring to the temporary hospital being put up at about that time at the Pensacola Navy Yard. Preparations for that move began by late August 1862.[39]

The removal of the Pilot Town hospital made it necessary to provide hospital beds for WGBS personnel serving on the lower Mississippi, so in March 1863 Whelan asked Surgeon General William Hammond of the army if naval patients might be accommodated in any of the army hospitals in New Orleans. Such patients, thought Whelan, would probably not cause much inconvenience because naval supply steamers offered frequent opportunities to transport patients north; thus, army accommodations would be used primarily for wounded rather than chronically disabled sailors. Hammond granted that permission, which applied to all army hospitals in the city, but specified that the admission of naval patients would not be allowed to prevent the reception of army patients. The army also offered to carry naval patients north on transport vessels. Whelan was willing to pay for the use of army hospitals in the amount and manner deemed proper by Hammond. By mid–June

1863, Fleet Surgeon Foltz reported that the army hospitals were filling up with soldiers wounded at the siege of Port Hudson and that it would thus be necessary to establish a naval hospital in the area. Whelan again encouraged sending naval patients north.[40]

During the summer of 1863, the army transferred a "partially arranged" and "unfurnished" building in New Orleans to the navy for use as a hospital. By late August 1863, the naval hospital, under the charge of Surgeon Jacob S. Dungan, was accepting patients. The hospital, which also served as a depot for medical supplies, appears to have been at the corner of Erato and New Levee streets.[41]

In June 1865, the hospital was ordered to be closed as soon as the WGBS was reduced to its minimum level. The facility was reported to have admitted 271 patients in 1863, 809 in 1864, and 642 in 1865.[42]

Mound City and Memphis

Before October 1862, naval personnel of the Western Gunboat Flotilla needing hospitalization were sent to army hospitals at Mound City and Cairo, Illinois. The transfer of the flotilla from the army to the navy presented the necessity and opportunity for the navy to control its own medical affairs, which implied a need for a naval hospital. There were also the practical considerations of the army hospitals running out of space and hospital ship USS *Red Rover* needing repairs over the winter and not being able to keep patients aboard. In late September 1862, Fleet Surgeon Edward Gilchrist, after consulting with Surgeon E.C. Franklin, director of the army hospital at Mound City, recommended that the navy rent the Mound City Hotel and use it as a hospital. Franklin believed that the building could accommodate about 250 patients, could be had for no more than $1,500 a year in rent, and could be occupied within two days after possession was transferred to the navy. Gilchrist agreed with Franklin and relayed the recommendation through official channels, and in a short time, BUMED chief Whelan approved rental of the hotel at $75 a month.[43]

Surgeon William Grier was assigned in late October to take charge of the hospital, and at about that time, the hospital began admitting men from squadron vessels and from the army's Mound City hospital, which had accommodated naval patients. In mid–December 1862, Grier reported having 203 patients and a number of civilian employees originally hired by Fleet Surgeon Gilchrist or by his authority. Those workers included a hospital steward, a matron, four nurses, a laundress, and nine African Americans—three washerwomen and six laborers. Other staff included two cooks and a master-at-arms from the squadron's receiving ship at Cairo and an apothecary from *Red Rover,* which was undergoing repairs. Finally, several convalescents were working at the hospital as nurses or kitchen assistants.[44]

Whelan thought the workers' wages were too high and instructed Grier to pay no more than what the navy was paying elsewhere. However, Whelan understood that the army was paying much less and directed Grier to try to hire help at army rates, especially if, as Whelan had heard, "no difficulty is experienced in procuring attendants for the army hospital contiguous to yours."[45]

In hopes of establishing a hospital that was more conveniently located (farther south) than the facility at Mound City, Surgeon Grier inquired in Memphis about buildings that might be used. He reported in February 1863 that the army was reluctant to give the navy possession of the only structure, the Gayoso Hotel, that might suffice. Surgeon Pinkney, who had become the Mississippi Squadron's fleet surgeon in December 1862, then visited with Major General Ulysses S. Grant, Commanding the Department of Tennessee. In early March 1863, Grant ordered the Commercial Hotel in Memphis to be vacated and turned over to the navy for hospital use—this under the assumption that it was owned by disloyal persons and thus liable to confiscation. Pinkney occupied the building, but Joseph J. Andrews, a "highly respectable gentleman of New York," successfully proved his loyalty and exclusive ownership of the hotel and claimed rent of $1,500 per month. Whelan recommended that a board—which eventually consisted of Flag Officer David D. Porter and Pinkney—determine a fair rent, and about a year after Andrews first claimed ownership of the hotel, an annual rent of $3,000 was established.[46]

The Mound City Naval Hospital was abandoned in March 1863, and Surgeon Grier took command of the Memphis Naval Hospital, also known as Pinkney Hospital, in May 1863. In October 1863, Acting Assistant Surgeon Hiram Beauchamp, assigned to the hospital, reported having 257 patients. Other medical officers serving there included Surgeon Henry F. McSherry and Assistant Surgeon Gustavus H.E. Baumgarten. According to one report, the Memphis hospital admitted 1,650 patients in 1863 and 852 during the first seven months of 1864.[47]

Pinkney, shortly after occupying the Commercial Hotel building, described it as capable of accommodating 550 patients comfortably and in generally good condition. It did, though, have an older section that was "considerably out of order" and needed a "good deal of repair." In December 1863, Surgeon Grier reported that he had occupied a building in the Memphis Navy Yard to accommodate African American patients.

"The mortality among this class of patients has been hitherto, proportionately, much greater than among the white patients," wrote Grier, "owing, without doubt, in some degree, to the limited and badly ventilated quarters necessarily assigned to them." (Grier may have been referring to the older portion of the hotel that needed repair.) The navy-yard building, about a half mile from the main naval hospital, had 62 beds and offered "very comfortable and well ventilated accommodation to that number of patients." Grier acknowledged that operating two facilities would incur some additional trouble and expense but that "the increased comfort and well being of the inmates will more than compensate these disadvantages."[48]

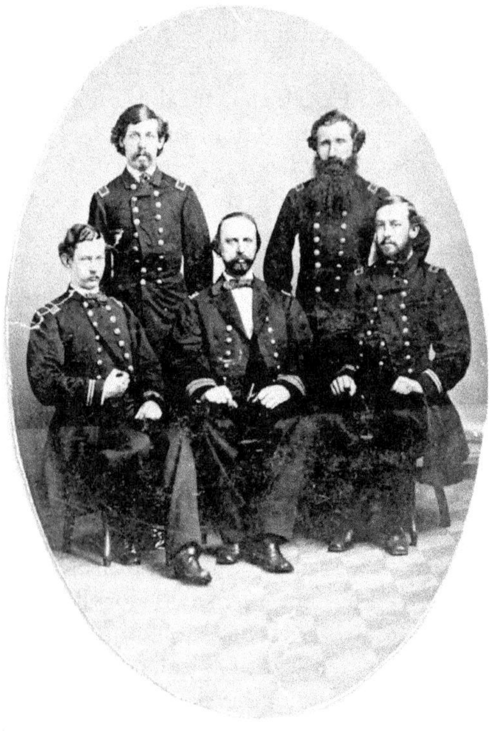

Officers associated with the temporary naval hospital in Memphis, also known as Pinkney Hospital. Standing, from left: Acting Assistant Surgeon Abner Thorp and Acting Assistant Paymaster Hugh Nott. Seated, from left: Assistant Surgeon Gustavus H.E. Baumgarten, Surgeon William Grier, and Acting Assistant Surgeon Joseph B. Parker (NHHC, image NH 53388).

A sampling of 300 Memphis Naval Hospital admission tickets for the third quarter of 1864 shows that about 16 percent were for patients identified as Negro, colored, or contraband, with almost all of them listed as members of ships' crews. This figure contrasts with the finding of one researcher that African Americans constituted 34 percent of enlisted men in the Mississippi Squadron. Much of the disparity is probably attributable to patients' race not being required, and usually not included, on tickets; medical officers rarely, if ever, noted that a patient was white. In any event, African Americans accounted for a substantial proportion of the Mississippi Squadron's hospitalized patients.[49]

Sufficient documentation has not been found

to establish that sickbays and shore hospitals were generally segregated. In July 1863, Flag Officer David D. Porter of the Mississippi Squadron encouraged the recruitment of contrabands because of the great frequency of sickness in the navy and the supposed ability of African Americans to better tolerate exposure to the Southern sun. Black sailors, ordered Porter, "can be exercised separately at great guns and small arms" and "in all cases they must be kept distinct from the rest of the crew." On one gunboat of the Mississippi Squadron, black sailors messed separately from white crewmembers and had their own mess cook. Surgeon Grier's statement that his African American patients had *necessarily be*en placed apart suggests that segregation was routine in naval hospitals.[50]

BUMED reported the Memphis hospital admitting 1,146 patients in 1864 and 594 in 1865. Orders were given to close the facility on August 1, 1865, and to inform the owner that he could resume its possession on the same day.[51]

Mare Island, California

The San Francisco Navy Yard, which served the Pacific Squadron, was located on Mare Island, about 23 miles from the city of San Francisco. At the beginning of the war, the receiving ship USS *Independence* provided the yard's only accommodations for the sick. There was general agreement that a hospital was needed on shore, and in 1863, Congress appropriated $25,000 to begin its construction.[52]

Various factors contributed to delays in beginning construction of a permanent hospital. The projected cost turned out to be much higher than first thought, and Whelan was apprehensive about whether the facility would be appropriately located and designed. Responsibility for construction, repair, and improvement of hospitals was to be transferred from the Bureau of Yards and Docks to BUMED on July 1, 1864. Whelan was quick to point out that naval officers and civil engineers, under the supervision of the Bureau of Yards and Docks, had built naval hospitals that cost a great deal but did not "present all the peculiar features which should characterize such institutions." Building proper hospitals, he wrote, was a specialty that considered problems that could only be "duly appreciated by minds familiar with the cause of disease, and the many, other than mere professional, means essential to cure, or preservation of health." Until BUMED had control of establishing a permanent hospital, Whelan seemed to favor other means of providing hospital facilities, such as erecting a frame building on *Independence* or sending patients to the marine hospital in San Francisco.[53]

The station's commandant and its medical officer, Captain Thomas O. Selfridge and Passed Assistant Surgeon William S. Bishop, feared that a permanent hospital would be a long time coming, so Selfridge ordered that an existing yard building, formerly a granary, be modified into a temporary hospital. That structure, with a capacity of 20–30 patients, was ready for occupancy by January 1864. In late 1865, BUMED chief Horwitz reported that the temporary hospital was sufficient for current needs and that plans for building a permanent facility had been suspended.[54]

The provision of temporary hospital facilities required BUMED to take advantage of assistance from multiple sources, including the Treasury and Interior Departments and the army. When existing buildings could not be occupied as hospitals, various obstacles sometimes delayed BUMED's attempt to build its own.

Chapter 14

Preexisting Hospitals and Sick Quarters

At the start of 1861, the USN had five hospitals: at (or near) Boston, New York, Philadelphia, Norfolk, and Pensacola. BUMED assigned medical officers to those hospitals and administered them, and the facilities did not organizationally belong to any particular naval squadron. The operation of hospitals was supported through the hospital fund, which consisted of mandatory monthly deductions of 20¢ from the salaries of all naval personnel, the transfer of pensions surrendered by patients residing in the Naval Asylum in Philadelphia, and the cost price of rations that were not being received by patients who were cared for and fed in naval hospitals.[1]

The January 1861 seizure and the May 1862 burning of the Pensacola Navy Yard and Naval Hospital meant that the permanent hospital building there was never used by the Union during the war. After Federal forces reoccupied the yard and its surroundings, a temporary hospital was erected on the grounds of the yard and served the needs of the WGBS. A replacement permanent hospital was rebuilt on the old site, outside of the yard, during the postwar years. Because establishment of the Boston, New York, Philadelphia, and Norfolk Naval hospitals predated the war, wartime developments involving those facilities, rather than their prewar histories, are emphasized here.

The navy also had sick quarters on the grounds of navy yards. A yard's surgeon was primarily responsible for issuing and accounting for medical supplies for naval vessels using the yard. He also used the sick quarters to provide medical care to sick or injured personnel and would presumably send patients who needed more intensive or prolonged care to a nearby naval hospital, which had its own medical staff. Before 1861, sick quarters were associated with yards in the vicinity of Portsmouth (New Hampshire), Boston, New York City, Philadelphia, Washington (DC), Norfolk, and Pensacola. Grouped with these yards, for statistical purposes, were medical facilities at the National Observatory in Washington (DC) and the Naval Academy.

Of the four categories used by BUMED in compiling sick reports—hospitals, navy yards, receiving ships, and squadrons or vessels at sea—hospitals tended to have the sickest patients, largely because they received many patients who could not get appropriate care elsewhere. This factor, the relatively high cost of hospital care, and the fact that hospitals reduced the medical burden of yards, receiving ships, and ships at sea help explain why BUMED paid considerable attention to increasing the number of hospital beds.

BUMED chief Whelan consistently urged medical officers to employ strategies to reduce the number of patients sent to hospitals. Patients with chronic ailments that clearly did not result from naval service should be discharged from the navy. Those with chronic disease unlikely to be cured, even if associated with naval service, should be discharged from the service and considered for a pension. Patients on receiving ships who were not seriously ill, so-called "walking cases," should be retained on shipboard. Nevertheless, hospitals continued to receive patients in those categories, perhaps because harried medical officers simply found it easier to transfer patients to hospitals than to initiate those other processes.

Boston

At the beginning of the war, the Boston Naval Hospital—located at Chelsea, Massachusetts, and often called by that city's name—could comfortably accommodate about 60 patients. In mid–1862, Congress appropriated funds for an extension of and repairs to the hospital, which were originally projected to be complete in late 1863 or early 1864 and have room for at least 200 patients. That prediction was too optimistic, for the extension—complete with "the most improved heating culinary and laundry works"—was not ready for occupancy until June 1865. Also added to the hospital grounds was a building, constructed by George H. Davies, for patients with smallpox. Before and during construction of the extension, patients who could not be accommodated at the naval hospital were accepted at the Boston Marine Hospital in Chelsea, which had room for 125–150 naval patients.[2]

The naval hospital was under the charge of Surgeon John L. Fox from April 1861 to July 1863. Fox was succeeded by Surgeon Joseph Beale, who served until July 1865. About 20 other medical officers served there during the war, with many assignments lasting only a few weeks. The

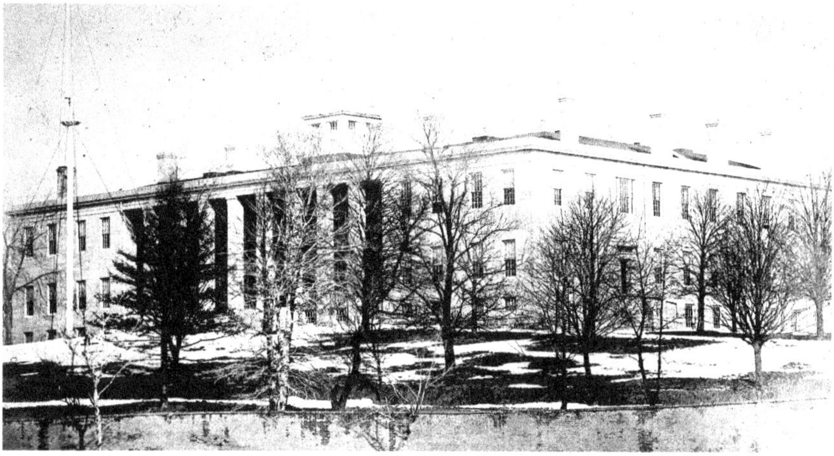

The New York Naval Hospital in Brooklyn, photographed in 1876 (NARA, identifier 71-NYA-1A-9).

hospital admitted 267 patients in 1861, 756 in 1862, 658 in 1863, 812 in 1864, and 546 in 1865.[3]

New York

In December 1861, Whelan advised Secretary Welles of the urgent need to expand the capacity of the New York Naval Hospital, located in Brooklyn. At the time, the hospital could suitably accommodate no more than 150 patients but contained 50 more than that. Captain Hiram Paulding, commandant of the New York Navy Yard, appointed a board of officers to examine local facilities that might house patients and recommended the yard's new Marine barracks, a portion of which received hospital patients by early 1862 and was attended by the medical officers who served in the permanent hospital.[4]

One proposal for providing additional room was to fit out USS *Savannah* as a stationary hospital ship, but the cost of doing so, dredging a channel to allow the vessel to be moved to a convenient site, and repairing the hospital wharf was far more than that of constructing a temporary building. In August 1862, Whelan reported that the Brooklyn hospital and "such other quarters as provided" nearby contained 277 patients. In late November 1862, Whelan contracted with George H. Davies to build a temporary structure on the hospital grounds with a capacity of 270 patients, to be completed within 40 days. Whelan reported in October 1863 that the addition had been promptly completed and furnished "excellent accommodations" for 200 patients. About a year later, Whelan wrote that accommodations at Brooklyn were "sufficient, though not more than sufficient," and that the average patient census was 262.[5]

The medical officer with the longest wartime tenure at the New York Naval Hospital was Surgeon Thomas L. Smith, who served from January 1862 to December 1865. About 50 different medical officers—mostly assistant surgeons assigned for a few weeks or months at a time—served at the hospital during the war. Admissions numbered 935 in 1861, 1,602 in 1862, 2,068 in 1863, 1,839 in 1864, and 1,853 in 1865.[6]

Philadelphia

BUMED's facility in Philadelphia consisted of a combined naval hospital and an asylum or home for disabled men of the navy and Marine Corps. In mid–1863, the residents of the asylum numbered about 125, while there were about 130 hospital patients, some of whom occupied the building's passages and corridors. Some of the room taken by hospital patients may have become available after Whelan recommended appropriating some of the asylum's nonessential space, which included four "smoking rooms" for asylum residents and rooms allotted to asylum officers—four assigned to the lieutenant, three assigned to but unoccupied rooms by the commander, three assigned to the chaplain, and another three assigned to the assistant surgeon. Whelan asked for and, in March 1864, received a $75,000 appropriation to build an extension to the structure. He quickly realized that the amount was much too small and postponed the start of construction "rather than have the grounds defaced and disfigured" when there was no certainty of work being completed in a reasonable time. Construction of the hospital improvements did not start until June 1866.[7]

The medical officers with the longest wartime postings to the hospital were Surgeons William Johnson (May 1861 to August 1863) and David Harlan (August 1863 to May 1865). About 20 other medical officers served, usually for short periods, at the facility during the war. The hospital admitted 210 patients in 1861, 616 in 1862, 938 in 1863, 746 in 1864, and 697 in 1865.[8]

Norfolk

The Norfolk Naval Hospital—sometimes referred to by other place names, such as Gosport or Portsmouth—and the neighboring navy yard were abandoned by Union forces in April 1861. Confederate forces used the facilities until abandoning them in early May 1862.

The hospital was quickly reclaimed by medical officers of the Union army, who used it for their sick and wounded but also accommodated some USN patients. A USN surgeon, who spoke with an army medical officer shortly after the hospital's repossession and saw part of the facility himself, described it: "Destitute of every thing except for a few bedsteads, the privy pipes from the water closets throughout the house are choked, and every part of the building except what we have cleaned is filled with filth and vermin."[9]

The hospital was filled with army patients throughout most of June and July 1862 as a result of heavy fighting near Richmond. Although there was agreement that the navy was rightfully entitled to resume control of the facility, the army had great need for it, and the navy was reluctant to insist on occupying it. In mid–June 1862, NABS Fleet Surgeon William Maxwell Wood reported the hospital "crowded to discomfort, with army patients," with more expected from the current battles. NABS Flag Officer Louis M. Goldsborough wrote that Wood, "does not feel himself warranted by any instructions he has, so far, received, to use [the hospital] to the disturbance of the army patients." Wood understood the situation but nevertheless urged taking control of the hospital: "The army has other resources, and we have not."[10]

Discussions took place between army and navy officials at Norfolk and Washington, D.C., through most of the summer. In late July, Whelan described Surgeon General Hammond of the army as ready to order "the removal of all the army patients, now in the building, if I would be so regardless of the greater necessities of the army, as to make such an untimely demand." A few days later, when some space became available, Whelan urged Wood to claim it: "If we can secure accommodation for seventy five sick at this time, it is important that such an opportunity of initiating our possession of our own property should not be neglected. We can never expect to obtain possession of the premises unless we avail ourselves of an occasion, when the army inmates are reduced in number."[11]

In early August 1862, Whelan took a firmer step toward obtaining the hospital by asking Hammond to order his medical officers stationed at the facility "to make such arrangements as will tend to the reception of a greater number of sick from the navy." Those naval patients came from vessels on the James River and at Hampton Roads and from elements of a mortar flotilla, recently arrived at Hampton Roads after service on the Mississippi. Patients from the mortar flotilla numbered 103 men who had been "confined on board small vessels of the most wretched description." Whelan reminded Hammond that he (Whelan) had, in the past, "foreborne to ask for more than a limited portion of the building" and asked the surgeon general to "excuse the request so unwillingly preferred." The army appears to have vacated the hospital around the end of August 1862.[12]

Surgeon Solomon Sharp was in charge of the hospital from September 1862 to October 1864 and was succeeded by Surgeon Andrew A. Henderson, who served there until mid–July 1867. About 16 other medical officers were assigned to the hospital during the war. In September 1862, Wood informed Whelan that the hospital would need a matron; a house steward; an apothecary steward; a dispensary boy; two white nurses and two African American laborers to each ward; one gardener and four African American laborers for the garden and grounds; one carpenter; one gatekeeper; four boatmen; eight washerwomen; and two cooks. Much of the labor was available locally, including African Americans, who could be had for a food ration and enough money to supply necessary clothing. Whelan advised Sharp to base his labor needs on a minimum of 200 patients.[13]

The hospital admitted 516 patients in 1862, 991 in 1863, 1,920 in 1863, and 1,087 in 1865. A structure for patients with smallpox was built on the hospital grounds by George H. Davies around spring 1864.[14]

Sick Quarters at the Portsmouth, New Hampshire, Navy Yard

The only navy-yard sick quarters to earn substantial attention from Whelan was the facility associated with the Portsmouth, New Hampshire, Navy Yard. Sick quarters there consisted of an old "inconvenient frame-house" that was much in need of repair, was "not creditable to the Government," did little more than offer "a cover for the sick," and was unable to accommodate a large number of patients. (The yard occupied an island in the Piscataqua River, within the boundaries of Maine. Although the closest town was Kittery, Maine, the yard was named for the city of Portsmouth, which was across the Piscataqua from Kittery.) The sick quarters, although sometimes called a hospital, did not qualify as a hospital per se, but Whelan proposed that a modest hospital be built—he thought simply replacing the old building would be most expedient—and asked for an appropriation in 1861 of $20,000 for that purpose. In light of the rapidly expanding naval force, erecting a hospital seemed prudent, especially since the navy's practice was to use its northernmost facility to receive vessels with epidemics, and the Portsmouth yard would fill that role. Whelan suggested that a wooden structure would suffice and could be built and put into service quickly. His efforts, though, undoubtedly caused more frustration than he anticipated.[15]

In July 1862, Congress responded to Whelan's request for funds by appropriating $14,500 for the purchase of 27 acres of land on Seavey's Island, which was next to the navy yard and accessible by a bridge, and $10,000 for construction of a hospital on the purchased property. Whelan saw no need for the land on Seavey's Island, considered $10,000 as inadequate for the building—"only sufficient to delay its completion," as he expressed it—and surmised that there was "an unfortunate commingling of public with private interests." Whelan claimed that nobody, to his knowledge, had recommended purchase of the land except its owners. Whelan knew the provisions of the appropriations legislation before it was enacted. He endeavored, unsuccessfully, to correct the situation by writing to one of the primary proponents of purchasing the property, Senator John P. Hale of New Hampshire, and a to a friend of the medical department, Senator James W. Grimes of Iowa.[16]

Various factors, including questions about gaining assent from the state of Maine, prevented the purchase of the land. In March 1864, Congress, after much debate, appropriated $25,000 for building the hospital, with no provisos concerning its location. Because of the long-standing disagreements about where the hospital should be built, Whelan, with Secretary Welles's approval, appointed a board of officers to address the question, and the panel recommended building within the navy yard's boundaries. Senator Hale and various colleagues—claiming to be insulted by Whelan's insinuations about private interests and by the board expressing an opinion contrary to their own—managed to get Congress to repeal the appropriation in July 1864. In response to that development, Whelan expressed hope that the increased capacity of other naval hospitals would make improvements at Portsmouth of less importance.[17]

In November 1865, BUMED chief Horwitz reported that during the summer of 1865, the sick-quarters building at the navy yard had been "thoroughly repaired, at a very trifling outlay" and would suffice for the navy's immediate (postwar) wants. The facility, which BUMED never had the opportunity to develop into a full-fledged hospital during the war, admitted 182 patients in 1861, 239 in 1862, 324 in 1863, 533 in 1864, and 317 in 1865. Through most of the war, the yard's medical concerns were managed by Surgeon M.G. Delaney.[18]

Naval Academy

The U.S. Naval Academy appeared regularly, as a navy yard, in BUMED's summaries of sick reports. The academy moved, for safety, from Annapolis to Newport, Rhode Island, in May 1861 and returned to Annapolis shortly after the war ended. Medical officers were responsible for caring for students and staff, but the academy never seemed to be a serious candidate to receive patients from outside the institution. While the academy was in Newport, its Annapolis buildings were used as a Union army hospital.[19]

Surgeon James C. Palmer was in charge of the Naval Academy sick quarters, usually called a hospital, from late 1860 to August 1863. He was succeeded, from August 1863 to October 1864 by Surgeon Samuel Jackson, who was followed by Surgeon R.C. Dean, who served there until late August 1866.[20]

BUMED was able to expand the capacity of its Boston and New York hospitals while claiming more space at the Philadelphia Asylum and Hospital. It reestablished control of the Norfolk Naval Hospital after prolonged negotiations with the army. Attempts to build a small hospital at the Portsmouth, New Hampshire, Navy Yard were stymied by Congress.

Chapter 15

Provisions for Disabled Naval Personnel

The navy offered a few options to assist personnel who were disabled and needed long-term care. The possibility of extended care often depended on whether the illness or injury arose as a consequence of naval duty, a fact that reinforced the importance of careful physical examination at naval rendezvous and elsewhere.

Naval Hospitals

According to Whelan, naval hospitals could retain patients until cured. Those with an uncurable condition stemming from "the performance of duty, or exposure incident thereto," were retained until a pension could be secured. Hospitals could also retain men, after the expiration of their term of service, for treatment and subsistence, although such patients would, of course, receive no salary. Unfortunately, men becoming ill after being discharged from the navy were ineligible for admission to a naval hospital, regardless of how long or recently they had served in the navy.[1]

Whelan noted the importance of determining "with some regard to the justice, and humanity of the case, how far, or to what extent, persons enjoy our hospital accommodations who have very questionable claims thereto." Hospitals should not, he said, retain patients whose disease was "the result of vicious habits" or who wished to be discharged. Also subject to discharge should be "persons manifesting chronic disease soon enough after enlistment to make it palpable that the origin was not an incident of the service." It was advisable for receiving ships to keep "walking cases" on board instead of transferring them to hospitals that were crowded with "large numbers of invalids returned from the blockading squadrons, whose hospital tickets [transfer papers] attest they are subjects of disease, not originating in the service."[2]

Having to deal with patients without legitimate claims to naval hospital services probably tested Whelan's sense of fairness and compassion. He may have taken some comfort in the fact that the government was "not altogether unmindful of those who have served it faithfully, or lost health, or limb, in its employ." Indeed, benefits could extend beyond treatment in a regular naval hospital.[3]

Naval Asylum

Long-standing legislation required the provision of a "permanent asylum for disabled or decrepid navy officers, seamen and marines" at a naval hospital. That facility turned out to be the Naval Asylum, which was erected around 1832 adjacent to the naval hospital in Passyunk Township, Philadelphia County. (In 1854, the city boundaries of Philadelphia were expanded to include all of Philadelphia County.) The completed asylum building contained space for the hospital, so the separate structure that had previously housed the hospital was demolished. Admission to the asylum, which was under the jurisdiction of the Bureau of Yards and Docks, required evidence of at least 20 years of naval service—with exceptions under extraordinary circumstances—and a naval surgeon's certification that the applicant was unable to support himself by manual labor. Applicants receiving a naval pension were required to relinquish it to be admitted.[4]

Each beneficiary of the asylum was assigned a modest room not much larger than a stateroom on a vessel. Medical attendance and three good meals a day were provided, and reading and smoking rooms were available. Monthly benefits included a clothing allowance of up to $3, a gratuity of $1 for good conduct and performance of occasional assigned duties, and one and one-half pounds of tobacco. The average occupancy of the asylum during the war was 125 beneficiaries.[5]

Captain Joseph Smith, chief of the Bureau of Yards and Docks, described in 1859 the asylum's inhabitants as mainly well-behaved. Although allowed to go into town, however, some would "go on debauches," return intoxicated, or smuggle liquor into the asylum. Many beneficiaries considered the asylum a government hotel with no obligation to do any work to support themselves or the facility. Smith believed that an alternative location, distant from the temptations of the city, would be advantageous but also suggested the possibility of giving beneficiaries a yearly stipend so they could reside elsewhere.[6]

In 1863, BUMED chief Whelan seemed to acknowledge the asylum's problems with discipline but concluded that its site had "been so

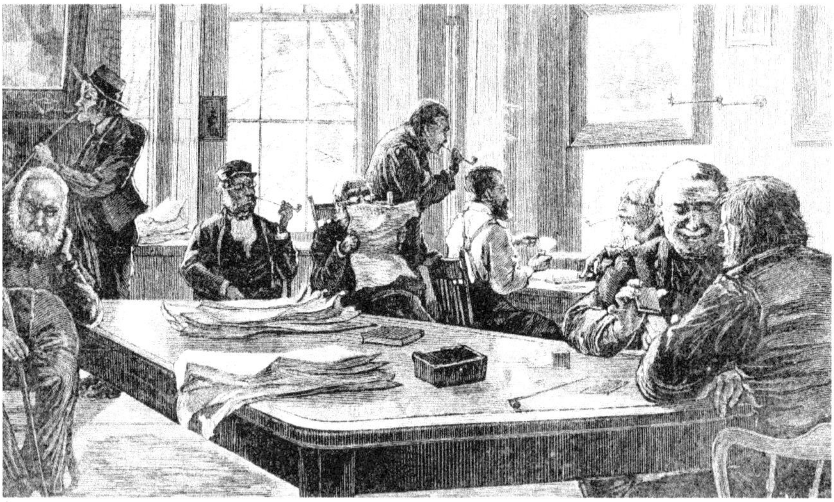

Postwar depiction of the reading room of the Philadelphia Naval Asylum. The same building also housed the naval hospital. Residents of the asylum, most of whom had served at least 20 years in the Navy, had certification of being unable to support themselves by manual labor (*Harper's Weekly*, February 23, 1878).

long occupied for the present purpose that it is too late to discuss its advantages or disadvantages." He, too, mentioned the possibility of providing a monetary allowance that could be used by beneficiaries to live elsewhere. A separate problem was that the facility was overcrowded because the war was creating large numbers of sick or injured sailors who had to be hospitalized there.[7]

Government Hospital for the Insane

In 1852, Congress furnished an appropriation for the establishment of "an asylum for the insane" in the neighborhood of Washington to care for mentally ill persons of the District of Columbia and of the army and navy. A site was selected within the District of Columbia but on the east side of the Anacostia River, outside of the city limits of Washington. The institution, under the supervision of the Department of the Interior, opened in 1855 as the Government Hospital for the Insane; that name was officially changed in 1916 to Saint Elizabeths Hospital.[8]

Naval personnel with mental illness could be admitted by order of the secretary of the navy and kept in custody until cured or removed by order of the secretary. At any time during the war, the facility contained, on average, about 17 hospitalized naval officers, naval enlisted men, or Marines, with the number increasing as the war progressed. The annual wartime number of patients arriving or leaving—because of cure, death, or desertion—averaged in the mid-teens. The hospital's board of visitors noted that the admission of naval patients rose from the beginning to the middle of the war but at a proportionately slower rate than the navy itself grew during the same interval. The board attributed that fact to the hardiness of seamen and the relatively modest change in lifestyle, compared with army recruits, experienced by civilian mariners who had joined the navy. (That explanation did not account for naval recruits who had never been at sea.) Furthermore, they observed, naval surgeons were quick to recognize "recurrent insanity" and to get the affected sailors discharged and admitted to institutions in their own community. Finally, wrote the board, the underlying reason behind the relatively small numbers of naval admissions was BUMED's "wise and efficient administration."[9]

In 1863, Whelan suggested creating a means to put aside a portion of the salary of officers hospitalized at the facility to pay for their clothing and other necessities. He cited the example of three officers without families whose salaries were either accumulating in the treasury or sent "under guardianship, to those who fail to supply many things ... essential to their comfort or well being, and which the asylum has no funds to provide." That recommendation led to a law enacted in 1864 that authorized and required the secretary of the navy, on the advice of the hospital's superintendent, to reserve a portion of the salary of a naval or Marine Corps patient to pay for items "needed for his personal use and comfort" in addition to the hospital's ordinary resources. The funds would be put into the hands of the superintendent to buy the necessary items and accounted for in quarterly statements. Whelan praised the legislation and hoped that it might "contribute somewhat to the ultimate recovery of the unfortunate class of patients for which the government has founded this most admirably conducted asylum."[10]

Artificial Limbs

In July 1862, Congress began appropriating funds for the purchase of artificial limbs "for soldiers and seamen disabled in the service of the United States." The army surgeon general, William Hammond at the time, was charged with directing the expenditure of the funds. Hammond quickly assembled a panel of medical experts to determine the type of devices that should be provided. One member of that group was

Surgeon Benjamin F. Bache, director of the navy's medical laboratory in Brooklyn. The program developed to a point at which approved limb manufacturers agreed to supply specified models of their limbs at an agreed-upon price, qualified recipients could select from those models of limbs, and the government covered the expense.[11]

The original law mentioned soldiers and seamen as its only beneficiaries; officers and, apparently, Marines were excluded. (In 1868, Congress expanded the possible beneficiaries to include officers in the "military or naval services" up to and including army captains and naval lieutenants. In 1879, the program was opened to all officers, soldiers, sailors, and Marines disabled in the service.) In May 1866, the surgeon general's office reported paying for about 3,800 legs and 2,200 arms and hands, with only 14 prostheses supplied to sailors. In late 1865, however, new BUMED chief Phineas J. Horwitz reported 71 artificial limbs being furnished to naval personnel. In light of the efforts made to acquaint naval amputees with the limbs program, wrote Horwitz, the modest number of recipients suggested that the number of sailors and Marines permanently maimed in the war was "almost incredibly small."[12]

Rather than exclude naval officers from the limbs program, the Navy Department, by its own authority, decided to pay for artificial limbs for officers. Because manufacturers offered upgrades to basic limb models offered in the program, the Navy Department sought to establish a limit to what it would pay, "beyond which the officer is expected to meet the cost of any extra arrangements, or ornamentation." If BUMED covered officers' costs at the same rate paid by the army—about $60 per prosthesis, as reported in 1866 by the surgeon general—and if about 15 percent of the 71 naval limb recipients were officers, then the Department's generosity toward officers cost BUMED approximately $640, about half the annual sea salary for an assistant surgeon.[13]

Pensions

Army, navy, and Marine Corps personnel disabled by wounds or disease during their service and in the line of duty were eligible for a pension. If wounds or disease resulted in death, pension payments could go to widows, children, dependent mothers, or orphan sisters of the deceased. Naval pensions were funded by the sale of prizes taken by the navy. Possibly because he spent so much time corresponding with the Pension Office, Whelan took special interest in the fairness of pension laws as they affected naval personnel, even though that subject did not fall within BUMED's purview.[14]

Whelan pointed out that a law enacted in July 1862, which specified the amounts of pension payments for various naval grades, made no provisions for the new grades of rear admiral, commodore, lieutenant commander, and ensign. The law also lowered a captain's monthly pension from its previous level, $50, to $30—an example, opined Whelan, of "a hitherto moderate allowance ... reduced with as little reason, perhaps, as it is increased in other instances." According to a July 1864 law, persons who were previously entitled to a lower payment were now entitled to monthly pensions of $20 if they had lost both feet "in the military service" or $25 if they had lost both hands. Many people, including those in the Pension Office, took *military service* to mean *army*—as was consistent with the era's phraseology—and believed that the new law did not apply to the navy. Thus, many navy men who had suffered identical loss of limbs were victims of "painful inequality" and continued to receive meager monthly payments of $8 or $10 instead of the higher amounts. Pension payments were generally much too low, argued Whelan, and should also be considered for cases other than death or totally disability, such as that of an officer "whose body bears honorable evidence that he has stood in the breach." Any modifications to pension laws in response to Whelan's observations were not made in his lifetime.[15]

Other Potential Options

Whelan contemplated the possibility of the navy establishing a program like the army's Invalid Corps—established in 1863 and later renamed the Veteran Reserve Corps (VRC)—in which disabled soldiers could assume duties in forts or arsenals or guard public buildings. Not only did the VRC provide useful employment, it relieved able-bodied soldiers from such duties so they could be transferred to fighting units. In mid–1864, Whelan speculated that naval shore stations could probably employ disabled sailors as watchmen, laborers in certain departments, permanent crewmembers on receiving ships, and in various other roles.[16]

Once the war ended, many VRC members showed little inclination to remain in the service, possibly because doing so was no longer contributing to the war effort. That sentiment, added to the government's need to reduce the military force and expenses, resulted in many VRC members being mustered out in late 1865 and 1866. The VRC was disbanded altogether in 1869 by the consolidation of its four regiments into other units. Had the USN formed a counterpart to the VRC, which it did not, that endeavor too would probably have had a short life.[17]

Late in the war, the U.S. Sanitary Commission established the Bureau of Employment for Disabled and Discharged Soldiers and Sailors. Its mission was to connect men who had served in the army or navy, especially those with disabilities, with willing employers. In March 1865, the effort gained the endorsement of President Lincoln, who promised to suggest to various government departments that they support the Bureau's purposes. The extent to which the USN participated is unknown.[18]

Most medical officers had little to do with the care of men with long-term disabilities other than participate in surveys and prepare documents that were used in pension decisions. BUMED chief Whelan, however, argued for fair treatment of the navy's disabled while being mindful of the need to control government spending.

Chapter 16

War's End

The end of the war prompted the navy to rid itself of numerous vessels and reduce the number of men serving. The estimated average naval force was about 44,000 men in 1864, 33,000 in 1865, and 17,000 in 1866. There was a corresponding reduction in the number of medical officers. In early 1865, about 436 medical officers were serving in both the regular and volunteer navy. That number dropped to about 252 at the end of 1865 and 199 at the end of 1866. Most of the reduction in the medical force was accounted for by the resignation or honorable discharge of acting assistant surgeons. To show the Navy Department's appreciation for volunteer officers, Secretary Welles ordered that those who were in the service on May 1, 1865, and were mustering out should receive a month of paid leave for every year they had served. In the regular navy, the number of full surgeons stayed fairly constant through 1866 at about the maximum number allowed, which was 80 after mid–1861. The number of assistant and passed assistant surgeons in the regular navy had peaked in late 1862 and early 1863 at the prescribed limit of 120, but that number fell to 111 by late 1864 and 80 by late 1865.[1]

As the war wound down, so did the health of BUMED chief Whelan. He wrote a last will and testament on March 1, 1865. Throughout the war, his assistant, Surgeon Phineas J. Horwitz, had occasional signed BUMED letters on Whelan's behalf, but by May 1, 1865, Whelan stopped affixing his signature altogether to official correspondence. On May 31, Horwitz informed the American Medical Association, of which Whelan was a vice president, that Whelan, "in consequence of severe indisposition," would be unable to attend the organization's meetings. Through about June 8, Horwitz signed documents that apparently reflected Whelan's intent.[2]

Among the last letters dictated by Whelan were instructions concerning the downsizing of squadrons. The Navy Department had determined that the NABS, for example, which consisted of about 120 vessels in early 1865, was to be reduced to one monitor, seven tugs, and 10 other steamers. Similar reductions from early 1865 levels were ordered for the other major squadrons: the SABS from about 80 vessels to six tugs and 15 other steamers; the EGBS from about 30 vessels to four tugs and 10 other steamers; the WGBS from about 75 vessels to one monitor, one Mississippi ironclad, six tugs, and 15 other vessels; and the Mississippi Squadron from about 90 vessels to 15 vessels in all. On June 5, Whelan directed Fleet Surgeons Lewis B. Hunter of the NABS, William Johnson of the SABS, and David Harlan of the EGBS to remove all medical articles that could be spared from ships that were proceeding north for decommissioning; those items could be used to replenish the supplies of remaining squadron vessels.[3]

Surgeon James C. Palmer of the WGBS was given special instructions on June 5. As soon as the squadron was reduced, he was to close the naval hospital at New Orleans and either transfer its government-owned property to the naval hospital at Pensacola or sell it and credit the proceeds to the naval hospital fund. One medical officer from the New Orleans hospital was to be transferred to Pensacola and the other sent north.[4]

On June 7, Whelan give similar orders to Fleet Surgeon Ninian Pinkney of the Mississippi Squadron. The naval hospital at Memphis was to be closed when the number of vessels was reduced, and any of its supplies not needed by the squadron's remaining vessels were to be disposed of by public sale, with the proceeds credited to the hospital fund. If the hospital could be vacated by August 1, the building's owner was to be notified that he could resume possession on that date. Medical supplies removed from vessels being decommissioned could be retained for the remaining vessels or sold, with the proceeds credited to the "surgeons' necessaries and appliances" portion of BUMED's budget. Instruments not needed in the remaining squadron were to be sent to the medical laboratory in Brooklyn. *Red Rover* should, for the time being, be retained to care for the sick of the squadron.[5]

Surgeon Thomas Dillard, stationed at the navy yard in Philadelphia, would be dealing with ships returning north to be decommissioned. On May 26, Whelan directed Dillard to pack up their medical supplies, "except the furniture and such articles as are obviously unfit for further use," and ship them to the medical laboratory. Dillard was to notify the surgeons of the Naval Asylum and Hospital in Philadelphia and the receiving ship *Princeton* that the large amounts of returned supplies at the yard were to be used, to the extent possible, to replenish their stock. Furniture from returning ships, except for a small amount kept for reissue to vessels fitting out at Philadelphia, was to be sold. Whelan specifically ordered the removal of "metallic bottle racks" from the dispensaries of vessels that were supplied with them; the racks were to be shipped to the medical laboratory. Those racks may have been the bottle clasps that, at $18 a set, had struck Whelan four years earlier as unnecessarily costly. Estimated values of items changing hands were to be reported to BUMED directly or entered on the proper routine forms. Thus, even in failing health, Whelan cared about details, knew with remarkable specificity what he wanted done, and was able to make his wishes known to Horwitz.[6]

At 3 a.m. on June 11, 1865, Surgeon William Whelan, chief of BUMED, died at his Washington, D.C., residence. Horwitz reported the death to Secretary Welles the next day. Newspapers reported that Whelan, who had not yet reached his 57th birthday, had succumbed to a protracted heart ailment, and medical officers surmised that his "untiring industry, and unremitting attention to the duties of his office, laid the foundation of the painful disease which terminated his life." Whether the injuries sustained in the 1855 train accident contributed to his death is unknown. Whelan's funeral was held at Saint Aloysius Church in Washington, D.C., with the burial taking place at Mount Olivet Cemetery.[7]

Upon Whelan's death, Surgeon Horwitz, as acting chief of BUMED, assumed Whelan's responsibilities. Secretary Welles appointed Horwitz as BUMED chief by mid–July 1865, but the position officially required presidential nomination and Senate confirmation. Consequently, on December 4, 1865, President Andrew Johnson nominated Horwitz to that post, to date from July 1, and the Senate confirmed the nomination on January 22, 1866. Horwitz's term in that position ended in 1869.[8]

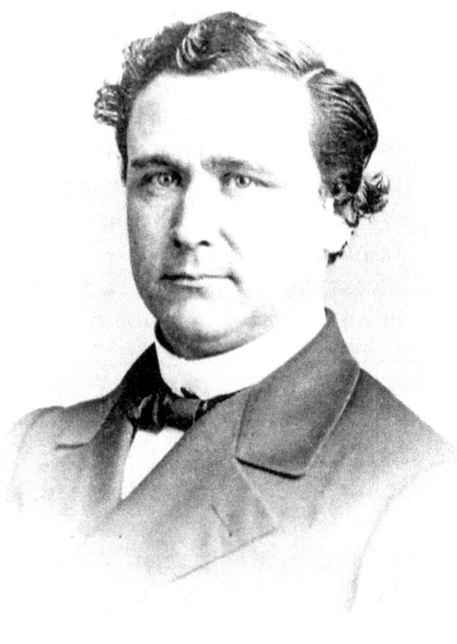

Surgeon Phineas J. Horwitz, who assisted Surgeon William Whelan in the BUMED office and then succeeded him as BUMED chief (NHHC, image NH 48901).

William Whelan's term as BUMED chief (1853–65) was the longest of any officer to ever head the bureau. The next three men to serve as BUMED chief after Horwitz's term—William Maxwell Wood, Jonathan M. Foltz, and James C. Palmer—had all been fleet surgeons during the war. In 1871, during Wood's term, Congress enacted a bill that bestowed on whoever led BUMED the title of surgeon general and the assimilated rank of commodore. The same legislation raised the assimilated ranks of other medical officers to about what they were from March 13, 1863—as ordered by then-Secretary Welles—to 1869, when revocation of that order reduced those assimilated ranks to what they had been from 1854 to 1863.[9]

After Palmer, the next seven BUMED chiefs, ending with William K. Van Reypen, were also Civil War veterans. In 1899, during Van Reypen's term, Congress granted the grade—not assimilated rank—of rear admiral to all officers appointed as bureau chiefs for as long as they held those offices. Accompanying that grade were the pay and allowances of a brigadier general in the army. All of Van Reypen's successors as BUMED chief entered the navy after the Civil War. Although they enjoyed a status never granted to Whelan, they lacked the benefit of having witnessed that officer's fight to obtain higher standing for all naval medical personnel.[10]

Conclusion

THE CIVIL WAR PUT TREMENDOUS pressure on the USN's medical department. The marked growth of the naval force, in personnel and vessels, created a demand for surgeons and medical assistants that was never fully met. Facilities in the North to treat the sick and wounded had to be expanded, and hospital arrangements had to be improvised in the South. The fact that the department managed as well as it did attests to the leadership of its chief, Surgeon William Whelan, and the hard work of its medical officers, surgeons' stewards, and nurses.

Whelan's personality and priorities seemed well-suited to the situation. He was proud of his officers, and he considered it his duty as their representative to advocate for higher salaries and enhanced status. Not only did the officers deserve those benefits, Whelan believed that the lack of adequate pay and prestige discouraged civilian physicians from applying for appointments as assistant surgeons. A constant wartime shortage of medical officers meant that many vessels large enough to warrant one had to manage with an enlisted medical caregiver only or with no medical personnel at all.

Whelan had mixed feelings about volunteer medical officers, who entered the navy through a casual evaluation process that used standards well below those used for regular-navy applicants. Given that line officers and Congress opposed higher pay and status for medical officers, Whelan acknowledged that the number of assistant surgeons could be bolstered only by making entry easier for applicants who had marginal qualifications and were unable to find decent employment elsewhere. Whelan thus characterized the quality of volunteer medical officers as indifferent, yet he came to realize that there were many gems among them and that their services were indispensable. His disappointment in the quality of officers extended to some in the regular service who were behaving in ungentlemanly ways. He attributed their presence to the wartime need to appoint all applicants who achieved a satisfactory score on the entrance examination, not just those deemed best in professional and personal quality, as was the prewar practice.

One of Whelan's key attributes was his sense of justice. Not only, he believed, did medical officers deserve better compensation, so did their assistants. Thus, Whelan argued for higher salaries for surgeons' stewards while, at the same time, being mindful of the need to control spending. The same need to balance fairness with economy characterized Whelan's attitude toward men who became disabled in the service of their country. Men who did not meet that criterion and imposed upon the government for benefits should be weeded out, but deserving men were entitled to a gesture of their country's gratitude, such as a pension, for faithful service.

Whether to allow applicants of foreign origin or parentage into the medical corps brought multiple facets of Whelan's personality and BUMED's needs into play. There was no arguing with the Navy Department's requirement that applicants must be American citizens by birth or naturalization. Beyond that, Whelan freely granted requests to be examined and left admission decisions with examining boards. If an applicant's command of English was not sufficient for him to perform a medical officer's duties, then he should, advised Whelan, be turned away, regardless of his background. He should also be turned away if his command of the language was deficient enough to make him subject to ridicule rather than respect. Thus, in the face of a serious manpower shortage, Whelan wished to protect the medical corps and the applicant himself from the scorn of other officers, especially those of the line, and of enlisted men. Disappointed applicants no doubt had Whelan's sympathies, but those with respectable professional qualifications could probably find employment—with higher pay—elsewhere.

Whelan's respect for economy and rationality was evident in his opposition to a proposed purchase of land near the Portsmouth, New Hampshire, Navy Yard on which to build a hospital. That proposal came from certain legislators and was clearly, in Whelan's mind, an example of special interests coming into play. He argued that the hospital could be built, and more conveniently situated, on land already owned by the government. That episode raised Whelan's indignation to a level that seemed second only to what he felt toward parties who blocked fair compensation for his officers.

The ability to communicate clearly and courteously served Whelan well. His letters were articulate and explanatory. They showed respect for divergent opinions and patience with correspondents who were ignorant of the navy's way to doing things. The BUMED chief was also well-informed. When advocating for higher status for medical officers, he cited the practices of other countries, and when asked about disinfecting solutions, he knew the properties of various available substances. He kept up on the medical literature and provided his regular-navy surgeons with a medical periodical.

Fleet surgeons were drawn from the most experienced medical officers who were fit to serve at sea. To the extent possible, Whelan regarded his senior officers as professional peers. He typically declined to question their judgment yet did not hesitate to gently chide them when necessary. He was apt to trust the opinions of officers facing on-the-spot decisions—in the ordering and storage of supplies, for example, or the establishment of temporary hospitals. In situations involving obeying the law, such as abolition of the spirit ration, he was firm but courteous.

Officers who examined recruits at rendezvous or evaluated assistant-surgeon applicants were given wide latitude in establishing their own standards. Those officers were generally experienced at their task and probably understood the navy's need for men as well as Whelan did. Although the BUMED chief could have dictated rigid standards, he was not onsite to judge the overall quality of applicants. He probably understood that the faith he placed in officers' hands would be repaid in loyalty and in the likelihood that his directives—when they absolutely had to be followed—would be obeyed.

Whelan showed particular gratitude for medical personnel who displayed a conspicuous regard for duty and patient care. Thus, when an assistant surgeon took it upon himself to submit suggestions about the proper outfitting of expeditions, or when other officers reported their observations about health on ironclads, Whelan was quick to express his written thanks. He was equally grateful to a medical officer who had been taken prisoner and opted to stay in captivity so he could care for fellow prisoners. Whelan, apparently without being asked, showed his concern for common sailors by suggesting improvements to the accommodations on receiving ships and recommending changes in the choice and preparation of items in the naval ration. He stated that his suggestions would not just promote health, they would improve sailors' spirits and comfort.

As a bureau chief, Whelan was obligated to control expenses. He demonstrated his own frugality by never asking for more assistance in the BUMED office. For two officers, two clerks, and a messenger—staffing identical to the prewar level—to manage the wartime multitude of paperwork is impressive indeed. The number of medical officers during the war was nearly triple what it been previously been. The whereabouts and assignments of those officers had to be tracked, and their submitted paperwork had to be examined. Many of those documents required correction or return because the new officers responsible for them did not know or care how to complete and submit them. Officers had to be hounded for overdue forms. Whelan needed complete and correct paperwork not only because he valued procedure, but because the details were needed for his own reports to Secretary Welles or for preparing budgets. The office also had correspondence to manage, assignments to recommend, and politicians to lobby. It is no wonder that Whelan's fellow officers believed that the chief's unremitting devotion to his duty contributed to his death.

Whelan positioned medical personnel as best he could, but surgeons and their assistants actually dealt with real and potential patients. Physicians of the time had little ability to cure disease, with one possible exception being the use of quinine for malaria. The illnesses that caused the most suffering and loss of manpower were infectious in origin. Although the role of microorganisms in diseases was not appreciated, medical officers did know that proper hygienic measures helped. Thus, their advice to keep vessels away from marshes, when followed, probably helped protect against malaria and other mosquito-borne diseases. Isolating ships infected with yellow fever or sending them north helped to prevent spread of the disease. Vaccinating against smallpox probably averted many cases of that sickness. Heeding advice to avoid drinking river water probably prevented many cases of diarrhea and dysentery. Although not an infectious disease, scurvy could be headed off if fresh fruits and vegetables were supplied in adequate amounts, as advised by medical officers. Surgeons reported poor ventilation and high temperatures as probable causes for some illness on ironclads, and resultant improvements in ventilation evidently improved the situation.

Treating disease, although often based on medical beliefs not accepted today, tended to keep patients alive and comfortable until the causative factors disappeared or self-limiting ailments followed their natural course. Medical officers treating injuries undoubtedly saved lives by arresting serious hemorrhage. Setting bones and applying splints helped injured sailors retain use of their limbs. Contrary to popular belief, major surgery, such as amputation—which itself was intended to improve the probability of survival—was almost always performed with the patient anesthetized with ether or chloroform. Other useful drugs included opiates, which were administered to help control pain, diarrhea, and coughing.

The medical laboratory in Brooklyn continued its prewar role as a central supply depot, but the wide dispersal of naval forces necessitated that some supplies be purchased locally by medical officers. The laboratory, ably managed by Surgeon Benjamin F. Bache, tested what it bought and manufactured many of its medicines, which were of high and dependable quality. That practice gave naval surgeons confidence in the uniformity of what they prescribed, a luxury not enjoyed by most civilian physicians, who had to be constantly on guard against impure drugs.

Surgeons and their assistants shared the same hazards, whether ashore or afloat, as the men whose health they were assigned to protect. Thus, medical personnel appear in accounts of men who became ill, were injured or died, or were taken prisoner. The undermanned medical department, led by the example of Surgeon Whelan, made the best of the situation and performed creditably.

Whelan held that "considering the nature of the service performed, the protracted exposure of ships' companies to unhealthy climates or localities, the novel character of many of the vessels, [and] the unremitted vigilance and labor imposed by blockade duty," there was good reason to expect a much higher rate of sickness in the navy. That it was not so high, he suggested, was a "satisfactory exhibit of the sanitary condition of the service" and "ample evidence of the efficiency and devotion of the medical corps."[1] Indeed, whether within or outside of BUMED's headquarters, the watchwords of the medical department were *efficiency* and *devotion*.

Appendix A: Numbers of Active-Duty Commissioned Medical Officers in the U.S. Navy

	Value in Indicated Year					
Variable	**1861**	**1862**	**1863**	**1864**	**1865**	**1866**
Surgeons, Regular Navy						
No. officers at start of year	69	76	80	80	80	80
No. new appointees	30	10	5	6	5	8
No. officers lost						
Resigned	6	1	0	1	2	1
Placed on retired list	10	3	4	1	2	5
Dismissed	6	0	1	0	0	0
Died	1	2	0	4	1	3
No. officers at end of year	76	80	80	80	80	79
Assistant Surgeons, Regular Navy						
No. officers at start of year	80	63	120	118	111	80
No. new appointees	48	73	17	17	4	16
No. officers lost						
Resigned	8	2	9	14	27	4
Promoted to surgeon	30	10	5	6	5	8
Placed on retired list	6	1	2	0	0	1
Dismissed	18	0	0	0	0	1
Died	3	3	3	4	3	2
No. officers at end of year	63	120	118	111	80	80

	Value in Indicated Year					
Variable	**1861**	**1862**	**1863**	**1864**	**1865**	**1866**
Acting (Volunteer) Assistant Surgeons						
No. officers at start of year	0	77	141	205	245	92
No. new appointees	88	100	120	118	60	11
No. officers lost						
Resigned	6	23	20	46	71	5
Honorably discharged	0	0	0	0	121	47
Appointed to regular navy	1	2	13	15	4	11
Dismissed	0	2	4	5[a]	4	0
Appointment revoked	4	7	10	0	10	0
Died	0	2	9	12	3	0
No. officers at end of year	77	141	205	245	92	40

[a]*Includes one desertion.*

Note: Table may include slight inaccuracies because of inconsistency and incompleteness of information in reference sources. Legislation enacted in July 1861 raised the maximum allowed number of medical officers in active service in the regular navy from 69 to 80 for surgeons and from 80 to 120 for assistant surgeons and passed assistant surgeons combined. There was no limit on the number of acting assistant surgeons or acting passed assistant surgeons. Numbers of regular assistant surgeons and acting assistant surgeons include passed assistant surgeons. Sources: *NDR*s (1861–67); Entry 43, RG 52; B.F. Tracy to Levi P. Morton, Dec. 3, 1889, S. Exec. Doc. 3, 51st Cong., 1st sess., 20–23 (1890); Callahan, *List of Officers*.

Appendix B: USN Fleet Surgeons During the Civil War

Home Squadron (existed prewar; reorganized as Coast Blockading Squadron, May 13, 1861)

Thomas Dillard, Sept. 20, 1860, to May 17, 1861

Atlantic Blockading Squadron (established May 13, 1861, as Coast Blockading Squadron; renamed May 17, 1861, as Atlantic Blockading Squadron; divided Oct. 29, 1861, into North and South Atlantic Blockading Squadrons)

Thomas Dillard, May 21 to Oct. 29, 1861

North Atlantic Blockading Squadron (established Oct. 29, 1861)

Thomas Dillard, Oct. 29, 1861, to Jan. 27, 1862
William Maxwell Wood, Jan. 27, 1862, to Feb. 29, 1864
John L. Fox, Mar. 10 to Dec. 17, 1864
Lewis B. Hunter, Jan. 3 to July 15, 1865

South Atlantic Blockading Squadron (established Oct. 29, 1861)

George Clymer, Sept. 21, 1861, to July 16, 1863
Wiliam Johnson, July 16, 1863, to June 22, 1865

Gulf Blockading Squadron (established May 6, 1861; divided Jan. 20, 1862, into East and West Gulf Blockading Squadrons)

Gustavus R.B. Horner, May 7, 1861, to Jan. 20, 1862

East Gulf Blockading Squadron (established Jan. 20, 1862)

Gustavus R.B. Horner, Jan. 20, 1862, to June 10, 1863
Edward Gilchrist, June 15, 1863, to May 22, 1865

West Gulf Blockading Squadron (established Jan. 20, 1862)

William Maxwell Wood, Jan. 2 to 27, 1862

Jonathan M. Foltz, Jan. 27 to Aug. 11, 1863
James C. Palmer, Aug. 8, 1863, to Aug. 25, 1865

West India Squadron (established May 17, 1861; discontinued Sept. 7, 1861; reestablished Sept. 8, 1862; discontinued Sept. 12, 1864)
Thomas Dillard, May 17 to 21, 1861
George Clymer, May 29 to Sept. 21, 1861

Mississippi River Squadron (established Oct. 1, 1862)
Edward Gilchrist, Aug. 13 to Dec. 12, 1862
Ninian Pinkney, Dec. 12, 1862, to June 28, 1865

Pacific Squadron (existed prewar)
Solomon Sharp, Apr. 9, 1859, to Oct. 11, 1861
Daniel Egbert, Aug. 8, 1861, to Feb. 27, 1862
John A. Lockwood, Feb. 27, 1862, to Apr. 19, 1864
Charles D. Maxwell, May 6, 1864, to June 4, 1866

East India Squadron (existed prewar)
Benjamin R. Tinslar, May 21, 1859, to Dec. 5, 1861

Africa Squadron (existed prewar)
Thomas L. Smith, Apr. 8, 1859, to Sept. 2, 1861

Mediterranean Squadron (existed prewar)
William S.W. Ruschenberger, Sept. 18, 1860, to July 9, 1861

Brazil Squadron (existed prewar)
Lewis B. Hunter, June 18, 1859, to Aug. 21, 1861

Note: Most dates are for assignment or detachment orders and do not necessarily indicate when officers were on duty. Some orders anticipated organizational changes or accounted for travel delays. The East India, West India, Africa, Mediterranean, and Brazil squadrons appear not to have had a fleet surgeon for most of the war. Source: Rolls 9 and 11, microfilm M330, RG 24.

Appendix C: Assistant Surgeon J.J. Magee's Report and Recommendations on Medical Officers' Participation in Expeditions

(From vol. 1 [Jan.–Mar.] for 1862, box 9, LRB)

U.S. Flag Ship Wabash
Port Royal S.C. Jan 23d. 1862

Sir.

In compliance with your request, I beg leave to submit the following statement of the Medical Arrangement for the boats of this ship which formed part of the recent combined Army and Naval Expedition to the Port Royal Ferry twelve miles from Beaufort.

The army division, under General Stevens, consisted of 2500 men; the naval, under Captain Rodgers, of four launches and the gig of this ship, with the gun-boats Seneca, Ottawa, Pembina, Ellen, and Hale.

The object of the expedition was to capture and destroy forts at the ferry and at Seabrook's plantation.

The Ottawa, Pembina, Hale, and launches from this ship went up Beaufort River, and through Brickyard Creek, into Coosaw River, the Seneca and Ellen went up Broad River, and met the others at the ferry.

The naval portion left Port Royal on the morning of the 31st of December, 1861. That of the army left Beaufort early on the 1st of January, 1862. They met near the ferry, soon after sunrise, and advanced together toward the fort, which they took at 2 P.M.

The enemy made little resistance. Towards evening they appeared in the rear of the fort; they were shelled by the gunboats and retreated precipitately.

On the 2nd of January the boat howitzers were landed to cover the return of the troops. When this was accomplished we re-embarked, and returned to Port Royal.

The only surgical appliances that could be taken, on account of limited space, were as follows, a capital amputating knife, capital saw, bullet forceps, pocket case, tourniquets Petit and field, ligatures, lint, adhesive plaster, isinglass plaster, sponge, suture needles, spirit lamp, tin cup, towels, bandages, muslin, cerate spread, needles, pins, catheters, scissors, artery forceps, twine, ferri-persulph sol [solution of persulphate of iron], tr. ferri chlor. [tincture of chloride of iron], spts. Terebinthinae [spirits of turpentine], spt. ammon. aromat. [spirits of ammonia], tr opii [tincture of opium], chloroforum [chloroform]; ol. olivae [olive oil], whiskey, wine, and preserved beef.

It would have been very difficult, if not impossible, to render any material assistance to the wounded in the crowded launch in which I was, the body of which was occupied by ammunition and provisions, the bow by the howitzer, and the stern by its carriage.

Permit me to offer a few suggestions in relation to the means and appliances by which, in my opinion, the sick and wounded on boat expeditions may have prompt treatment.

When an expedition of any magnitude is to be fitted out, the officer in command would much facilitate its medical equipment by stating to the Fleet Surgeon or senior medical officer, the nature and extent of the service likely to be performed, in time for him to direct the medical outfit accordingly.

System is as necessary in preparing attendance and comfort for the wounded as it is in any department of the service. From the want of it, especially in neglecting to assign to each attendant his particular duty, the surgeon could accomplish little towards alleviating the suffering of the wounded.

This is particularly applicable to detachments operating on land, where, for want of proper organization, the medical officer, instead of attending to a particular company at a designated place, endeavors to attend to the whole detachment in various places.

There are several circumstances, which, under the mode now adopted of placing the medical officer in an already over-crowded launch, modify and limit the necessary provision for the proper treatment of the sick and wounded; to wit, want of sufficient space, limited means of transportation, and want of protection from inclemency of the weather. These are serious difficulties, but they may be easily obviated by having a Floating Relief, or a boat especially assigned to the Surgeon and fitted out under his supervision. This is an indispensable part of the medical outfit. It should be of a size sufficient to perform the probable duties, and furnished to secure the ease and tranquility of the sick and wounded as far as possible. It should have an awning (if tented, so much the better), with side-curtain, and be fitted with removable thwarts, so that, in cases of necessity, mattresses could be laid on the bottom of the boat as well as on the thwarts, which in this case would have to be raised to the gunwale of the boat in order to give sufficient space beneath.

The Relief could be served by extra men or supernumeraries, part of whom would repair to their stations when the expedition arrived at its destination.

It is impossible to state precisely the medicines and instruments that may be required in a boat expedition; as they will be varied according to its object, to climate and other circumstances.

The following list may serve as an approximation to what is most likely to be required. It is prepared as an allowance for one hundred men for a week; viz.,

Capital Amputation Knife, one
Bullet Forceps, one
Artery Forceps, one
Catlin, one
Capital Saw, one
Pocket Case, one
Tourniquets, Petit, six
Tourniquets, Field, fifteen
Needles, Suture, six
Scissors, two
Catheters, diff sizes, three
Adhesive Plaster, two yds
Isinglass Plaster, qrt yd
Ligatures, fifty
Patent Lint, one lb.
Bandages, twenty
Muslin, five yds.
Towels, six
Sponges, six
Basins, two
Splints, padded, one set
Needles, Pins, Twine
Cups, drinking, two
Nursery Lamp, one
Small Blank Book, one
Lead Pencil, one
Mattresses, five
Cots, five
Mag. Sulph [sulphate of magnesia], one lb.
Per-Sulph Ferri sol., ℥ij [two ounces]
Tr. Ferri. Chlor., ℥ij
Terebinth. Spts., ℥iv [four ounces]
Chloroforum, ℥iv
Ammon Spts Aro, ℥ij
Tinct. Opii, ℥iv
Ol. Olivae, ℥ij
Pil. Cath. Comp. [compound cathartic pills], fifty
Pil. Quiniae [pills of sulphate of quinia] gr. v. [5 grains], fifty
Whiskey, two bots.
Wine, two bots.
Alcohol, six ounces
Beef Preserved, five lbs.
Blankets, five
Stretchers, two

If the expedition is to remain long absent the supply of materials for dressings must be increased.

A box not more than two feet in length, one foot wide, and six inches deep, will contain the medicines and the small surgical appliances above enumerated. It may be divided into three compartments; one partition extending crosswise six inches from one end, the other parallel with the side and six inches from it, would make a very convenient division. The smallest compartment is intended for the amputating instruments, which may [be] tightly packed in a part of the lint to prevent them from injury; a piece of serge or cloth should be fastened around the edge, upon which the lid should close tightly to exclude moisture. A good lock is necessary. A strap should be provided by which it may be carried. The smaller articles of the case, such as catheters, scissor, pencil &c may be fastened to the inside of the lid by loops of sheepskin or tape.

If the expedition were intended to operate on land, a small tent would be indispensable, especially if the boats could not be reached over night; this might easily be extemporized by stretching one of the lighter sails over any material suitable for tent poles. The tent is best pitched on rising ground near a stream.

Besides the Surgeon and Surgeon's Steward, four men, instructed in applying the tourniquet, in carrying the wounded, and in performing services connected with their comfort, should be ready to render any assistance required.

In case the expedition is made up of detachments from several vessels, each one, sending one hundred or more men, should send a Medical Officer.

The respective duties of each Surgeon will be designated by the Senior Surgeon.

It is undeniable that there is little room for the Surgeon in a launch containing those things prescribed by the Ordnance Manual, and less for instruments and other appliances for the comfort of the wounded. Even if there were room to carry him, there is no place in which to lay an injured man, or perform the most trifling operation, in a boat where firing is going on and where the men are running backwards and forwards with ammunition. Hence the necessity for a Floating Relief, which is free to move from launch to launch as may be required, and in which the wounded would be comparatively well attended. This would not only disencumber the launches, but it would give room for the Surgeon properly to attend to the wounded.

If the expedition land with the view of operating a short distance from the boats, the Surgeon would render more efficient service by remaining in the boat, and receiving the wounded, carried by men detailed for that purpose, than by passing from place to place in the field of action. If there were two Surgeons, one could land with the detachment, and be stationed in the rear; while the other remained in the boat to receive those severely injured.

Should it be necessary to leave the boats some distance, the Surgeon must take as few impediments as possible: the box containing instruments &c is small and easily carried; to this might be added a few blankets and a small tent if no means of shelter were near.

Operations during the battle ought, if possible, to be limited to arresting hemorrhage, alleviating pain, sustaining under the effects of shock, and dressing wounds, reserving capital operations till its termination, at which time the surgeons could see the cases together and have sufficient assistance so much needed in performing delicate operations.

I have seen nothing in the books on this subject; but having to prepare the medical outfit of expeditions, the more I have reflected on it, the greater has seemed its importance; and although I am conscious of not having exhausted the subject; yet I hope the foregoing remarks will not be unacceptable to you,

I am very respectfully your obedient servant
J. J. Magee
Asst. Surgeon U.S.N.

Surgeon of the Fleet
George Clymer
U.S. Flag Ship Wabash,
Port Royal, S.C.

Appendix D: Acting Assistant Surgeon J.W. Sherfy's Account of His Captivity, 1863–64

(From vol. 4 [Apr.] for 1864, box 27, LRB)

Champaign City, Champaign Co., Illinois.
April 25, 1864

Sir:

I transmitted to you from the U.S. Ship "Morning Light," through the Fleet Surgeon, early in January 1863, the Annual Report for 1862, and the Report for the last quarter of the same year, both of which I hope reached you and were found correct.

On the 21st January, 1863, the "Morning Light" was captured off Sabine Pass, Texas, by Rebel "Cotton Clads," after a most gallant, tho' unsuccessful resistance of nearly three hours, and all the Surgical Instruments, Medicines, Stores, Furniture, Books, &c., belonging to my department fell into the hands of the enemy.

Inclosed is a copy, from memory, of the Report of the casualties of the fight, presented to Act. Mast. John Dillingham, late commander of the ship, at Houston, Texas. Upon some frivolous pretext, I was afterwards arrested, and the original copies taken from me. Also a report of the engagement from Capt. Dillingham to Rear Admiral Farragut, which I had been requested to convey to the Fleet for him should I be released before the other prisoners.

The wounded were conveyed to Sabine City, where everything was done that could be to alleviate their sufferings. The citizens, especially the ladies, were exceedingly kind and attentive. They were in a few days, removed to Houston.

Patrick Turbin was buried in the city cemetery, the day following the engagement, with military honors, and the same interment and courtesy was exhibited in the case of Albert W. Marshall, who died of his wounds six days after.

The case of McArthur is of some interest. A fragment of shell broke the left humerus two inches below the shoulder joint, making a large flesh wound on the anterior portion of the arm. It was determined by the Rebel Surgeons, of whom three were present, that immediate amputation was necessary, with little prospect of the patient's recovery. They yielded however to reasons presented by me why the arm should not be removed. The case seemed a fair one for exsection of the shoulder joint. At the Houston General Hospital the operation was successfully performed, and in a few weeks, with careful attendance and nursing, he recovered, and now has quite a serviceable arm, minus two and a half inches of the humerus. The case attracted a great deal of attention.

Inclosed are "Certificates of Death" for all who died under my own care while I remained in Texas, among the prisoners from various commands, and of all others so far as I could obtain a list of them, from the Rebel Surgeons in charge. It was impossible to make out these certificates in due form at the proper time, and it is equally impossible now to procure the endorsements of the different officers, and the filling of the usual conditions in ordinary cases, and I must claim your indulgence while I do the best that can be done under the circumstances. The Paymaster left the "Morning Light" a few days before its capture, and his clerk and the commander are yet prisoners.

At Houston we joined the officers captured at Galveston. Repeated assurances had been given us, that in a very short time, the men and non-combatants should be sent forward for exchange, or paroled and sent into the Federal lines. This was delayed from time to time, intentionally or otherwise, we could not decide, until the raid of Gen. Banks up the Teche, and the subsequent investment of Vicksburg and Port Hudson rendered it impossible, had not exchanges already ceased. Every day gave birth to new promises of release, only to disappoint us, and we remained in this state of uncertainty and suspense, nearly five months. We were then sent to "Camp Groce," near Hempstead, fifty miles North West of Houston, the officers, surgeons excepted, having been transferred to the Huntsville Penitentiary, where they remained two months, and were then sent to Camp Groce.

Here we remained from the 14th of June until the 9th of December, when we were removed to "Camp Instruction," 10 miles of Shreveport, La.—the officers being detained at Camp Ford, near Tyler, Texas.

While at Houston, I was permitted to visit daily the Prisoners in the Barracks and Hospital, and to superintend their treatment. With rare exceptions my suggestions were respected, and the patients treated as well as their own. The Medical Authorities were humane and attentive—any deviation from kind treatment, attributable to the inadvertence or ill will of subordinates, being promptly checked when observed.

The funeral of James Duffy, who died here, was superintended by the Catholic Clergyman, who took charge of the body, and gave it a respectable interment in the Catholic cemetery, with the rites and services of that church.

We got along comparatively well in Houston, but in Camp Groce, it was quite different. Here began our troubles, which pass description. The men were with rare exceptions, unacclimated, & this fact, in connexion with their imprudence, their coarse and unvarying subsistence, plentiful enough generally, such as it was, and the almost total want of the ordinary comforts of life, made them a fearful prey to disease.

The location was naturally unhealthy, the water bad, and the camp, for the greater part of the time without efficient police, was horribly filthy. Within a week after our arrival there were thirty cases, and they steadily increased, until there were not well men enough to take care of the sick! We numbered about one-hundred and thirty, with occasional additions until the 14th of September, when two-hundred-and fifty men and twenty-one officers from the "Sachem" and

"Clifton" were sent in, increasing our number to four hundred. With the exception of these officers, who were quartered separate from the main body, no intercommunication permitted, and who were prescribed for by Dr. Nestelle [Acting Assistant Surgeon D.D.T. Nestell] of the Clifton, who was confined with them, the entire number was under my own personal charge.

The only medicines I had during the first month were contained in a small pocket case! After the most urgent entreaties, a requisition of the Post Surgeon was filled. We made application to the authorities for permission to send to the Federal Fleet off Galveston, for medicines, and such provisions as could not be obtained in camp for the sick, but it was peremptorily refused. A few months later, the application was renewed, but was again refused. We purchased by voluntary contributions, from time to time, nearly eight hundred dollars worth of medicines. But frequently we were almost destitute of everything, and were compelled to resort to every botanic remedy of the neighborhood, ringing the changes upon herbs, barks, roots, &c, to the end of the list. I used nearly three bushels of Cotton Seed, in the cure of intermittents (as set forth in the U.S Dispensatory), and found it efficient in numerous instances.

Positive orders forbade the sending of any of our sick, to the Houston General Hospital, and an attempt was made by the Post Surgeon to supply the wants of the patients by commuting a number of their rations, and this to some extent relieved them. But yet, the few comforts provided were entirely insufficient. Many died solely in consequence of the inadequate supply of medicines, the improper diet, and from the absence of comfortable quarters and the care it was impossible to secure under the circumstances. If such negligence or refusal to provide for the most common necessities of the sick were intentional on the part of the Rebel Authorities, I cannot call it justly my any milder epithet than down right murder!

The most faithful and patient exertions were made by our people to alleviate by kind attentions the sufferings of the sick, and these good offices to a considerable extent mitigated the severity of their unhappy condition.

During these six months my labors were excessive. I made daily a morning and evening visit, and frequent calls at any hour both day and night. I kept a journal and prepared monthly reports, made up many of the prescriptions, distributed the sick ration, and maintained a constant watchfulness as to the condition of the camp and the men. Being without authority I had to depend upon voluntary assistants, and the co-operation, when it could be obtained, of the Rebel Officers, whose indifference, want of system, and in some cases inability to do what was needed, were the cause, intentional or otherwise, of a large proportion of our discomforts and suffering. In this connexion I must not fail to mention that the Confederate Surgeons were generally disposed to do all in their power to oblige us, and to co-operate with me in my efforts in behalf of the Prisoners. The same may be said of some of the officers in whose immediate keeping we were.

I send you abstracts of such copies as I was able to preserve of the monthly reports to the medical director. It may be observed that while the immediate treatment of our people was courteously granted me, as the only Federal Surgeon able to perform so heavy a task (Dr. Cummings being an invalid some months before his death, and Dr. Nestelle confined with the officers captured with him), the labor was accomplished under the supervision of the Rebel Surgeons, and the Reports made out according to the regulations of their Army, which required only the number of cases, the diseases, and deaths. The "sick days" were not called for. These will give you a pretty accurate conception of the vast amount of sickness that prevailed. After the first month, the number daily on the list ranged from fifty to one hundred and ten! There was no separate apartment for the patients, though repeated efforts were made by me to have a portion of the Barracks appropriated exclusively for the worst cases.

Those who died at Camp Groce were buried immediately adjoining the grounds in a spot appropriated for that purpose, though not inclosed. Their graves were marked by head and foot boards, with name, age, and date of death. I send you a complete list of all who died in Texas and Louisiana from the various commands of the Navy and Army to which they were attached.

Dr. A.I. [Ariel L.] Cummings, Surgeon of the 42d Regt. Mass. Vols., captured at Galveston, Jan. 1st 1863, died on the 9th of September, of acute dysentery. The greatest respect was shown to his remains, which were interred with Masonic honors, those of that Fraternity, both Confederate and Federal uniting cordially in the ceremonies.

The noncommissioned officers and privates were paroled on the 18th November to be sent to Shreveport for immediate exchange. We were detained till the 9th December. I was permitted to accompany them in my official capacity. The commissioned officers, including Dr. Nestelle, of the "Clifton" were not paroled, but sent to "Camp Ford" near Tyler, Texas, with the gloomy prospect of remaining there until the close of the war.

Charles Tweedy, ordinary seaman, of the Morning Light, and Joseph Parker, of the 42d Regt. Mass. Vols., private, both suffering with chronic dysentery, and unable to be removed, were left in camp. I was afterwards informed that both died at the hospital in Hempstead.

Lt. Col. A.J.H. Duganne, 176th N.Y. Vols. with Remittent Fever, was also left behind. I afterwards leaned that upon his recovery he was removed to "Camp Ford."

Alpheus Todd, Lds., Clifton, died on the 11th day of the march, Dec. 20, '63, of chronic dysentery and was as decently interred as possible, by the public highway, between Jacksonville and Larissa, near the line of Smith and Cherokee Counties, Texas.

Wm S. O'Brien, died of chronic dysentery in the Hospital at Tyler, Dec 27th. He had been left there on the 23rd, being unfit to travel.

I cannot speak too condemnatory of the harsh treatment of the prisoners on the march. Our men had suffered so severely from sickness and other causes that a large number were utterly unfit to be removed without transportation. Of twenty-eight who were thus disabled, nearly two-thirds were compelled to travel on foot. Sixteen, twenty, or twenty five miles was the usual days march—rarely less. Consequently a great number gave out, and when the evening camping ground was reached, these poor fellows were scattered along the road for miles, and were only brought in by the most laborious efforts of the guard and myself. The transportation was utterly insufficient. By frequently changing the sick from the wagon to the road and back again, thus relieving the most tired ones, they were with great effort brought on; though I cannot describe the sufferings of these men, in their struggles to keep up, wearily toiling on with trembling steps, till nature could endure no more, and they sank down utterly exhausted in the road. To stimulate the weak ones harsh appeals were not wanting, and bitter epithets and vile upbraidings were freely resorted to by a few of the guard. One heartless wretch who I am sorry to say wore the form of a man, finding that abuse and curses did not succeed, cut a large switch, and when he saw a prisoner falling behind, he mercilessly applied it over his shoulders! It is due to Lt. Kellom, then in command, who was never wanting in kindness and did all in his power to favor us on the route, to say that upon this cruelty being represented to him, the villain's conduct met the severest condemnation, and he was detailed for other duty than guarding the prisoners. I am glad to say too that there were many instances of sympathy from the guard. Often they dismounted and gave their horses to the weary men, and did all they could to assist them forward. The authorities at Houston, and not the escort, were responsible for the limited transportation furnished. I had by request sent them a list of patients amounting to sixty, twenty-eight of whom I judged to be entirely disabled. Yet only about a dozen could be carried during the first days of the march, and at no time more than one-half the number that should have been.

At Tyler, we rested two days, during which the officers came up, and we were, contrary to promises repeated made at Camp Groce, detained at "Camp Ford."

Capt. Davis relieved Lt. Kellom, and the escort numbered fifty instead of twenty-five. And now began a scene of irregularity and confusion, and consequent suffering, that cannot be portrayed. Whatever of system had been introduced (and there had been considerable) was utterly discarded. The authority that had been given me to superintend the transportation of the sick and their baggage, was taken away, and the men even counseled to use violence if I interposed. The able bodied were rushed on to the end of the day's march in the most disorderly manner. The command extended along the road in varying groups for six miles or more. Well men rode or crowded the wagons with their baggage, while the sick men walked, and carried what they had or threw it away. If our sufferings were great before, they were now much more. Arriving at "Camp Instruction" (a bitter "school of adversity" it proved to be) after a heavy march through a driving rain, on the last day, Dec. 30, no arrangement having been made for our reception, we were turned loose in the woods! It became intensely cold, and continued so for weeks. For thirty years previous there had not been such a severe winter in Louisiana and Texas as the last one, and the deaths of three of our men at Shreveport shortly after our arrival, I believe to be solely attributable to hard marching and subsequent exposure.

There were already at Camp Instruction four hundred prisoners, captured principally at Morganza, and the quarters were scarcely sufficient for their accommodation. Our men, thus turned out unguarded, immediately inaugurated a series of stampedes, in squads of from two to twenty, so that in a short time, nearly two hundred were missing. Probably one-tenth of these succeeded in reaching our lines. The country was alive with "fugitive Yankee," with rebel cavalry in hot pursuit! Those recaptured were imprisoned in Shreveport, Alexandria, and other places.

Those who did not attempt their escape were ordered into camp, closely guarded, and informed that they could either build "huts," or go without! Dissatisfaction grew apace, with murmurings loud and deep. Some yielded however, and quite a motley village soon sprang up, the logs being carried from the woods half a mile distant. Only the strong men could accomplish so heavy a task. I found it necessary to engage in such work myself, and the result was one of the most comfortable houses in the camp.

As I have before said, we were sent forward with repeated assurances of immediate exchange. These promises were not fulfilled, and there seemed to be little prospect that they would be soon. Without any authority or facilities for treating the sick, now exclusively under control of the Confederate Surgeons, who, I believe, aimed to treat them as well as their own soldiers, I felt myself at liberty to ask to be sent into the Federal lines. About the same time the late commanding officer of the "Morning Light" wrote me from "Camp Ford" urging this step, with the hope that I might accomplish something toward effecting the release of our people in Louisiana and Texas, by representing their condition to the Federal Authorities, and stating the willingness of the insurgents to deliver them over, as soon as arrangements could be effected. The request was granted, and I left Shreveport on the 17th of February, and after some detention on the way, during which I was treated most courteously by the rebel authorities, I entered our lines near Franklin, La., on the 9th of March, having been a prisoner nearly fourteen months.

I represented the condition of our people to Maj. Gens. Banks and Franklin, and others, who I tho't could effect something towards their release. Since my arrival here I have, by order of Rear Admiral Farragut, reported in full concerning them and myself, to the Secretary of the Navy, whose orders I now await.

While at Sabine City, the Insurgent Commander of the expedition against us proffered to send me to the Federal Fleet under flag of Truce, But I could not reconcile it with my convictions of duty to abandon my fellow prisoners, especially the wounded, who urgently requested me to remain, and I respectfully declined his offer. I believe that without exception the officers and men will testify to the faithfulness with which I applied myself to serve them not only professionally, but in every way that presented itself during our unexpectedly prolonged and unhappy captivity, and to me a most laborious one. I worked incessantly, not only for my own command, but impartially for all, whether officer, soldier, or sailor. I lost but eleven days from sickness during the whole time.

I do not regret the severe and trying ordeal through which I have passed. The consciousness of performing my duty and the conviction that I was of great service to my fellow prisoners, sustained me when surrounded by the most untoward circumstances under which a medical officer ever labored.

At New Orleans I conferred with Fleet Surgeon Palmer, who advised me to report to you direct, as soon as I could conveniently, and to inform you fully of the circumstances of the captivity, concerning myself and those who had been under my care. I have acted on this instruction, and I trust this report will be found neither too elaborate in detail, nor devoid of any essential particulars. I have felt it due me to address you without reserve, and I hope my course throughout will be fully approved by you.

I have the honor to be,
Very Respectfully
Your Obedient Servant,
J. W. Sherfy
A.A. Surgeon, U.S.N.
Late of the U.S.S. Ship "Morning Light"

Surgeon W. Whelan, U.S.N.
Chief of Bureau Med. & Surg.
Navy Department
Washington, D.C.

Appendix E: Squadrons' Most Common and Most Deadly Sickbay Admission Diagnoses

table on the following pages

	No. Deaths/No. Cases in Indicated Squadron								
Admission Diagnosis	**Potomac Flotilla (1861–65)**	**Atl. Blkg. (1861)**	**NABS (1861–65)**	**SABS (1861–65)**	**Gulf Blkg. (1861)**	**EGBS (1862–65)**	**WGBS (1862–65)**	**Mississippi (1862–65)**	**Overall Mortality**
Most Common									
Intermittent fever	1/460	0/93	7/3,218	1/1,552	0/233	1/460	8/5,734	26/10,352	44/22,111 (0.20%)
Acute diarrhea	0/487	0/204	1/2,580	0/1,944	2/218	0/576	7/3,840	26/5,504	50/15,353 (0.33%)
Catarrh	0/391	0/401	0/2,345	1/2,477	0/311	0/531	1/1,717	0/968	2/9,141 (0.02%)
Remittent fever	1/197	0/17	6/894	7/663	0/44	7/824	49/2,360	132/3,625	202/8,624 (2.34%)
Acute bronchitis	0/175	0/59	2/1,242	7/1,214	0/106	4/216	2/990	6/941	21/4,943 (0.42%)
Acute rheumatism	0/178	0/112	3/1,199	4/1,282	1/115	0/322	1/943	5/772	14/4,923 (0.28%)
Contusion	0/59	0/121	0/940	5/910	0/118	0/245	5/891	2/376	12/3,660 (0.33%)
Chronic rheumatism	0/66	0/51	0/833	1/1,140	0/42	0/225	0/713	0/576	1/3,646 (0.03%)
Acute dysentery	0/83	0/58	6/566	10/846	2/50	1/237	16/1,076	19/689	54/3,605 (1.50%)
Furuncle	0/76	0/48	0/659	0/1,397	0/70	0/393	0/747	0/181	0/3,571 (0%)
Contused wound	0/51	0/98	2/706	0/708	0/68	1/145	3/595	10/366	16/2,737 (0.58%)
Constipation	0/184	0/64	1/801	0/533	0/52	0/265	0/422	0/366	1/2,657 (0.04%)

Cutaneous abscess	0/88	0/52	0/707	0/695	0/59	0/208	2/480	0/252	2/2,541 (0.08%)
Adynamia	0/30	0/10	1/361	2/459	0/10	0/54	5/351	9/886	17/2,161 (0.79%)
Gonorrhea	0/76	0/46	0/590	0/374	0/24	0/83	0/444	0/490	0/2,127 (0%)
Chronic diarrhea	0/52	0/6	2/233	1/129	0/0	0/33	7/318	108/1,305	118/2,076 (5.68%)
Primary syphilis	0/81	0/60	0/498	0/375	0/23	0/59	0/640	0/330	0/2,066 (0%)
Tonsillitis	0/53	0/52	0/595	0/566	0/50	0/148	0/324	0/235	0/2,023 (0%)
Gunshot wound	5/28	0/10	108/409	84/337	2/27	12/73	152/588	85/498	448/1,970 (22.74%)
Continued fever	0/87	0/10	2/483	1/417	0/21	1/112	0/414	6/385	10/1,929 (0.52%)
Associated with Most Deaths[a]									
Pneumonia	2/36	1/13	21/317	23/281	1/225	7/61	17/188	54/509	126/1,630 (7.73%)
Pulmonary tuberculosis	2/27	1/16	9/274	14/340	0/18	3/68	9/236	57/321	95/1,300 (7.31%)
Typhoid fever	3/25	2/19	15/182	17/114	1/3	6/18	20/113	82/278	146/752 (19.41%)
Yellow fever	0/2	0/0	1/13	0/4	1/1	33/345	95/348	2/22	132/735 (17.96%)
Drowning	57/57	0/0	62/62	134/134	0/0	5/5	195/195	117/117	570/570 (100%)

[a]*Includes diagnoses associated with the most deaths not already included among the 20 most common diagnoses.*

Note: The order of diagnoses is based on the denominator in the "Overall Mortality" column (number of cases for all squadrons combined). Common terms have been substituted for some medical terms used in the navy's nomenclature of diseases. The table includes all diagnoses associated with 44 or more deaths and accounts for 72.42% (104,310 of 144,038) of reported treated cases and 82.11% (2,079 of 2,532) of reported deaths. Blkg = Blockading. NABS = North Atlantic Blockading Squadron, SABS = South Atlantic Blockading Squadron, EGBS = East (or Eastern) Blockading Squadron, WGBS = West (or Western) Blockading Squadron. Compiled from Horwitz, BUMED Report (Oct. 26, 1867), 220–302.

Chapter Notes

Works, designators, and institutional authors frequently cited in the notes are identified by the following abbreviations and short forms:

BUMED Report: Report of the Bureau of Medicine and Surgery (various authors, dates, and sources)
LRB: Letters Received (Bureau of Medicine and Surgery), Jan. 1857–Feb. 1885, Entry 7, RG 52
LSB: Letters Sent (Bureau of Medicine and Surgery), Sept. 1842–Feb. 1886, Entry 1, RG 52
NDR: Navy Department. *Register of the Commissioned...* (various titles, dates, and publishers)
ORN: *Official Records of the Union and Confederate Navies in the War of the Rebellion*
RG: Record Group, National Archives and Records Administration

Foreword

1. A.A. Henderson to William W. McKean, Oct. 22, 1861, roll 119, microfilm M89, RG 45.

Introduction

1. Welles, Report of the Secretary (Dec. 2, 1861), 3, 11; Welles, *Report of the Secretary* (1864), xxiii; Welles, *Report of the Secretary* (1865), xii, xiii.

2. The acronym BUMED, although not employed during the Civil War era, is used here for convenience and in deference to the Navy Department, which uses it consistently, even when referring to the bureau's origin and early operations.

Chapter 1

1. Munden and Beers, *The Union*, 439; Act of Aug. 31, 1842, ch. 286, 5 Stat. 579 (1850).

2. Navy Department, *Instructions for the Government* (1844), 5; Paulin, "Half Century," 1319; Gideon Welles to William Whelan, numerous letters, 1861–65, roll 2, microfilm M480, RG 45; Whelan to Welles, numerous letters, 1861–65, rolls 16–21, microfilm M518, RG 45.

3. Tenney, *Military and Naval History*, 804; "William Whelan"; *Catalogue of Medical Graduates*, 83; Entries for Whelan, rolls 4, 5, 7, and 11, microfilm M330, RG 24.

4. "A New Chief of the Naval Bureau of Surgery, &c," *Evening Star* (Washington, D.C.), Sept. 26, 1853, 2; Entry for Bureau of Medicine and Surgery, p. 1, entry 41, RG 52; Whelan nomination, Dec. 13, 1853, and confirmation, Jan. 23, 1854, *S. Exec. Journal*, 33rd Cong., 1st sess., 9:168–69, 215 (1887); *NDR* (for 1853), 46–49.

5. "Shocking Railroad Accident," *Plattsburgh (NY) Republican*, Sept. 1, 1855, 2; Tenney, *Military and Naval History*, 804.

6. *NDR* (to Sept. 1, 1862), 24–25; Whelan nomination, July 12, 1862, and confirmation, July 17, 1862, *S. Exec. Journal*, 37th Cong., 2nd sess., 12:399–400, 434 (1887); Whelan to Welles, July

23, 1863, roll 17, microfilm M518, RG 45; Entry for Wm. Wheelan [*sic*] family, City of Washington, District of Columbia, dwelling 1368, family 1421, roll 102, microfilm M653, RG 29.

7. Welles, *Diary*, 1:335–36.

8. Act of Aug. 31, 1842, ch. 286, §§ 4–6, 5 Stat. 579, 580 (1850); *NDR* (for 1848), 14; *NDR* (for 1853), 16; *NDR* (for 1859), 14; Act of Mar. 3, 1853, ch. 97, § 3, 10 Stat. 189, 209–10 (1855).

9. *NDR* (1865), 10, 46–47; Whelan to Welles, May 24, 1861, roll 16, microfilm M518, RG 45; Act of July 16, 1862, ch. 183, § 18, 12 Stat, 583, 586–87 (1865).

10. Whelan, BUMED Report (Nov. 4, 1864), 1188.

11. George Clymer to Whelan, May 23, 1862, vol. 2 (Apr.–June) for 1862, box 10, LRB.

12. Clymer to Whelan, May 23, 1862, vol. 2 (Apr.–June) for 1862, box 10, LRB; Whelan to Clymer, June 4, 1862, vol. 23, LSB; Whelan to B.F. Wilson, Oct. 26, 1861, vol. 22, LSB.

13. Whelan to Ninian Pinkney, July 31, 1863, vol. 25, LSB.

14. Mills, *Guide to the Capitol*, 53, 56–57; Wineberger, *Department Directory*, 53–57; Welles to Whelan, May 30, 1861, roll 2, microfilm M480, RG 45.

Chapter 2

1. Act of May 24, 1828, ch. 121, § 1, 4 Stat. 313 (1846). Although the prewar requirements for promotion to passed assistant surgeon included five years of service, two of which were to be served at sea, the need for five years of total service, if ever enforced, was dropped during the war. "Regulations for Admission and Promotion"; *NDR* (to Jan. 1, 1863), 46.

2. Paullin, "Naval Administration," 1469–70.

3. *NDR* (for 1861), 38–39.

4. *NDR* (for 1861), 42–45, 152; William Whelan to J.H. Gunning, Apr. 22, 1865, vol. 30, LSB.

5. *NDR* (for 1859), 52–53; *NDR* (for 1860), 53–54; *NDR* (for 1861), 44–45; *NDR* (to Jan. 1, 1863), 46–47.

6. Act of Aug. 4, 1842, ch. 121, 5 Stat. 500 (1850); Homans, *Register*, 10, 12, 13; Thomas Harris, BUMED Report (Nov. 6, 1846), 594; Thomas Harris, BUMED Report (Oct. 30, 1848), 938–39; Homans's 1842 *Register* lists 69 assistant and passed assistant surgeons as of September 15, 1842, but four appointments made earlier in 1842 reduce the number to 65 on January 1. Thomas Harris's Nov. 6, 1846, BUMED report places the authorized number of assistant and passed assistant surgeons at 67, and his 1848 report shows 80 assistant and passed assistant surgeon serving.

7. *NDR* (to Jan. 1, 1863), 109, 113–14; Gideon Welles to Lewis W. Minor, May 7, 1861, to D.B. Conrad, May 10, 1861, and to Charles F. Fahs, Nov. 13, 1861, roll 390, microfilm T829, RG 45; Dudley, *Going South*, 4, 13; Hasegawa, *Confederate Navy Medical Corps*, 189–90; Act of July 31, 1861, ch. 31, 12 Stat. 284 (1865); Whelan, BUMED Report (June 10, 1861), 108. A few more medical officers left the USN in 1862 or 1863 to join the Confederate States Navy.

8. Act of Feb. 21, 1861, ch. 49, §§ 3–4, 12 Stat. 147, 150 (1865); Act of Aug. 3, 1861, ch. 42, §§ 21–22, 12 Stat. 287, 290–91 (1865); Act of Dec. 21, 1861, ch. 1, 12 Stat. 329 (1865).

9. Whelan to Welles, April 20, 1861, roll 273, microfilm M148, RG 45.

10. Whelan to Welles, April 20, April 30, May 24, and June 4, 1861, roll 15, microfilm M518, RG 45; *NDR* (to July 1, 1867), 45–46; B.F. Tracy to Levi P. Morton, Dec. 3, 1889, S. Exec. Doc. 3, 51st Cong., 1st sess., 20–23 (1890); *NDR* (to Jan. 1, 1863), 109, 114; *NDR* (to Jan. 1, 1865), 118; Death notice for William Whelan.

11. *NDR* (for 1861), 40; *NDR* (to Aug. 31, 1861), 25–26, *NDR* (to Sept. 1, 1862), 27–28; *NDR* (to Jan. 1, 1863), 48–51, 109, 113–14; *NDR* (to Jan. 1, 1864), 44–45, 50–51, 112, 113; *NDR* (to Jan. 1, 1865), 48, 52–55, 116, 118; Statements for multiple officers, pp. 4, 12, 426, 427, entry 43, RG 52; Bertolette, Gibbs, King, and Leach nominations, May 28, 1862, and confirmations, June 18, 1862, *S. Exec. Journal*, 37th Cong., 2nd sess., 12:306, 350 (1887). There may be slight inaccuracies in the reported numbers of medical officers because of inconsistencies in reference sources.

12. Dow, "Volunteer Navy"; Whelan memorandum, May 11, 1861, vol. 22, LSB; Welles, Report of the Secretary (Dec. 2, 1861), 18–19; Act of July 24, 1861, ch. 13, 12 Stat. 272 (1865); *NDR* (to Aug. 31, 1861), 43; *NDR* (to Sept. 1, 1862), 87–88; *NDR* (to Jan. 1, 1863), 148–49, 166–71; *NDR* (to Jan. 1, 1864), 15–61, 192–201; *NDR* (to Jan. 1, 1865), 172–75, 217–27; Statements for numerous officers, pp. 1–434, entry 44, RG 52.

13. Adams, *Doctors in Blue*, 47, 174–76; Hasegawa, *Matchless Organization*, 112, 148; Hasegawa, *Confederate Navy Medical Corps*, 69–75.

14. Whelan to Alfred Holt, Oct. 18, 1861, vol. 22, LSB; Statements for numerous officers, pp. 1–434, entry 44, RG 52; Whelan to S.W. Kellogg, Apr. 6, 1865, and Whelan to Welles, Jan. 20, 1865, vol. 30, LSB; J.E. Dow, "Volunteer Navy," 572; *NDR* (to Jan. 1, 1866), 145–46; *NDR* (to Jan. 1, 1867), 136–37.

15. Act of February 15, 1879, ch. 83, 20 Stat. 294 (1879). Callahan, *List of Officers*; *NDR* (to July 1, 1881), 64.

16. Welles, Report of the Secretary (Dec. 2, 1861), 18–19; *NDR* (to Jan. 1, 1863), 170; *NDR* (to Jan. 1, 1864), 196; *NDR* (to Jan. 1, 1865), 222.

17. Whelan, BUMED Report (Nov. 4, 1864), 1184; Whelan, BUMED Report (Oct. 23,1863), 1064; Whelan to Henry B. Morrell and M.G. Delaney, June 24, 1864, vol. 27, LSB; Whelan to William McMillan, Jan. 17, 1865, vol. 29, LSB; P.J. Horwitz to George W. Webb, June 29, 1865, vol. 30, LSB.

18. Whelan to Alexander H. Rice, Mar. 5, 1864, vol. 26, LSB.

19. Whelan memorandum, Apr. 26, 1864, vol. 26, LSB; Act of Mar. 3, 1865, ch. 124, § 6, 13 Stat. 539 (1866); M.S. Thompson, *General Orders and Circulars*, 27–28.

20. Callahan, *List of Officers*, 99, 512, 547.

Chapter 3

1. "Regulations for Admission and Promotion"; "Naval Medical Board," *Pennsylvanian* (Philadelphia), Apr. 5, 1858, 3; "A Naval Medical Board," *Public Ledger* (Philadelphia), Mar. 8, 1859, 3; "Naval Medical Board," *Daily National Intelligencer* (Washington, D.C.), Feb. 8, 1860, 3; Entries for Special Duty, pp. 218, 410–11, entry 41, RG 52; Whelan, BUMED Report (Oct. 23, 1863), 1064.

2. William Whelan to Isaac Toucey, Feb. 12, 1861, and Whelan to Gideon Welles, May 6, 1861, roll 16, microfilm M518, RG 45; Whelan to Welles, Mar. 4 and July 31, 1862, roll 17, microfilm M518, RG 45; Whelan to Welles, Nov. 7, 1862, and Feb. 16, 1863, roll 18, microfilm M518, RG 45; Whelan to Welles, Aug. 20 and Dec. 10, 1863, roll 19, microfilm M518, RG 45; Whelan to Welles, May 4, 1864, roll 20, microfilm M518, RG 45; Entries for Special Duty, pp. 218, 410–11, entry 41, RG 52; Whelan to 10 periodicals, May 7, 1861, vol. 22, LSB; "Medical News"; "Naval Medical Board," *American Medical Times*; "The Naval Medical Examining Board," *New York Herald*, Oct. 8, 1861, 3.

3. "Regulations for Admission and Promotion"; "The Naval Medical Examining Board," *New York Herald*, Oct. 8, 1861, 3; "Naval Medical Board," *American Medical Times*; Whelan to Editor, *National Intelligencer*, Mar. 4, 1862, vol. 23, LSB; Whelan to J. Stevens, Feb. 26, 1863, vol. 24, LSB; Navy Department, *Regulations for the Government*, 1, 39.

4. "Regulations for Admission and Promotion"; Whelan to 10 editors, May 7, 1861, and Whelan to D.H. Lovejoy, Sept. 21, 1861, vol. 22, LSB; Whelan to James M. Greene, Mar. 9, 1863, vol. 24, LSB; Whelan to Green, May 6, 1864, vol. 27, LSB.

5. Dunham, "Homoeopathy in the Army"; "The Naval Medical Examining Board," *New York Herald*, Oct. 26, 1861.

6. William Maxwell Wood to Whelan, July 19, 1862, vol. 3 (July–Aug.) for 1862, box 11, LRB.

7. Slawson, "Medical Training"; Gradijan, "Navy Surgeons."

8. Horner, *Diseases and Injuries of Seamen*, 26–27, 33–36; Whelan to James M. Greene, Aug. 20, 1863, vol. 25, LSB.

9. Horner, *Diseases and Injuries of Seamen*, 26–27, 33–36; Whelan to S. Barrington, May 22, 1861, vol. 22, LSB; Finding aid and examination papers of Robert R. Gibbes, Examination Papers Collection, National Library of Medicine.

10. Whelan to Barrington, May 22, 1861, vol. 22, LSB.

11. Whelan to Barrington, May 22, 1861, vol. 22, LSB, Greene to Whelan, Dec. 24, 1863, vol. 11 (Dec.) for 1863, box 23, LRB; "Philadelphia School of Anatomy."

12. Whelan to Barrington, May 22, 1861, vol. 22, LSB.

13. Horner, *Diseases and Injuries of Seamen*, 26–27; Gradijan, "Navy Surgeons"; "Regulations for Admission and Promotion."

14. Gradijan, "Navy Surgeons"; Whelan, BUMED Report (Nov. 4, 1864), 1185.

15. Whelan to Samuel Barron, May 29, 1861, vol. 22, LSB; Whelan to Welles, June 10, 1861, roll 16, microfilm M518, RG 45; *NDR* (to Jan. 1, 1863), 46–49.

16. Dow, "Volunteer Navy"; Whelan to Alfred Holt, Oct. 18, 1861, vol. 22, LSB; Pray, *Civil War Journal*, Jan. 28, 1862.

17. Gradijan, "Navy Surgeons"; Boyer, *Naval Surgeon*, 5–7; Whelan to Welles, June 22, 1862, roll 17, microfilm M518, RG 45; Statement for Lucien H. Kendall, p. 200, entry 44, RG 52.

18. Whelan memorandum, May 11, 1861, vol. 22, LSB. BUMED evidently produced a circular outlining the requirements for applicants for acting assistant surgeon, but it has not been found. Whelan to Charles F. Crebore, Aug. 13, 1861, vol. 22, LSB.

19. Whelan to Crebore, Aug. 13, 1861, and Whelan to S. Chester Smith, Oct. 24, 1861, vol. 22, LSB; Whelan to L.J. Jones, Feb 2, 1864, vol. 26, LSB.

20. Pray, *Civil War Journal*, Jan. 28, 1862; Welles to Daniel D.T. Nestell, Jan. 6 and Feb. 19, 1862, and Nestell appointment, Jan. 25, 1862, Daniel D.T. Nestell Papers, Nimitz Library.

21. Batten, *Reminiscences*, 9; B.F. Bache and Thomas J. Turner to Welles, Sept. 18, 1862, roll 301, microfilm M148, RG 45; W.S.W. Ruschenberger and S.F. Coues to Welles, Aug. 9, 1862, roll 297, microfilm M148, RG 45; Whelan to Welles, Aug. 23, 1862, vol. 22A, LSB; Whelan, BUMED Report (Nov. 4, 1864), 1184.

22. Whelan to E.S. Ruggles, Dec. 9, 1861, vol. 22, LSB; Whelan to J.M. Warner, Mar. 18, 1863, vol. 24, LSB; Whelan to James M. Barnard, Sept. 29, 1863, vol. 25, LSB; "Dr. William Argyle Watson," *Providence (RI) Sunday Journal*, July 28, 1901, 2; Newman, *Smoots of Maryland and Virginia*, 41; Bache and Turner to Welles, July 21, 1862, roll 296, microfilm M148, RG 45; Statements for James Kinnier, Samuel Clement Smoot, and William Argyle Watson, pp. 200, 332, 405, entry 44, RG 52.

23. Whelan, BUMED Report (Nov. 4, 1864), 1185–86; Statements for numerous officers, pp. 1–434, entry 44, RG 52.

24. Gatewood, "William Longshaw, Jr."; Whelan, BUMED Report (Nov. 4, 1864), 1185; Statements for numerous officers, pp. 1–434, entry 44, RG 52.

25. Whelan to Green, Aug. 20, 1863, vol. 25, LSB.

26. Whelan to J.J. Magee, Feb. 20, 1862, vol. 23, LSB; Whelan to C.J. Cleborne, Aug. 24, 1863, and Whelan to John Paul Quinn, Sept. 25, 1863, vol. 25, LSB.

27. *NDR* (for 1861), 151; Navy Department, *Instructions for the Government* (1857); Whelan to Barrington, May 22, 1861, vol. 22, LSB.

28. John A. Dahlgren, General Order, Nov. 18, 1863, and Welles to William Longshaw, Jr., Dec. 1, 1863, *ORN*, ser. 1, 15:120; Welles to Longshaw, Mar. 8, 1864, vol. 26, LSB; James Parker to Joseph Lanman, Jan. 15, 1865, *ORN*, ser. 2, 11:495–97.

29. Act of Mar. 3, 1865, chap. 124, § 6, 13 Stat. 539 (1866); M.S. Thompson, *General Orders and Circulars*, 27–28; *NDR* (to Jan. 1, 1866), 124; *NDR* (to Jan. 1, 1867), 124.

30. Whelan to Ninian Pinkney, Mar. 30 and Apr. 28, 1865, vol. 30, LSB.

Chapter 4

1. Navy Department, Code of Regulations, 27; B.F. Gibbs to William Whelan, June 30, 1863, vol. 6 (July) for 1864, box 18, LRB.

2. Whelan, BUMED Report (Oct. 23, 1863), 1061–64; Whelan, BUMED Report (Nov. 4, 1864), 1183–86; Paullin, "Naval Administration, 1842–1861," 1465–68; Ruschenberger, *Brief History*.

3. Navy Department, *General Regulations* (1841), 1–2; *NDR* (for 1860), 149;

Act of Aug. 5, 1854, ch. 268, § 4, 10 Stat. 583, 587 (1855).

4. Act of July 16, 1862, ch. 183, § 1, 12 Stat. 583 (1865); Whelan to J.W. Grimes, July 8, 1862, vol. 22A, LSB.

5. Whelan to Grimes, July 8, 1862, vol. 22A, LSB; Slawson, "Medical Training," 18–19.

6. Propositions regarding assimilated rank, and regulations respecting relative rank of line and staff officers, as approved by Secretary of the Navy, Mar. 13, 1863, vol. 25, LSB; Whelan to Louis M. Goldsborough, Nov. 25, 1862, vol. 22A, LSB; Navy Department, *Instructions for the Government* (1864), 47–48; *NDR* (to Sept. 1, 1862), 3–4; "Important Naval Regulations," *New York Times*, Apr. 19, 1863, 3.

7. Welles, *Diary*, 3:570–71.

8. Whelan to J.M. Foltz, June 3, 1863, vol. 25, LSB.

9. Whelan, BUMED Report (Oct. 23, 1863), 1164; *NDR* (for 1861), 16–25; *NDR* (to Sept. 1, 1862), 11–17; *NDR* (to Jan. 1, 1863), 108–16.

10. Entries for William Johnson and John A. Dahlgren, roll 9, microfilm M330, RG 24; *NDR* (to Jan. 1, 1865), 3–5, 12–13, 26–27, 30–31, 40–41, 56–57, 66–67, 124, 140, 249; Whelan to Grimes, Feb. 3, 1865, vol. 30, LSB; Act of Apr. 21, 1864, ch. 63, § 7, 13 Stat. 53, 54 (1866).

11. Whelan, BUMED Report (Oct. 23, 1863), 1161–63; Whelan to Gustavus G. Fox, Nov. 26, 1862, roll 18, microfilm M518, RG 45; Paullin, "Naval Administration, 1842–1861," 1465–68.

12. Whelan, BUMED Report (Nov. 4, 1864), 1185.

13. Whelan, BUMED Report (Nov. 4, 1864), 1185; War Department, *Revised Army Regulations*, 544; *NDR* (to Sept. 1, 1862), 3–4; Act of Mar. 3, 1835, ch. 27, 4 Stat. 755 (1846); Whelan, BUMED Report (Oct. 29, 1860), 378.

14. Whelan to Gideon Welles, Jan. 20, 1865, vol. 29, LSB.

15. Whelan to Welles, Jan. 20, 1865, vol. 29, LSB.

16. Medical Department of the Navy, Jan. 24, 1865, *Cong. Globe*, 38th Cong., 2nd sess., 393 (1865); Whelan to W.N. Pindell, Jan, 18, 1865, to James Anderson, Jan 21, 1865, to N. Pinkney, Jan. 26, 1865, and to A.H. Rice, Jan. 27, 1865, vol. 29, LSB; Whelan to Rice, Feb. 2, 1865, to Grimes, Feb. 3, 1865, to Charles Sumner, Feb. 4, 1865, and to W.D. Kelley, Feb. 13, 1865, vol. 30, LSB.

17. Whelan to Kelley, Feb. 13, 1865, vol. 30, LSB.

18. Whelan to Rice, Feb. 2, 1865, to Grimes, Feb. 3, 1865, and to Kelley (including private memorandum), Feb. 13, 1865, vol. 30, LSB.

19. Whelan to Kelley (private memorandum), Feb. 13, 1865, vol. 30, LSB.

20. Whelan to Welles, Feb. 27, 1865, vol. 30, LSB.

21. M.S. Thompson, *General Orders and Circulars*, 75–77; Paullin, "Half Century of Naval Administration," pt. 3, 746–47.

22. Ruschenberger, *Brief History*, 15, 85.

23. Whelan to N. Pinkney, Apr. 11, 1865, vol. 30, LSB.

24. George H. Cooke to Theodorus Baily, May 11, 1863, enveloped labeled "Proposed new naval regulations with special reference to assimilated rank, together with opinions of numerous officers thereon, 1863," box 276 (subject NI), entry 502, RG 45; M.S. Thompson, *General Orders and Circulars*, 9.

25. General Order, July 31 1862, roll 2, microfilm M977, RG 45; Whelan to Welles, July 25, 1863, vol. 25, LSB; "Changes in Navy Uniform"; Navy Department, *Uniform for Officers*; Tily, *Uniforms of the United States Navy*, 116–35.

Chapter 5

1. Navy Department, *Instructions for the Government* (1857), 8; Horner, *Diseases and Injuries of Seamen*, 14–15; Earp, *Yellow Flag*, 19.

2. Navy Department, *Instructions for the Government* (1857), 8; William Whelan to Gideon Welles, June 12, 1861, vol. 22, LSB; *NDR* (for 1861), 6; Horner, *Diseases and Injuries of Seamen*, 14–15; Woodward, *Hospital Steward's Manual*, 16.

3. Whelan to Welles, June 12, 1861, vol. 22, LSB.

4. Navy Department, *Instructions for the Government* (1864), 44–46; Whelan to James M. Greene, Dec. 11, 1861, vol.

22, LSB; One- and three-year shipping articles, 1864, and shipping articles, U.S. Navy, 1861–1865, box 356 (subject NR), entry 502, RG 45.

5. Welles, General Order No. 36.

6. Whelan to W. Johnson, May 16, 1864, vol. 27, LSB.

7. Whelan to E. Gilchrist, Sept. 16, 1863, vol. 25, LSB; Whelan to Robert J. Richards, July 6, 1864, vol. 27, LSB.

8. Whelan to Welles, Nov., 1864, roll 21, microfilm M518, RG 45; M.S. Thompson, *General Orders and Circulars*, 25; Whelan to Daniel Egbert, Jan. 5, 1863, vol. 24, LSB.

9. Whelan to A.H. Rice, Feb. 2, 1865, vol. 30, LSB.

10. Whelan to James M. Greene, Dec. 11, 1861, vol. 22, LSB; Dodson, "Apothecary in our Navy."

11. Navy Department, *Instructions for the Government* (1857), 8; Whelan to C. Evesfield, Apr. 4, 1865, vol. 30, LSB.

12. Navy Department, *Instructions for the Government* (1857), 8; E. Cutbush, George Davis, Samuel R. Marshall, and Thomas Ewell, Report on Naval Hospitals, Mar. 16, 1812, 24 *Annals of Cong.* 2150–56 (1853); Whelan to L.J. Williams, May 19, 1863, vol. 24, LSB; Whelan memorandum, May 23, 1861, vol. 22, LSB; Articles of agreement for R.H. Cooper, Aug. 4, 1863, vol. 2, entry 45, RG 52; Articles of agreement for Du Fay Bowman, July 26, 1864, vol. 3, entry 45, RG 52; Whelan to W. Smith, June 10, 1863, vol. 25, LSB.

13. P.J. Horwitz to J.C. Palmer, June 30, 1865, vol. 31, LSB; Articles of agreement for Du Fay Bowman, July 26, 1864, vol. 3, entry 45, RG 52. Although the official name of the city of New Bern appears to have been Newbern during the Civil War, *New Bern* is used in this book by default. "How to Spell the Name 'Newbern,'" *State Chronicle* (Raleigh, NC), July 23, 1891, 4.

14. Whelan to E.C. Doran, Aug. 9, 1864, vol. 28, LSB; Whelan to commander, Naval Station, Pensacola, FL, June 13, 1864, folder 2, box 206 (subject MA), entry 502, RG 45; Joseph Smith, Report of the Chief of Bureau of Yards and Docks, 629–35; Whelan, BUMED Report (Nov. 4, 1864), 1190–92.

15. Entries 45 and 45A, RG 52.

16. Entry for Cornelius Hale, New York, week of Oct. 19, 1861, roll 16, microfilm M1953, RG 24; Entries for Hale, USS *Isaac Smtih*, vol. 193, entry 132, RG 24; Entry for Hale, USS *Morse*, vol. 287, entry 132, RG 24.

Chapter 6

1. *NDR* (to Jan. 1, 1863), 42–51, 148–49, 174–209.

2. Welles, Report of the Secretary (1862), 25–26.

3. Navy Department, Code of Regulations, 24–25.

4. G.V. Fox to Samuel L. Breese, Sept. 14, 1861, Gideon Welles to F.H. Gregory, Oct. 6, 1862, and A Table Showing the Number of Persons for the War Complements of the Different Classes of Vessels of the Navy of the United States, Jan. 20, 1838, envelope 2 (General, U.S. Navy, Complements Allowed to Various Vessels, 1861–1865), box 236 (subject NA), entry 502, RG 45; Complement of Officers and Crew Allowed to Vessels of Each Class, ca. 1840, and Complements of Officers and Crew, July 20, 1854, folder labeled "Correspondence Relative to Complements on Board Various Vessels, 0–1859," box 220 (subject NA), entry 502, RG 45; Horner, *Diseases and Injuries of Seamen*, 13.

5. Navy Department, *Allowances*, 156–59; *NDR* (to Jan. 1, 1863), 178, 192.

6. *NDR* (to Jan. 1, 1864), 178–209.

7. Welles, Report of the Secretary (July 4, 1861), 89; : Gideon Welles to S.H. Stringham, May 1 and 17, 1861, *ORN*, ser. 1, 5:619–20, 635; Welles to S.F. Du Pont, Sept. 18, 1861, *ORN*, ser. 1, 12:208; Welles to L.M. Goldsborough, Oct. 12, 1861, *ORN*, ser. 1, 6:313–14; Welles to S.P. Lee, July 26, 1864, *ORN*, ser. 1, 10:307; Welles to Charles Wilkes, and Welles to Goldsborough, July 6, 1862, *ORN*, ser. 1, 7:548.

8. Welles to S.H. Stringham, May 1, 1861, *ORN*, ser. 1, 5:619–20; William Mervine to Welles, May 11, 1861, roll 118, microfilm M89, RG 45; Welles to F.B. Ellison, T.D. Shaw, and L.C. Sartori, May 17, 1861, *ORN*, ser. 1, 4:175; Welles to William W. McKean, Jan. 20, 1862, *ORN*, ser. 1, 17:56–57.

9. Welles to McKean, Jan. 20, 1862, *ORN*, ser. 1, 17:56–57.

10. Welles to David G. Farragut, Jan. 9, 1862, *ORN*, ser. 1, 18:5.

11. Act of July 16, 1862, ch. 185, 12 Stat. 587 (1865); George D. Wise to M.C. Meigs, Sept. 14, 1863, in Meigs, *Report of the Quartermaster General*, 800–801; Adjutant General's Officer, War Department, General Orders No. 150, Oct. 1, 1862, *ORN*, ser. 1, 23:388–89; Kenney, "From the Log of the Red Rover," 36–37; John Rodgers to Welles, Aug. 9, 1861, *ORN*, ser. 1, 22:297–98; A.H. Foote to Meigs, Nov. 14, 1861, *ORN*, ser. 1, 22:429; Foote to Welles, Feb. 11, 1862, with enclosure, *ORN*, ser. 1, 22:550–51; Navy Department, Code of Regulations, 42; Entry for Edward Gilchrist, roll 9, microfilm M330, RG 24; Whelan to Gilchrist, Aug. 26, 1862, vol. 22A, LSB.

12. Porter, *Naval History*, 677–78; *NDR* (to Jan. 1, 1863), 207–8; *NDR* (to Jan. 1, 1864), 240–48; *NDR* (to Jan. 1, 1865), 277–79.

13. *NDR* (to Jan. 1, 1864), 205–9; Munden and Beers, *The Union*, 486–87; William, Seligman and Co.; Duncan, Sherman and Co.; J.D. Jones, et al., Petition to Salmon P. Chase, Apr. 17, 1861, *ORN*, ser. 1, 1:8; Welles to G.J. Pendergrast, May 17, 1861, *ORN*, ser. 1, 5:636; Pendergrast to Welles, Sept. 7, 1861, *ORN*, ser. 1, 6:183; Welles to Charles Wilkes, Sept. 8 and 9, 1862, *ORN*, ser. 1, 1:470–71, 473; Welles to James L. Lardner, Sept. 12, 1864, *ORN*, ser. 1, 3:212.

14. *NDR* (to Jan. 1, 1863), 178–209; Whelan to Welles, Nov. 16, 1863, roll 19, microfilm M519, RG 45; Whelan to Welles, Aug. 31, 1864, roll 20, microfilm M518, RG 45; Whelan to Welles, Welles, Mar. 8, 1865, RG 45, M518, roll 21; Whelan to J.M. Foltz, Sept. 30, 1862, vol. 22A, LSB.

15. Navy Department, Code of Regulations, 12, 126–131, 425–30. The 1858 Code of Regulations, proposed by a panel of officers after a previous set of regulations was ruled invalid by the attorney general, was never enacted by Congress but still reflected naval practices of the time. The 1858 code was also the basis of the 1862 regulations of the Confederate States Navy. Confederate States Navy, *Regulations*.

16. *NDR* (to Jan. 1, 1863), 181, 208; Navy Department, *Dictionary of American Naval Fighting Ships*, 2:63, 298; Navy Department, Code of Regulations, 24–26; Whelan to A.H. Rice, Feb. 2, 1865, vol. 30, LSB.

17. Whelan to J.N. Warner, Mar. 18, 1863, vol. 24, LSB; *NDR* (to Jan. 1, 1863), 148–49, 184, 190, 213–31.

18. N. Pinkney to Whelan, Sept. 22, 1863, vol. 8 (Sept.) for 1863, box 23, LRB; Muster rolls of USS *Covington*, vol. 94, entry 132, RG 24. During part of 1864, when it carried 62 men, excluding officers, *Covington* had an acting assistant surgeon. *NDR* (to Jan. 1, 1864), 232.

19. N. Pinkney to Whelan, Sept. 22, 1863, and David D. Porter, General Order No. 80, Aug. 19, 1863, vol. 8 (Sept.) for 1863, box 20, LRB; Whelan to Pinkney, Sept. 28, 1863, vol. 25, LSB.

20. Navy Department, *Allowances*, 156–59; Whelan to A.H. Rice, Feb. 2, 1865, vol. 30, LSB.

21. Whelan to Welles, May 3 and 21, 1861, roll 16, microfilm M518, RG 45.

22. Robert Means Thompson and Wainwright, *Correspondence of Fox*, 2:268–71; Entries for various officers, rolls 9 and 11, microfilm M330, RG 24; *NDR* (to Jan. 1, 1863), 42–43.

23. Navy Department, Code of Regulations, 125–26; Act of May 24, 1828, ch. 121, § 2, 4 Stat. 313 (1846); Horner, *Diseases and Injuries of Seamen*, 19–20; Whelan memorandum to J.W. Grimes, Feb. 3, 1865, vol. 30, LSB; James C. Palmer to Whelan, Nov. 5, 1863, vol. 10 (Nov.) for 1863, box 22, LRB.

24. George Clymer to Whelan, Jan. 31, 1862, vol. 1 (Jan.–Mar.) for 1862, box 9, LRB; *NDR* (for 1860), 111–20.

25. Whelan to J.M. Foltz, May 22, 1863, vol. 24, LSB; Entry for steam sloop *Hartford*, p. 285, entry 41, RG 52; *NDR* (to Jan. 1, 1863), 178.

26. *NDR* (to Jan. 1, 1863), 174–77; Roberts, "Naval Station."

27. Navy Department, *Regulations for the Government*, 156–57.

28. Whelan to R.T. Maccoun, May 30, 1863, vol. 24, LSB; Whelan to W.M. Wood, July 17, 1863, vol. 25, LSB.

29. Entries for Isaac Brinkerhoff and Gilchrist, rolls 7 and 9, microfilm M330, RG 24; Entries for Navy Yard, Portsmouth, NH, and Naval Rendezvous, Philadelphia, pp. 3, 24, entry 41, RG 52; *NDR* (for 1860), 46–47.

30. *NDR* (to Jan. 1, 1865), 48–51; Statement for numerous officers, entry 43, RG 52.

31. Entries for numerous officers, entry 41, RG 52; Register of Volunteer Officers ("Acting Volunteer Officers"), May 1861–June 1866, pp. 475–507, entry 164, RG 45.

32. Entries for Naval Hospitals, Boston (Chelsea) and Norfolk, VA, pp. 13, 43, entry 41, RG 52.

33. B.F. Gibbs to Welles, Oct. 24, 1862, roll 305, microfilm M148, RG 45; J.R. Tryon to Welles, June 27, 1864, roll 360, microfilm M148, RG 45; Thomas J. Turner to Whelan, Feb. 11, 1864, roll 348, microfilm M148, RG 45; Entry for Gibbs, roll 9, microfilm M330, RG 24; Entries for Tryon and Turner, roll 11, microfilm M330, RG 24; Act of Mar. 3, 1851, ch. 34, § 1, 9 Stat. 621 (1851).

34. George Clymer to Whelan, July 27, 1863, vol. 6 (July) for 1863, box 18, LRB.

35. Navy Department, *Instructions for the Government* (1864), 44.

36. Whelan to Vincent Falon, June 13, 1864, vol. 27, LSB; Proceeding of a Naval Court of Inquiry, case 4313, roll 167, microfilm M273, RG 125.

37. Proceeding of a Naval Court of Inquiry, case 4313, roll 167, microfilm M273, RG 125.

38. Proceedings of a Naval General Court Martial, case 4010, roll 147, microfilm M273, RG 125.

Chapter 7

1. Orison Blunt to Horatio Seymour and Frederick Townsend, Aug. 22, 1864, *New York Daily Transcript*, Sept. 1, 1864, 2; David D. Porter, Announcement, Nov. 25, 1862, *Cleveland Daily Plain Dealer*, Dec. 2, 1862, 5; John J. Glasson, Announcement, Jan. 1, 1863, *Whalemen's Shipping List and Merchants' Transcript* (New Bedford, MA), Apr. 28, 1863, 1; Provost Marshal General's Office, Circular No. 13; "Singular Proceeding," *Eastern Argus* (Portland, ME), Jan. 29, 1863, 2. The only medical officer known to have been assigned to the Portland rendezvous, Surgeon Charles Chase, was there during the second quarter of 1861. Entry for Portland Rendezvous, p. 197, entry 41, RG 52.

2. Numerous entries, pp. 5–398, entry 41, RG 52; Navy Department, *Instructions for the Government* (1857), 10–11, 50; Horner, *Diseases and Injuries of Seamen*, 28–42.

3. William Whelan to W.E. Taylor, Aug. 22, 1864, vol. 28, LSB.

4. Horner, *Diseases and Injuries of Seamen*, 28–30.

5. Charles Chase to Whelan, Dec. 29, 1863, vol. 11 (Dec.) for 1863, box 23, LRB; John J. Abernethy to Whelan, May 26, 1864, vol. 5 (May) for 1864, box 28, LRB.

6. Navy Department, *Regulations for the Government*, 180–81, 184; Navy Department, *Instructions for the Government* (1864), 50; Negus, "Conduct Unbecoming," 40.

7. Edward Shippen to Whelan, May 23, 1864, and Solomon Sharp to Whelan, May 15, 1864, vol. 5 (May) for 1864, box 28, LRB; Whelan to Sharp, May 17, 1864, vol. 27, LSB.

8. "Recruiting for the Navy"; "Recruiting—The Difficulties That Beset It," *New York Times*, Aug. 25, 1864, 5; "Naval Recruiting," *New York Times*, Aug. 31, 1864, 4; Negus, "Conduct Unbecoming."

9. Proceeding of a Naval Court of Inquiry, case 4335, roll 169, microfilm M273, RG 125.

10. Whelan to Taylor, Aug. 22, 1864, vol. 28, LSB.

11. Entries for Naval School, p. 222, entry 41, RG 52; Navy Department, *Regulations of the U.S. Naval Academy*, 11.

12. Navy Department, *Regulations of the U.S. Naval Academy*, 11–12; Navy Department, *Official Register*, 33–35; Whelan memorandum to Welles, Jan. 9, 1863, vol. 24, LSB.

13. Navy Department, *Regulations of the U.S. Naval Academy*, 61; Whelan to Welles, May 26, 1864, vol. 27, LSB; Navy Department, *Official Register*, 35.

14. Navy Department, Code of Regulations, 164–65; Navy Department, *Regulations for the Government*, 184.

15. Navy Department, Code of Regulations, 36–37, 126, 171.

16. Whelan, BUMED Report (Oct. 23, 1863), 1065.

17. Navy Department, *Instructions for the Government* (1857), 8.

18. Whelan to L.B. Hunter, Mar. 3, 1865, vol. 30, LSB.

Chapter 8

1. William Whelan to Gideon Welles, July 24, 1862, roll 17, microfilm M518, RG 45; Whelan to Welles, Feb. 8, 1864, vol. 26, LSB.

2. Act of Mar. 3, 1843, ch. 83, 5 Stat. 615 (1850); Act of Mar. 3, 1845, ch. 77, § 3, 5 Stat. 790, 794 (1850); Ruschenberger, "Naval Laboratory"; Whelan to James C. Dobbin, Oct. 19, 1853, with Dobbin's endorsement, roll 11, microfilm M518, RG 45. Bache was a great-grandson of Benjamin Franklin and a cousin of physician Franklin Bache, coauthor of the *Dispensatory of the United States*, a standard reference book issued to naval vessels. Parton, *Life and Times of Benjamin Franklin*, 629–30.

3. Whelan, BUMED Report (Nov. 4, 1864), 1178; Entry for Edward R. Squibb, roll 7, microfilm M330, RG 24; *NDR* (to Jan. 1, 1864), 44–45.

4. Freedley, *Leading Pursuits*, 113–35.

5. Whelan to J.W. Grimes, Mar. 21, 1864, vol. 26, LSB.

6. Whelan to J.W. Grimes, Mar. 21, 1864, vol. 26, LSB; Navy Department, *Allowances*, 128; Whelan to J.M. Foltz, Feb. 3, 1863, vol. 24, LSB; George Winston Smith, *Medicines for the Union Army*, 15–16.

7. Whelan to Welles, Jan. 14, Sept. 7, Nov. 4, and Dec. 24, 1864, roll 21, microfilm M518, RG 45; Churchman, "Use of Quinine."

8. Whelan to Welles, [June 3, 1861?], vol. 22, LSB; George Winston Smith, *Medicines for the Union Army*, 24–25; Whelan to Welles, roll 16, microfilm M518, RG 45.

9. Charles A. Nichols to Whelan, Oct. 7, 1863, vol. 9 (Oct.) for 1863, box 21, LRB.

10. Navy Department, *Instructions for the Government* (1857), 11–17; Navy Department, *Instructions for the Government* (1864), 3, 12–19; Navy Department, *Allowances*, 127–32; Whelan to Grimes, Mar. 21, 1864, vol. 26, LSB.

11. Whelan to Welles, Feb. 8, 1864, vol. 26, LSB.

12. Navy Department, *Allowances*, 130–32; Whelan to W.S.W. Ruschenberger, Aug. 28, 1861, and to B.F. Bache, Aug. 31, 1861, vol. 22, LSB. Surgeon's Steward C. Marion Dodson described dispensary bottles on USS *Pocahontas* being held in place by iron clamps screwed into a wall or partition, an arrangement that removed the need for a large number of shelves and prevented the bottles from falling when the ship rolled. Earp, *Yellow Flag*, 13.

13. Whelan to J.C. Palmer, July 29, 1864, vol. 27, LSB; Whelan to J.M. Foltz, May 22, 1863, and to B.F. Gibbs, May 23, 1863, vol. 24, LSB; Whelan to J.C. Palmer, Aug. 10, 1863, vol. 25, LSB; Entries for *Bermuda*, *Circassian*, and *Union*, pp. 202, 224, 360, entry 41, RG 52.

14. Whelan to E. Gilchrist, Aug. 26, 1862, vol. 22A, LSB; William Maxwell Wood to Whelan, July 13, 1863, vol. 6 (July) for 1863, box 18, LRB; Whelan to C.D. Maxwell, July 21, 1864, and to J.C. Palmer, July 29, 1864, vol. 27, LSB.

15. Whelan to J.W. Grimes, Mar. 21, 1864, vol. 26, LSB; Whelan to William Grier, Dec. 19, 1862, vol. 22A, LSB.

16. Whelan to William Grier, Dec. 19, 1862, vol. 22A, LSB.

17. Whelan to J.C. Palmer, Aug. 10, 1863, vol. 25, LSB.

18. James E. Yeatman to George Wise, June 9, 1862, box 208 (subject ME), entry 502, RG 45; Yeatman to George H. Bixby, Dec. 16, 1863, George H. Bixby Papers, Abraham Lincoln Presidential Library; Whelan to James M. Barnard, Sept. 22, 1863, vol. 25, LSB; Whelan to J.L. Fox, June 3, 1864, vol. 27, LSB.

19. Foltz, *Surgeon of the Seas*, 212; E. Boylston Jackson to William W. McKean, Mar. 21, 1862, and Herman P. Babcock to John L. Fox, Aug. 16, 1864, folder for 1860–70 (hospital supplies for ships and stations), box 208 (subject ME), entry 502, RG 45.

20. Whelan to James M. Greene, Aug. 6, 1862, vol. 22A, LSB; Greene to Whelan, July 26, 1862, vol. 3 (July–Aug.) for 1862, box 11, LRB.

21. J.M. Foltz to Whelan, Jan. 9, 1863, vol. 1 (Jan.–Feb.) for 1863, box 14, LRB; Whelan to Foltz, Feb. 6, 1863. vol. 24, LSB. In October 1863, Foltz complained to Secretary Welles of his long sea duty with the WGBS and separation from this family and asked to be posted to duty at Philadelphia. The letter was referred to Whelan, who reported that Foltz had

been with the squadron no longer than some other squadron medical officers. Before his service in the Gulf, Foltz had been posted to Philadelphia for almost seven years. After his October 1863 request, Foltz was assigned to serve on a medical examining board. Foltz to Gideon Welles, Oct. 2, 1863, with endorsement by Whelan, roll 337, microfilm M148, RG 45.

22. Whelan to B.F. Gibbs, May 23, 1863, vol. 24, LSB; George Clymer to Whelan, Feb. 22, 1862, vol. 1 (Jan.–Mar.) for 1862, box 9, LRB.

23. Whelan to N. Pinkney, July 31, 1863, vol. 25, LSB.

24. B.F. Gibbs to Whelan, June 20, 1863, vol. 6 (July) for 1863, box 18, LRB.

Chapter 9

1. Navy Department, Code of Regulations, 125–31.

2. Navy Department, Code of Regulations, 125; William Whelan to W.S.W. Ruschenberger, Aug. 23. 1861, vol. 22, LSB; Horner, *Diseases and Injuries of Seamen*, 48–49.

3. Navy Department, *Ordnance Instructions*, pt. 1, pp. 7, 15, 30–31; Robert Means Thompson and Wainwright, *Correspondence of Fox*, 1:299–300.

4. Navy Department, Code of Regulations, 128.

5. Ericsson, "Monitors," 284; Plans for *Milwaukee*-Class Monitors, NAID 158704479, Alphabetical Series of Ship Engineering Drawings, RG 19.

6. Horner, *Diseases and Injuries of Seamen*, 11, 13–14; Hunter, *Year on a Monitor*, 178; True, "Life aboard a Gunboat," 38.

7. C. Eversfield to Whelan, Apr. 1, 1862, vol. 2 (Apr.–June) for 1862, box 10, LRB; Augustus S. Baldwin to Gideon Welles, Mar. 6, 1862, *ORN*, ser. 1, 1:338–40.

8. Navy Department, Code of Regulations, 129; Navy Department, *Instructions for the Government* (1857) 7–8, 28–30, Whelan to B.F. Wilson, Oct. 20, 1861, vol. 22, LSB.

9. George Clymer to Whelan, Feb. 23, 1862, vol. 1 (Jan.–Mar.) for 1862, box 9, LRB; Henry O. Mayo to Charles Steedman, Sept. 4, 1863, folder 2, box 206 (subject MA), entry 502, RG 45; W.L. Wheeler to Clymer, July 4, 1863, vol. 6 (July) for 1863, box 18, LRB.

10. Whelan memorandum to Welles, Feb. 3, 1862, vol. 23, LSB; Welles, General Order, Feb. 7, 1862, Navy Department, *Instructions for the Government* (1864), 47.

11. Ruschenberger, Review, 415–17; Hunter, *Year on a Monitor*, 53; Navy Department, *Ordnance Instructions*, pt. 1, pp. 30–31, 39.

12. James H. Conley to R. Wainwright, Apr. 28, 1862, H.R. Exec Doc. 1, 37th Cong., 3rd sess., 293–94 (1862); Foltz, *Surgeon of the Seas*, 245; George U. Morris to William Radford, Mar. 9, 1862, *ORN*, ser. 1, 7:21; "The Fight in Hampton Roads: Statement of the Pilot of the Cumberland," *World* (New York), Mar. 11, 1862, 1.

13. Ruschenberger, Review, 416; Navy Department, *Ordnance Instructions*, 98.

14. Ruschenberger, Review, 416.

15. Ruschenberger, Review, 416–17; Whelan to Clymer, Feb. 24, 1862, vol. 23, LSB.

16. Theodorus Bailey to Gideon Welles, Apr. 21, 1863, H.R. Exec. Doc. 1, 38th Cong., 1st sess., 286–87 (1863); John Dillingham to D.G. Farragut, Nov. 28, 1862, H.R. Exec. Doc. 1, 38th Cong., 1st sess., 298 (1863); D.G. Farragut, General Order No. 9, July 6, 1864, in Welles, *Report of the Secretary* (1864), 507; Navy Department, *Ordnance Instructions*, pt. 2, pp. 6, 9; Ruschenberger, Review, 416.

17. J.J. Magee to George Clymer, Jan. 23, 1862, vol. 1 (Jan.–Mar.) for 1862, box 9, LRB; Whelan to Clymer, Feb. 24, 1862, vol. 23, LSB.

18. *NDR* (to Jan. 1, 1863), 116, 171; *NDR* (to Jan. 1, 1864), 113, 201–202; *NDR* (to Jan. 1, 1865), 118, 226; *NDR* (to Jan. 1, 1866), 101, 170.

19. Pension application of Maria S. Whitney, case no. 18721, fiche 05142, microfilm M1274, RG 15; "Dreadful Marine Disaster," *New York Times*, Aug. 26, 1863, 1; Boyer, *Naval Surgeon*, 47. Chloroform could produce "intoxicating qualities equal to, or surpassing those of alcohol " and could result in habitual use that assumed "the character of a baneful luxury." Daniel B. Smith, "Certain

Compounds of Carburetted Hydrogen"; Sansom, *Chloroform*, 257.

20. William Mervine to Gideon Welles Aug. 8, 1861, *ORN*, ser. 1, 16:610–12; Edward Gilchrist to Whelan, Aug. 19, 1863, vol. 7 (Aug.) for 1863, box 19, LRB.

21. Joseph E. De Haven to James F. Armstrong, and W. Gaines Bruce to De Haven, May 22, 1863, *ORN*, ser. 1, 9:37; S.F. Du Pont to Welles, Feb. 3, 1863, *ORN*, ser. 1, 13:577–78; *NDR* (to Jan. 1, 1864), 113.

22. James Parker to Joseph Lanman, Jan. 16, 1865, *ORN*, ser. 1, 11:495–97; David D. Porter to Welles, Feb. 1, 1865, *ORN*, ser. 1, 11:448–49; Selfridge, "Navy at Fort Fisher," 661. Rear Admiral Porter's communication to Secretary Welles erroneously stated that USN Acting Assistant Surgeon John Blackmer died in a manner similar to Longshaw during the Fort Fisher assault. That was incorrect; Blackmer died in 1895. "Career of Dr. John Blackmer," *Worcester (MA) Daily Spy*, Apr. 17, 1895, 3.

23. G.H. Scott and W.F.A. Torbert, report of a court of inquiry, Jan. 24, 1865, *ORN*, ser. 1, 16:178–80; Entry for Henry A. Danker, roll 11, microfilm M330, RG 24.

24. W.H. Pierson to J.A. Dahlgren, Sept. 10, 1864, *ORN*, ser. 1 15:481–88.

25. "The Captured Gunboat Granite City," *Boston Evening Transcript*, June 21, 1864, 2; Entry for Edmund C. Ver Meulen, roll 11, microfilm M330, RG 24.

26. "List of Officers and Men Paroled from the Harriet Lane," and D.G. Farragut to Welles, Feb. 26, 1863, *ORN*, ser. 1, 19:443–44, 453.

27. J.W. Sherfy to Welles, Apr. 12, 1864, *ORN*, ser. 1, 19:558–62; Sherfy to Whelan, Apr. 25, 1864, vol. 4 (Apr.) for 1864, box 27, LRB.

28. Sherfy to Welles, Apr. 12, 1864, *ORN*, ser. 1, 19:558–62; Sherfy to Whelan, Apr. 25, 1864, vol. 4 (Apr.) for 1864, box 27, LRB.

29. D.F. [D.D.T.] Nestell, "Captivity in the South," *Philadelphia Inquirer*, Mar. 14, 1864, 2; Pledge, Feb. 2, 1864, Daniel D.T. Nestell Papers, Nimitz Library; Sherfy to Whelan, Apr. 25, 1864, vol. 4 (Apr.) for 1864, box 27, LRB. Nestell misrepresented Sherfy's name as "Shulz."

30. Charles Rivers Ellet to David D. Porter, Feb. 21, 1863, H.R. Exec. Doc. 1, 38th Cong., 1st sess., appendix pp. 437–40 (1863); D.G. Farragut to Welles, Feb. 26, 1863, *ORN*, ser. 1, 19:453; *Portrait and Biographical Record*, 379–80.

Chapter 10

1. Navy Department, *Instructions for the Government* (1864), 10, 14, 16, 50.

2. "Position of the Society"; Howard, *Improved System*, 293–94, 337–38.

3. Boyer, *Naval Surgeon*, 260; Wood and Bache, *Dispensatory*, 914–24, 1091–95; Warner, *Therapeutic Perspective*, 96–97, 124–27, 220–27.

4. Hammond, Circular No. 6.

5. William Whelan to N. Pinkney, July 31, 1863, vol. 25, LSB.

6. Tickets for John L. Brandt, July 14, 1864, Memphis, TN, 1863–64, and for Edward B. Edson, Feb. 1, 1862, Chelsea, MA, 1862, entry 25, RG 52; Hasegawa, "We Got Up," 294; Hasegawa, *Confederate Navy Medical Corps*, 147; Fuller, *Rheumatism, Rheumatic Gout, and Sciatica*, 108–14; Channing, "Alkaline Treatment of Rheumatism."

7. Hepworth, *Whip, Hoe, and Sword*, 296–97; Ticket for Michael O'Hearn, Jan. 25, 1862, Chelsea, MA, 1862, and for David Wilson, Apr. 16, 1863, New York, NY, 1863, pt. 1, entry 25, RG 52; Salter, *Asthma*, 265; Yeoman, *Catarrh*, 81; Paoli, "Double Pneumonia"; Wood, *Treatise on Practice of Medicine*, 2:29–30.

8. Bradshaw, *Anatomy of Dyspepsia*, 86; Flint, "Conservative Medicine," 1044; Ticket for William Jennings, Sept. 12, 1863, Norfolk, 1861–64, pt. 2, entry 25, RG 52.

9. Whelan to W.S.W. Ruschenberger, Sept. 3, 1861, vol. 22, LSB; Whelan to Pinkney, July 31, 1863, vol. 25, LSB; Wood and Bache, *Dispensatory*; Ellis, *Medical Formulary*; Griffith, *Universal Formulary*.

10. Whelan to B.F. Gibbs, May 23, 1863, vol. 24, LSB; Whelan to W.C. Foster, June 18, 1863, vol. 25, LSB.

11. Sayre, "Oakum as a Substitute for Lint"; Whelan to A. Hutchins, S.D. Flagg, and S.R. Forman, Sept. 16, 1862, and to James M. Green, Sept. 17, 1862, vol. 22A, LSB. Surgeon W.S.W. Ruschenberger,

serving at the Boston Navy Yard, had read the article before receiving it from Whelan and wrote to a medical journal stating that the oakum article's "assumptions are untenable, and its arguments illogical." He told Whelan he would nevertheless obey his directive to issue oakum in place of lint. Ruschenberger to Whelan, Sept. 27, 1862, vol. 4 (Sept.–Oct.) for 1862, box 12, LRB; Ruschenberger, "Oakum as a Substitute for Lint."

12. Whelan to C.D. Maxwell, July 21, 1864, vol. 27, LSB; Garratt, *Medical Electricity*, 11–12; Mitchell, Morehouse, and Keen, *Gunshot Wounds*, 136–42.

13. Act of Aug. 29, 1842, ch. 267, §§ 1, 5, 5 Stat. 546, 547 (1850); Act of July 14, 1862, ch 164, § 4, 12 Stat. 561, 565 (1865); Gideon Welles, Circular Letter, Sept. 16, 1862, roll 2, microfilm M977, RG 45; Welles, General Order no. 29, Feb. 1, 1864; roll 1, microfilm M984, RG 45.

14. P. Drayton to S.F. Du Pont, Apr. 14, 1862, *ORN*, ser. 1, 12:741–42; Drayton to Du Pont, May 11, 1862, *ORN*, ser. 1, 13:3–4.

15. Navy Department, *Instructions for the Government* (1857), 13; Navy Department, *Instructions for the Government* (1864), 13; Navy Department, *Allowances*, 128.

16. Wood and Bache, *Dispensatory*, 62–67; Merritt, "Quinine as a Prophylactic"; Derby, "Use of Quinine."

17. Charles Wilkes to Gideon Welles, Aug. 15, 1862, *ORN*, ser. 1, 7:651–52; William Maxwell Wood to S.P. Lee, Sept. 13, 1863, folder for 1811–88 (treatment, methods of), box 217 (subject MT), entry 502, RG 45.

18. Whelan to G.R.B. Horner, Nov. 19, 1862, vol. 22A, LSB; John J. Abernethy to Whelan, Mar. 7 1863, vol. 2 (Mar.) for 1863, box 15, LRB; Whelan to Abernethy, Mar. 9, 1863, vol. 24, LSB.

19. Whelan to James Suddards, July 26, 1862, RG 52, enty1, vol. 22A.

20. Whelan to J.L. Fox, June 3, 1864, vol. 27, LSB; George Clymer to Whelan, July 27, 1863, vol.6 (July) for 1863, box 18, LRB.

21. Whelan memorandum, Aug. 4, 1863, vol. 25, LSB; Whelan to Suddards, July 26, 1862, vol. 22A, LSB.

22. Whelan to J.C. Palmer, July 29, 1864, vol. 27, LSB; Whelan to G.R.B. Horner, Nov. 19, 1862, vol. 22A, LSB.

23. Whelan to S. Sharp, July 1, 1863, vol. 25, LSB; Act of Mar. 3, 1851, ch. 34, § 1, 9 Stat. 621 (1851).

24. Whelan memorandum to Gideon Welles, Mar. 7, 1864, vol. 26, LSB.

25. Whelan to Welles, Dec. 31, 1864, vol. 29, LSB.

26. Whelan to Welles, Dec. 31, 1864, vol. 29, LSB; "Professor Morgan's Plan."

27. Whelan to Welles, Dec. 31, 1864, vol. 29, LSB.

28. Whelan to Welles, Dec. 26, 1861, and to Clymer, Dec. 28, 1861, vol. 23, LSB.

29. J.C. Spear to William Maxwell Wood, July 29, 1862, vol. 3 (July–Aug.) for 1862, box 11, LRB; Sherman, *Memoirs*, 391; Wood to Welles Aug. 2, 1862, *ORN*, ser. 1, 7:616–18.

30. Whelan to Bailliere Brothers, July 27, 1863, vol. 25, LSB; Farquharson, "Scurvy in the Navy"; Act of July 18, 1861, ch. 7, 12 Stat. 264 (1865).

31. Wood to Welles Aug. 2, 1862, *ORN*, ser. 1, 7:616–18; Whelan to Welles, Aug. 5, 1862, vol. 22A, LSB.

32. Samuel W. Abbott to Clymer, July 1, 1863, C. Ellery Stedman to Clymer, July 1 and 14, 1863, W.L. Wheeler to Clymer, July 4, 1863, and Clymer to Whelan, July 10, 1863, vol. 6 (July) for 1863, box 18, LRB; Holden, "Inquiry."

33. Abbott to Clymer, July 1, 1863, Stedman to Clymer, July 1 and 14, 1863, and Wheeler to Clymer, July 4, 1863, vol. 6 (July) for 1863, box 18, LRB.

34. Wheeler to Clymer, July 4, 1863, vol. 6 (July) for 1863, box 18, LRB; Tryon, "Naval Architecture and Sanitation."

35. Clymer to Whelan, Mar. 26, 1863, vol. 2 (Mar.) for 1863, box 15, LRB; Whelan to Clymer, Apr. 4, 1863, vol. 24, LSB; Condy, *Disinfection*, 81–88.

36. Whelan to Clymer, Apr. 4, 1863, vol. 24, LSB; Wheeler to Clymer, July 4, 1863, vol. 6 (July) for 1863, box 18, LRB.

37. Stedman to Clymer, July 1 and 14, 1863, and Wheeler to Clymer, July 4, 1863, vol. 6 (July) for 1863, box 18, LRB; Tryon, "Naval Architecture and Sanitation"; Holden, "Inquiry."

38. William F. Jeffers to L.M. Goldsborough, May 22, 1862, *ORN*, ser. 1, 7:410–13; G.H. Perkins to D.G. Farragut, Oct. 13, 1864, *ORN*, ser. 1, 2:681–82.

39. Horwitz, BUMED Report (Nov. 1, 1865), 390; Moss, *Edgar Holden*, 110.

40. The possibility of a toxin introduced during construction was raised by two of the author's consultants: F. Terry Hambrecht, MD, and Jonathan O'Neal, MD.

41. Horwitz, BUMED Report (Nov. 1, 1865), 389–92, 410–21; Wheeler to Clymer, July 4, 1863, vol. 6 (July) for 1863, box 18, LRB.

Chapter 11

1. James C. Palmer, General Order, Jan. 6, 1864, vol. 5 (May) for 1864, box 28, LRB.

2. George Clymer to William Whelan, July 20, 1863, vol. 6 (July) for 1863, box 18, LRB; Horwitz, BUMED Report (Oct. 25, 1867), 254.

3. Clymer to Whelan, July 20, 1863, vol. 6 (July) for 1863, box 18, LRB.

4. John A. Dahlgren to Gideon Welles, July 20, 1863, *ORN* ser. 1, 14:376.

5. C. Ellery Stedman to Clymer, July 14, 1863, vol. 6 (July) for 1863, box 18, LRB.

6. D.G. Farragut to Welles, June 3, 1862, *ORN*, ser. 1, 18:577–79; Chatelain, "Turnover and Turmoil off Charleston"; Dahlgren to Wells, Sept. 2, 1863, roll 144, microfilm M89, RG 45.

7. Whelan, BUMED Report (Nov. 4, 1864), 1176; Horwitz, BUMED Report (Nov. 1, 1865), 385; *Statistics of the United States*, 44–47, 212–14; Kennedy, *Population of the United States*, 592–97. In 1863 and 1864 combined, 2,421 deaths were reported from squadrons, hospitals, receiving ships, and navy yards combined. Those deaths accounted for 73% of the 3,310 reported deaths from all causes for the entire navy during the same years.

8. Whelan, BUMED Report (Oct. 28, 1862), 897–98; Whelan, BUMED Report (Oct. 23, 1863), 1054–55; Whelan, BUMED Report (Nov. 4, 1864), 1175–76; Horwitz, BUMED Report (Nov. 1, 1865), 384–85; Horwitz, BUMED Report (Nov. 1, 1866), 195–96.

9. Whelan, BUMED Report (Oct. 28, 1862), 897–98; Whelan, BUMED Report (Oct. 23, 1863), 1054–55; Whelan, BUMED Report (Nov. 4, 1864), 1175–76; Horwitz, BUMED Report (Nov. 1, 1865), 384–85, 387; Horwitz, BUMED Report (Nov. 1, 1866), 195–96; Bollet, *Civil War Medicine*, 257.

10. Whelan, BUMED Report (Oct. 23, 1863), 1055; Whelan, BUMED Report (Nov. 4, 1864), 1176; Horwitz, BUMED Report (Nov. 1, 1865), 386.

11. Horwitz, BUMED Report (Oct. 25, 1867), 220–302.

12. Horwitz, BUMED Report (Oct. 25, 1867), 220–302.

13. Horwitz, BUMED Report (Oct. 25, 1867), 220–302. Computation of per-man figures for the war requires averaging of estimated average yearly complements. The latter must be weighted when figures were not collected for entire years.

14. Horwitz, BUMED Report (Oct. 25, 1867), 220–302; William Maxwell Wood to William Whelan, July 13, 1863, vol. 6 (July) for 1863, box 18, LRB.

15. Horwitz, BUMED Report (Oct. 25, 1867), 220–302.

16. "Treatment of Malarial Disease," in *Medical and Surgical History*, vol. 1, pt. 3, 176–82; Wood, *Treatise on Practice of Medicine*, 1:273.

17. Horwitz, BUMED Report (Oct. 25, 1867), 220–302; Keen, "Surgical Reminiscences," 109; Billings, "Medical Reminiscences,"116; Bollet, *Civil War Medicine*, 276; Hospital Surgeon, "Hints and Observations," 263–65.

18. Horwitz, BUMED Report (Oct. 25, 1867), 220–302; Bollet, *Civil War Medicine*, 272–77.

19. Horwitz, BUMED Report (Oct. 25, 1867), 220–302.

20. Theodorus Bailey to Gideon Welles, July 27, 1864, *ORN*, ser. 1, 17:737–39; "Gen. Butler on Yellow Fever"; Bollet, *Civil War Medicine*, 296–304.

21. Theodore P. Greene to Welles, Aug. 16, 1864, William J. Eldredge to Welles, Aug. 24, 1864, and William L. Martine to Welles, Sept. 28, 1864, *ORN*, ser. 1, 17:746–47; 748–49, 761–62; T. Bailey, Stations of vessels comprising the East Gulf Blockading Squadron, May 1, 1864, *ORN*, ser. 1, 17:691; Navy Department, *Dictionary of American Naval Fighting Ships*, 6:149; Welles, *Report of the Secretary* (1864), ix.

22. Theodorus Bailey to Welles, July 27, 1864, and Eldredge to Welles, Aug. 24, 1864, *ORN*, ser. 1, 17:737–39, 748–49;

Horwitz, BUMED Report (Oct. 25, 1867), 273.

23. Bartlett, *History, Diagnosis, and Treatment*, 561–73; "Proceedings of Societies," 57.

24. Martine to Welles, Sept. 28, 1864, *ORN*, ser. 1, 17:761–62; Lee, "Remarks on Disinfectants."

25. Horwitz, BUMED Report (Oct. 25, 1867), 220–302; Private Diary of Commander H.H. Bell, entry for July 13, 1862, *ORN*, ser. 1, 18:715; D.G. Farragut to Theodore P. Greene, Oct. 15, 1864, *ORN*, ser. 1, 21:687; R.O. Mason to Whelan, Dec. 31, 1863, vol. 11 (Dec.) for 1863, box 23, LRB.

26. D.C. Peters, "Extract from a Narrative of his Services in the Medical Staff," *Medical and Surgical History*, vol. 1, pt. 1, appendix, 234–35; Wood, *Treatise on Practice of Medicine*, 1:444–47.

27. Edward Shippen to Whelan, May 9, 1864, vol. 5 (May) for 1864, box 28, LRB; Whelan to H. M Welles, Aug. 8 1864; vol. 28, LSB.

28. Horwitz, BUMED Report (Oct. 25, 1867), 220–302.

29. Wood, *Treatise on Practice of Medicine*, 1:386–90.

30. Horwitz, BUMED Report (Oct. 25, 1867), 220–302.

31. Horwitz, BUMED Report (Oct. 25, 1867), 220–302; Bollet, *Civil War Medicine*, 365.

32. Wood to Welles Aug. 2, 1862, *ORN*, ser. 1, 7:616–18; Ticket for Joseph Colton, July 30, 1863, June–Dec. 1863, New Orleans, entry 25, RG 52.

33. Wood, *Treatise on Practice of Medicine*, 1:615–16; Boyer, *Naval Surgeon*, 82, 298.

34. Horwitz, BUMED Report (Oct. 25, 1867), 220–302; Wood, *Treatise on Practice of Medicine*, 1:805.

35. Horwitz, BUMED Report (Oct. 25, 1867), 220–302; Wood, *Treatise on Practice of Medicine*, 2:22–26.

36. Wood, *Treatise on Practice of Medicine*, 2:90–96; Cotton, *Consumption*, 201–40.

37. Horwitz, BUMED Report (Oct. 25, 1867), 220–302; Bollet, "Rheumatic Diseases "; Bollet, *Civil War Medicine*, 307–12; Watson, *Principles and Practice of Physic*, 1056–70.

38. Fuller, *Rheumatism*, 108, 113–14; Wood, *Treatise on Therapeutics*, 2:337, 349–50, 392–95.

39. Horwitz, BUMED Report (Oct. 25, 1867), 220–302.

40. Horwitz, BUMED Report (Oct. 25, 1867), 220–302.

41. Bumstead, *Pathology and Treatment*, 55–78; Horwitz, BUMED Report (Oct. 25, 1867), 220–302.

42. Bumstead, *Pathology and Treatment*, 394–421, 508.

43. Horwitz, BUMED Report (Oct. 25, 1867), 220–302.

44. McQuillen, "Dentists in the Army and Navy"; Boyer, *Naval Surgeon*, 115.

45. John P. Kennedy to Thomas Harris, Feb. 16 and 24, 1853, RG 45, M480, roll 1; Harris to Kennedy, Feb. 21 and 25, 1853, roll 11, microfilm M480, RG 45.

46. Harris to Kennedy, Feb. 25, 1853, roll 11, microfilm M518, RG 45; Field, *Dental Education at the Crossroads*, 39–40.

47. S.H. Stringham to Welles, May 8, 1861, *ORN*, ser. 1, 5:625–26.

48. E. Orville Matthews to H. Paulding, June 22, 1863, *ORN*, ser. 1, 2:298–99.

49. Wilson, *Naval Hygiene*, 37–38; Horner, *Diseases and Injuries of Seamen*, 151–52.

50. Horwitz, BUMED Report (Oct. 25, 1867), 220–302.

51. Horwitz, BUMED Report (Oct. 25, 1867), 220–302; Ticket for H.E. Pinkham, Aug. 7, 1864, Pensacola, 1864, entry 25, RG 52.

52. Horwitz, BUMED Report (Oct. 25, 1867), 220–302. Dunglison's medical dictionary equates *submersio* with submersion (plunging in a liquid) and applies *asphyxia immersorum* to drowning. Harris's medical dictionary also equates *submersio* with submersion but adds, "the act of plunging under water; drowning." Dunglison, *Medical Lexicon*, 878; Chapin A. Harris, *Dictionary of Medical Terminology*, 709.

53. Whelan to Henry Wilson, Feb. 2, 1863, vol. 24, LSB; Hasegawa, *Mending Broken Soldiers*, 3.

Chapter 12

1. Time Table of the U.S. Supply Steamer Newberne, ca. Nov. 1863, vol. 10 (Nov.) for 1863, box 22, LRB; *NDR* (to

Jan. 1, 1864), 158. The steamer's name appears as *Newberne, Newbern, New Berne*, and *New Bern*.

2. D.G. Farragut to Gideon Welles, Aug. 5, 1864, James E. Jouett to Farragut, Aug. 8, 1864, Alexander Asboth to George B. Drake, Aug. 6, 1864, and Abstract Log of the U.S.S. *Seminole*, Aug. 6, 1864, *ORN*, ser. 1, 21:405–406; 442–43; 522, 852–53.

3. Dixon, "White Lily," 7.

4. Thomas Dillard to L.M. Goldsborough, Oct. 9, 1861, folder 2 (hospital administration), box 206 (subject MA), entry 502, RG 45. In Dillard's October 9 letter, he referred to Goldsborough as the flag officer of the NABS, although the division of the Atlantic Blockading Squadron into the NABS and SABS was not considered official until October 29, 1861. *ORN*, ser. 1, 6:313–14.

5. Statistical Data of Ships: United States Vessels, *ORN*, ser. 1, 2:44; "Important from Fortress Monroe," *New York Herald*, Nov. 13, 1861, 5.

6. Tickets for John H. Davis, Dec. 1861, Thomas J. Dumont, Dec. 26, 1861, and John Devine, Apr. 5, 1862, Norfolk, 1861–64, entry 25, RG 52; Gideon Welles to Goldsborough, June 17, 1862, folder 2 (hospital administration), box 206 (subject MA), entry 502, RG 45; William Whelan to Solomon Sharp, June 20, 1862, vol. 23, LSB; William Maxwell Wood to G.J. Van Brunt, Mar. 10, 1862, *ORN*, ser. 1, 7:12; Goldsborough to Welles, May 21 and Aug. 1, 1862, *ORN*, ser. 1, 7:406–407, 608.

7. Goldsborough to Welles, Aug. 1, 1862, *ORN*, ser. 1, 7:406–407; Goldsborough to Welles, July 4, 1862, roll 158, microfilm M89, RG 45; Wood to Whelan, May 20 and June 13, 1862, vol. 2 (Apr.–June) for 1862, box 10, LRB; Wood to S.P. Lee, Nov. 5, 1863, vol. 10 (Nov.) for 1863, box 22, LRB.

8. George Clymer to Whelan, Feb. 22, 1862, vol. 1 (Jan.–Mar.) for 1862, box 9, LRB; Augustus S. Baldwin to S.F. Du Pont, Apr. 19, 1862, *ORN*, ser. 1, 1:349–52; G.V. Fox to L.M. Goldsborough, Dec 3, 1861, *ORN*, ser. 1, 6:462.

9. Tickets for William S. Kimball, Apr. 30, 1862, and for John P. Mullen, July 20, 1864, Port Royal, SC, entry 25, RG 52; Entry for Dec. 24, 1863, Logbook of USS *Vermont*, Dec. 18, 1863–July 29, 1864, and USS *New Hampshire*, July 30, 1864–Oct. 8, 1864, entry 118, RG 24; Entries for USS *Vermont*, p. 81, entry 41, RG 52; Whelan, BUMED Report (Oct. 23, 1863), 1060; W. Johnson to Whelan, Oct. 21, 1863, vol. 9 (Oct.) for 1863, box 21, LRB.

10. Gideon Welles to John A. Dahlgren, July 25, 1864, *ORN*, ser. 1, 15:579; Dahlgren to Welles, June 29 and July 9, 1864, *ORN*, ser. 1, 15:545–46, 564–65; S.C. Rowan to William Johnson, Mar. 21, 1864, *ORN*, ser. 1, 15:371; USS *New Hampshire*, report of sick for second and third quarters, 1864, South Atlantic Blockading Squadron, entry 25, RG 52; Entries for USS *Vermont* and *New Hampshire*, pp. 81, 393, entry 41, RG 52; Tickets for George E. Gross, July 29, 1864, and Peter Heath, Mar. 22, 1865, Port Royal, SC, entry 25, RG 52; Whelan, BUMED Report (Nov. 4, 1864), 1182.

11. USS *Home*, report of sick for second through fourth quarters, 1864, and first quarter, 1865, South Atlantic Blockading Squadron, entry 25, RG 52; Tickets for Alexander J. Mulholland, July 20, 1864, George J. Houghton, Dec. 10, 1864, and James M. Watrous, Oct. 6, 1864, Port Royal, SC, entry 25, RG 52; Whelan, BUMED Report (Nov. 4, 1864), 1182.

12. James C. Palmer to H.K. Thatcher, Apr. 19, 1865, *ORN*, ser. 1, 22:132–33; Theodorus Bailey, Stations of Vessels Composing the East Gulf Blockading Squadron, August 1, 1863, *ORN*, ser. 1, 17:524; Charles Steedman to D.D. Porter, Dec. 30, 1864, and J.F. Schenck to Porter, Jan. 17, 1865, *ORN*, ser. 1, 11:327–28, 534; Whelan to J.L. Fox, May 20, 1864, vol. 27, LSB; William W. McKean to Welles, May 26, 1862, *ORN*, ser. 1, 17:252.

13. Testimony of George N. Hollins, Extract from report of evidence..., *ORN*, ser. 1, 22:842. More has been written about *Red Rover* than any other Civil War hospital ship. Kenney, "From the Log of the Red Rover"; Fowler, "Relief on the River."

14. A.M. Pennock to Charles H. Davis, May 10, 1862, Davis to Pennock, May 12, 1862, and George D. Wise to A.H. Foote, May 25, 1862, *ORN*, ser. 1, 23:89–90, 91–92, 105–107; Wise to M.C. Meigs, Sept. 14, 1863, in Meigs, *Report of the Quartermaster General*, 800–801.

15. Pennock to Davis, June 10, 1862, and Wise to Foote, June 12, 1862, *ORN*, ser. 1, 23:148–49, 153–54; Fowler, "Relief on the River"; *Report of the Western Sanitary Commission*, 17–20.

16. Forman, *Western Sanitary Commission*, 54; Lyman, *Historical Sketch*, 13–18; ZB file for George H. Bixby, Navy Department Library; Bixby to Davis, June 3, 1862, *ORN*, ser. 1, 23:114; Navy Department, Code of Regulations, 42; Statement for George H. Bixby, p. 30, entry 44, RG 52.

17. List of Officers and Men on USN Str. *Red Rover*, roll 18, microfilm T829, RG 45; Davis to Welles, June 20, 1862, *ORN*, ser. 1, 23:177–78; Kenney, "From the Log of the Red Rover," 35, 40–41.

18. Davis, General Order, June 14 1862, *ORN*, ser. 1, 23:206–207.

19. Kenney, "From the Log of the Red Rover."

20. Davis to Wise, June 14, 1862, *ORN*, ser. 1, 23:207–208.

21. Davis to Bixby, June 24, 1862, *ORN*, ser. 1, 23:179; James M. Barnard to Whelan, Dec. 29, 1863, vol. 11 (Dec.) for 1863, box 23, LRB. Bixby, a skilled photographer, recorded numerous images of naval vessels, including *Red Rover*. Toll et al., "George Holmes Bixby."

22. Act of July 16, 1862, ch. 185, 12 Stat. 587 (1865); Wise to Meigs, Sept. 14, 1863, in Meigs, *Report of the Quartermaster General*, 800–801; Porter, General Order No. 80, Aug. 19, 1863, vol. 8 (Sept.) for 1863, box 20, LRB; Kenney, "From the Log of the Red Rover," 36, 47.

23. Wise to Bixby, Sept. 16, 1862, George H. Bixby Papers, Abraham Lincoln Presidential Library; Davis to Bixby, June 24, 1862, *ORN*, ser. 1, 23:179; A.M. Pennock to Davis, June 10, 1862, *ORN*, ser. 1, 23:148–49; David D. Porter to Welles, June 1, 1863, with enclosure, *ORN*, ser. 1, 25:145–46; Porter to Welles, May 21, 1864, with enclosure, *ORN*, ser. 1, 26:319–20.

24. Kenney, "From the Log of the Red Rover"; Porter, General Order no. 30, Jan. 7, 1863, *ORN*, ser. 1, 24:100; Porter, Special Order, June 23, 1863, *ORN*, ser. 1, 25:91–92; Statistical Data on Ships, *ORN*, ser. 2, 1:189.

25. Lieber, *Instructions for the Government of Armies*, 34; Woolsey, "Naval War Code"; Stockton, *Laws and Usages*, 14–17. In an 1885 book of anecdotes, Porter wrote that the Mississippi Squadron's fleet surgeon, Ninian Pinkney, asked that *Red Rover* be equipped with a gun for defense and signal purposes. According to the account, Porter believed a gun unnecessary because no civilized nation would fire on a hospital vessel, but he appeased the unwitting Pinkney by having what appeared to be a 32-pounder rifle—actually an imitation made of wood—placed on the vessel's bow. One reviewer of Porter's book referred to the anecdotes as sailors' yarns that should not be judged by the same standard of accuracy applied to "deliberate historical statements." Porter, *Incident and Anecdotes*, 202–3; Review of *Incidents and Anecdotes*.

26. Statement for George Hopkins, p. 158, entry 44, RG 52; Edward Gilchrist, Adrian Hudson, and Bixby to D.D. Porter, Nov. 16, 1862, roll 307, microfilm M148, RG 45; Ninian Pinkney to Whelan, Sept. 22, 1863, vol. 20, vol. 8 (Sept.) for 1863, box 23, LRB; ZB file for George Hopkins, Navy Department Library; Hopkins to W.H. Macomb, [Nov. 1, 1864?], *ORN*, ser. 1, 11:24; Entry for Pinkney, roll 9, microfilm M330, RG 24. In his 1885 book, Porter wrote that he considered Pinkney to be the de factor commander of *Red Rover*, since that vessel's captain was directed to obey all of Pinkney's commands. Porter, *Incidents and Anecdotes*, 202–3.

27. Kenney, "From the Log of the Red Rover," 48; Dixon, "White Lily," 7; Fowler, "Relief on the River."

28. Porter to A.M. Pennock, Dec. 12, 1862, *ORN*, ser. 1, 23:624; K.R. Breese to Porter, May 6, 1863, *ORN*, ser. 1, 24:654–55; Le Roy Fitch to Porter, Sept. 8, 1864, *ORN*, ser. 1, 26:553–54; Porter, General Order No. 199, May 27, 1864, *ORN*, ser. 1, 26:329–30; Horwitz, BUMED Report (Nov. 1, 1865), 384; Horwitz, BUMED Report (Nov. 1, 1866), 195.

Chapter 13

1. William Whelan to Gideon Welles, Mar. 22, 1862, vol. 23, LSB.

2. Thurm, *For the Relief of the Sick and Wounded*, 423, 466–69; Whelan to J.L. Fox, July 28, 1862, vol. 22A, LSB.

3. Austin, "Historical Sketch," 274–76; Whelan, BUMED Report (Nov. 4, 1864), 1180; Horwitz, BUMED Report (Nov. 1, 1865), 388.

4. Report of the Board of Visitors, Oct. 1, 1861; Report of the Board of Visitors, Oct. 1, 1862; Otto, *St. Elizabeths Hospital*, 74; Whelan, BUMED Report (Oct. 23, 1863), 1060; Whelan, BUMED Report (Nov. 4, 1864), 1182.

5. Report of the Board of Visitors, Oct. 1, 1861; Whelan to Welles, June 8, 1861, roll 16, microfilm M518, RG 45; Entry for temporary hospital, Washington, p. 46, entry 41, RG 52; F.M. Gunnell to Whelan, Oct. 12, 1863, vol. 9 (Oct.) for 1863, box 21, LRB.

6. Whelan, BUMED Report (Oct. 23, 1863), 1060, 1070; Whelan, BUMED Report (Nov. 4, 1864), 1182; Act of Mar. 14, 1864, ch. 30, 13 Stat. 22, 26 (1866); Act of Mar. 2, 1865, ch. 74, §§ 1, 6, 13 Stat. 462, 465, 467 (1866); Whelan to Ammi B. Young, Oct. 14, 1864, vol. 28, LSB.

7. Horwitz, BUMED Report (Nov. 1, 1865), 389; Horwitz, BUMED Report (Nov. 1, 1866), 201; "The Naval Hospital," *National Republican* (Washington, D.C.), Nov. 14, 1866, 3.

8. Gideon Welles to L.M. Goldsborough, June 18, 1862, folder 2 (hospital administration), box 206 (subject MA), entry 502, RG 45.

9. William Maxwell Wood to Whelan, Oct. 15, 1862, vol. 4 (Sept.–Oct.) for 1862, box 12, LRB; Wood to Whelan, July 26, 1862, vol. 3 (July–Aug.) for 1862, box 11, LRB.

10. Wood to Whelan, June 21, 1862, vol. 2 (Apr.–June) for 1862, box 10, LRB; Whelan to Solomon Sharp, June 20, 1862, vol. 23, LSB.

11. Whelan to Wood, Oct. 1, 1862, vol. 22A, LSB; Wood to Whelan, Oct. 15, 1862, vol. 4 (Sept.–Oct.) for 1862, box 12, LRB.

12. Wood to Whelan, Oct. 9, 1862, vol. 4 (Sept.–Oct.) for 1862, box 12, LRB; Whelan to Wood, Oct. 14, 1862, vol. 22A, LSB; "The Beaufort Hospital and Sisters of Mercy," *Newbern (NC) Weekly Progress*, Oct. 26, 1862, 2; Whelan to J.L. Fox, May 20, 1864, vol. 27, LSB. A listing of medical officers' assignments suggests that USS *Louisiana* served as a hospital ship while near Washington, North Carolina. Entry for USS *Louisiana*, p. 243, entry 41, RG 52.

13. Wood to Whelan, Oct. 9, 1862, vol. 4 (Sept.–Oct.) for 1862, box 12, LRB.

14. Wood to Whelan, Oct. 9, 1862, vol. 4 (Sept.–Oct.) for 1862, box 12, LRB; Wood to Whelan, July 13, 1863, vol. 6 (July) for 1863, box 18, LRB.

15. C.W. Flussser to Stephen C. Rowan, Aug. 22, 1862, *ORN*, ser. 1, 7: 666–68; George W. Gale to Wood, Sept. 21, 1862, and Wood to Whelan, Oct. 9, 1862, vol. 4 (Sept.–Oct.) for 1862, box 12, LRB; Wood to Whelan, July 13, 1863, vol. 6 (July) for 1863, box 18, LRB.

16. Wood to Whelan, Oct. 9, 1862, vol. 4 (Sept.–Oct.) for 1862, box 12, LRB.

17. Ticket for Edmund Danner, Oct. 15, 1862, Norfolk, 1861–64, pt. 1, entry 25, RG 52; Wood to Whelan, July 13, 1863, vol. 6 (July) for 1863, box 18, LRB; J.L. Fox to William H. Macomb, Aug. 16, 1864, folder 2 (hospital administration), box 206 (subject MA), entry 502, RG 45.

18. Wood to Whelan, Aug. 31, 1863, vol. 7 (Aug.) for 1863, box 19, LRB; Fox to Macomb, Aug. 16, 1864, folder 2 (hospital administration), box 206 (subject MA), entry 502, RG 45.

19. Macomb to Gideon Welles, Oct. 6, 1864, *ORN*, ser. 1, 10: 529–30; Herman P. Babcock to A.C. Rhind, with endorsement, Mar. 18, 1865, folder 2 (hospital administration), box 206 (subject MA), entry 502, RG 45.

20. Whelan, BUMED Report (Nov. 4, 1864), 1175; Horwitz, BUMED Report (Nov. 1, 1865), 384.

21. William Johnson to Whelan, Oct. 21, 1863, vol. 9 (Oct.) for 1863, box 21, LRB.

22. Johnson to Whelan, Oct. 21, 1863, Johnson to Dahlgren, Oct. 19, 1864, and Dahlgren to Johnson, Oct. 20, 1863, vol. 9 (Oct.) for 1863, box 21, LRB.

23. Dahlgren to Welles, Aug. 4, 1864, roll 149, microfilm M89, RG 45.

24. Johnson to Whelan, Mar. 17, 1864, vol. 3 (Mar.) for 1864, box 26, LRB; Whelan to Welles Apr. 11, 1864, vol. 26, LSB.

25. Whelan to Johnson, Apr. 23, 1864, vol. 26, LSB; "Sale of Lands for Unpaid Direct Taxes in Insurrectionary Districts, State of South Carolina." *Free South* (Beaufort, SC), Jan. 10, 1863, 3; Act

of Aug. 5, 1861, ch. 45, 12 Stat. 242 (1865); Act of June 7, 1862, ch. 98, 12 Stat. 422, 425 (1865); Act of Feb. 6, 1863, ch. 21, 12 Stat. 640 (1865).

26. Johnson to Whelan, Mar. 18, 1864, vol. 3 (Mar.) for 1864, box 26, LRB; Johnson to Whelan, Apr. 22, 1864, vol. 4 (Apr.) for 1864, box 27, LRB; Whelan to Welles, Apr. 11, 1864, vol. 26. LSB; Whelan to Johnson, June 10, 1864, and Whelan to George H. Davies, July 22, 1864, vol. 27, LSB; Whelan to Johnson, Aug. 25 and Sept. 17, 1864, vol. 28, LSB; William Lowber to Dahlgren, July 13, 1864, roll 149, microfilm M89, RG 45. The extent to which the hospital building was prefabricated in the North is not clearly indicated in Whelan's and Johnson's correspondence.

27. Whelan, BUMED Report (Nov. 4, 1864), 1182; Horwitz, BUMED Report (Nov. 1, 1865), 384, 389; Horwitz, BUMED Report (Nov. 1, 1866),195, 201.

28. Whelan to Welles, Dec. 4, 1861, vol. 22, LSB; Whelan to unidentified recipient, Apr. 2, 1862, vol. 23, LSB; William W. McKean to Welles, Mar. 24, 1862; W.F. Cornick, Extracts from a Narrative of His Services, *Medical and Surgical History*, vol. 1, pt. 1, p 246.

29. Whelan to David Thacker Lewis, Apr. 12, 1862, and to John Conrad, June 12, 1862, vol. 23, LSB; Tickets, Key West, 1859–70, entry 25, RG 52.

30. G.R.B. Horner to James L. Lardner, Aug. 1, 1862, roll 198, microfilm M89, RG 45; Lardner to Welles, Aug. 1, 1862, and Horner to Theodorus Bailey, Dec. 24, 1862, *ORN*, ser. 1, 17: 294, 340.

31. Death notice, *North American and United States Gazette* (Philadelphia), Sept. 25, 1863, 2; Tickets, Key West, 1859–70, entry 25, RG 52.

32. Theodorus Bailey to Welles, July 27, 1864, *ORN*, ser. 1, 17:737–39.

33. Tickets, Key West, 1859–70, entry 25, RG 52.

34. Whelan to G.R.B. Horner, May 23, 1862, vol. 23, LSB; B.F. Gibbs to Welles, Oct. 24, 1862, roll 305, microfilm M148, RG 45; D.G. Farragut to N.P. Banks, Jan. 27, 1863, *ORN*, ser. 1, 21:62; Horwitz, BUMED Report (Nov. 1, 1866), 202; James C. Palmer to Whelan, Mar. 17, 1864, vol. 3 (Mar.) for 1864, box 26, LRB.

35. W. Smith to Whelan, May 27, 1863, and B.F. Gibbs to Smith, May 12, 1863, vol. 4 (May) for 1863, box 16, LRB; Whelan to W. Smith, June 10, 1863, and to J.C. Palmer, Aug. 10, 1863, vol. 25, LSB.

36. J.M. Foltz to Whelan, June 19, 1863, vol. 5 (June) for 1863, box 17, LRB; Palmer to Whelan, Mar. 17, 1863, vol. 3 (Mar.) for 1864, box 26, LRB; Whelan, BUMED Report (Nov. 4, 1864), 1181.

37. Beale, BUMED Report (Nov. 1, 1875), 101.

38. D.G. Farragut to Welles, Apr. 8, 1862, *ORN*, ser. 1, 18:109; "The Expedition Against New Orleans," *Boston Morning Journal*, Apr. 30, 1862, 4; "From the Mortar Fleet," *Evening Post* (New York), Apr. 29, 1862, 4.

39. "Below New-Orleans," *New York Times*, June 23, 1862, 8; John H. Clark to Welles, June 2, 1862, roll 293, microfilm M148, RG 45; C.H. Burbank to Medical Examining Board, Sept. 14, 1863, American Civil War Medical Antiques, Douglas Arbittier, accessed Nov. 19, 2024, https://www.medicalantiques.com/civilwar/Navy_surgeon_applications/Burbank_charles_H.htm; Farragut to P.C. Johnson, Aug. 22, 1862, *ORN*, ser. 1, 27:454–55.

40. Whelan to W.A. Hammond, Mar. 5, 1863, and to J.M. Foltz, May 22, 1863, vol. 24, LSB; Foltz to Whelan, June 19, 1863, vol. 5 (June) for 1863, box 17, LRB; Whelan to Foltz, June 27, 1863, and to J.C. Palmer, Aug. 10, 1863, vol. 25, LSB.

41. Whelan to Palmer, Aug. 10, 1862, vol. 25, LSB; Whelan to A.H. Rice, Feb. 17, 1864, vol. 26, LSB; Ticket for Patrick B. Carrick, July 20, 1863, New Orleans, 1863, entry 25, RG 52; Entry for New Orleans Hospital, p. 384, entry 41, RG 52; Advertisement for surgeon's steward, *Era* (New Orleans), May 1864, 3; Earp, *Yellow Flag*, 39. Despite hospital tickets showing admissions in late August 1863 and Whelan writing the same month about the facility's recent transfer to the navy, Whelan reported in November 1864 that the hospital opened in December 1863. There is no indication that the various references were to different buildings. Whelan, BUMED Report (Nov. 4, 1864), 1181–82.

42. Whelan, BUMED Report (Nov. 4, 1864), 1175; Horwitz, BUMED Report (Nov. 1, 1865), 384, 389; Horwitz, BUMED Report (Nov. 1, 1866), 195.

43. Kenney, "From the Log of the Red Rover," 40–41; A.M. Pennock to Charles H. Davis, Sept. 24, 1862, Edward Gilchrist to Pennock, Sept. 24, 1862, and E.C. Franklin to Gilchrist, Sept. 24, 1862, *ORN*, ser. 1, 23:375–76.

44. Entry for William Grier, roll 9, microfilm M330, RG 24; Tickets for George Brand, Oct. 18, 1862, and Josef Bahr, Oct. 16, 1862, Mississippi Squadron, entry 25, RG 52; William Grier to Whelan, Dec. 12, 1862; Ninian Pinkney to Whelan, Sept. 22, 1863, vol. 8 (Sept.) for 1863, box 20, LRB; *NDR* (to Jan. 1, 1863), 203.

45. Whelan to Grier, Dec. 12, 1862, vol. 22A, LSB.

46. Kenney, "From the Log of the Red Rover," 44–45; Pennock to D.D. Porter, Feb. 15, 1863, and N. Pinkney to Porter, Mar. 3, 1863, *ORN*, ser. 1, 24:416, 448; Whelan memorandum, June 27, 1863, and Whelan to Joseph J. Andrews, June 8, 1863 vol. 25, LSB; Whelan to Welles, June 27, 1863, roll 19, microfilm M518, RG 45; Whelan to Grier, May 27, 1864, vol. 27, LSB.

47. Whelan, BUMED Report (Oct. 23, 1863), 1060; Whelan, BUMED Report (Nov. 4, 1864), 1175, 1181; Hiram Beauchamp to Whelan, Oct. 3, 1863, vol. 9 (Oct.) for 1863, box 21, LRB; Entry for Mound City and Memphis Hospitals, p. 394, entry 41, RG 52. In its tables of hospital admissions, BUMED provided numbers for the hospital at Mound City, but not Memphis, through the end of the war, even though the former was closed in March 1863. The figure of 1,650 admissions at Memphis during 1863 (from the text of Whelan's Nov. 4, 1864, BUMED report) seems not to jibe with the 1,090 admissions at Mound City during 1863 (from a table in the same report).

48. Whelan to Welles, June 8, 1863, vol. 25, LSB; Grier to Whelan, Dec. 16, 1863, vol. 11 (Dec.) for 1863, box 23, LRB.

49. Tickets 1–300, 1863–64, pt. 1 (third quarter 1863), Memphis, entry 25, RG 52. No ticket for an African American patient clearly indicated admission to the navy-yard portion of the hospital. A notation for Coleman Sanders, a contraband who died of meningitis one day after admission, included "navy yard," but this could have referred to his workplace (ticket 223, third quarter 1863); Reidy, "Black Men in Navy Blue," 158.

50. Porter, General Order no. 76, July 26, 1863, *ORN*, ser. 1, 25:327–28; True, "Life aboard a Gunboat," 38.

51. Horwitz, BUMED Report (Nov. 1, 1865), 384, 389; Horwitz, BUMED Report (Nov. 1, 1866). 195. The admission figures appear in tables under a heading for the Mound City hospital, which ceased to exist in March 1863. The number are assumed to apply to the Memphis hospital.

52. Farenholt, "Historical Sketch"; Act of Mar. 3, 1863, ch. 118, 12 Stat. 814, 817 (1865).

53. Farenholt, "Historical Sketch"; Snyder, *Mare Island Naval Hospital*, 22–26; Whelan, BUMED Report (Oct. 23, 1863), 1057, 1060–61; Whelan to W.S. Bishop, May 13, 1863, vol. 24, LSB.

54. Farenholt, "Historical Sketch"; Snyder, *Mare Island Naval Hospital*, 22–26; Bishop to Whelan, Oct. 19, 1863, vol. 9 (Oct.) for 1863, box 21, LRB; Horwitz, BUMED Report (Nov. 1, 1865), 389.

Chapter 14

1. Whelan, BUMED Report (Oct. 22, 1861), 511.

2. Whelan, BUMED Report (Oct. 22, 1861), 511; Whelan, BUMED Report (Oct. 28, 1862), 900; Whelan, BUMED Report (Oct. 23, 1863), 1058; Whelan, BUMED Report (Nov. 4, 1864), 1180; Horwitz, BUMED Report (Nov. 1, 1865), 388; William Whelan to George H. Davies, June 7, 1864, vol. 27, LSB; Whelan to Gideon Welles, Mar. 28, 1862, vol. 23, LSB. Davies constructed multiple temporary structures for BUMED.

3. Entries for Boston Naval Hospital, pp. 11–13, entry 41, RG 52; Whelan, BUMED Report (Oct. 28, 1862), 897; Whelan, BUMED Report (Oct. 23, 1863), 1054; Whelan, BUMED Report (Nov. 4, 1864), 1175; Horwitz, BUMED Report (Nov. 1, 1865), 384; Horwitz, BUMED Report (Nov. 1, 1866), 195. The figures for 1865 are suspect. Horwitz reported in November 1865 that 903 patients had been treated at the hospital during the year, but his November 1866 report

showed 546 patients being admitted in 1865.

4. Whelan to Welles, Dec. 23, 1861, and Whelan memorandum, Feb. 1, 1862, vol. 23, LSB; Whelan, BUMED Report (Oct. 28, 1862), 900.

5. P.J. Horwitz telegram to Whelan, Mar. 20, 1862, and Whelan to Welles, Mar. 20, 1862, vol. 23, LSB; Whelan memorandum, Aug. 15, 1862, and Whelan to Welles, Nov. 20, 1862, roll 18, microfilm M518, RG 45; Whelan, BUMED Report (Oct. 23, 1863), 1058; Whelan, BUMED Report (Nov. 4, 1864), 1180.

6. Entries for New York Naval Hospital, pp. 19–21, 396–97, entry 41, RG 52; Whelan, BUMED Report (Oct. 22, 1862), 897; Whelan, BUMED Report (Oct. 23, 1863), 1054; Whelan, BUMED Report (Nov. 4, 1864), 1175; Horwitz, BUMED Report (Nov. 1, 1865), 384; Horwitz, BUMED Report (Nov. 1, 1866), 195.

7. Whelan to Welles, Mar. 28, 1862, vol. 23, LSB; Whelan, BUMED Report (Oct. 23, 1863), 1058–59; Whelan, BUMED Report (Nov. 4, 1864), 1181; Horwitz, BUMED Report (Nov. 1, 1866), 201.

8. Entries for Philadelphia Naval Hospital, pp. 26–28, entry 41, RG 52; Whelan, BUMED Report (Oct. 22, 1862), 897; Whelan, BUMED Report (Oct. 23, 1863), 1054; Whelan, BUMED Report (Nov. 4, 1864), 1175; Horwitz, BUMED Report (Nov. 1, 1865), 384; Horwitz, BUMED Report (Nov. 1, 1866), 195.

9. C.H. Wheelwright to James L. Lardner, May 18, 1862, and William Maxwell Wood to Whelan, May 19, 1862, vol. 2 (Apr.–June) for 1862, box 10, LRB.

10. Wood to Whelan, June 13, 1862, vol. 2 (Apr.–June) for 1862, box 10, LRB; Wood to Whelan, July 26, 1862, vol. 3 (July–Aug.) for 1862, box 11, LRB.

11. Whelan to Welles, July 7, 1862, and Whelan to Wood, July 22 and 26, 1862, vol. 22A, LSB.

12. Whelan to W.A. Hammond, Aug. 5, 1862, vol. 22A, LSB.

13. Entries for Norfolk Naval Hospital, pp. 42–44, entry 41, RG 52; Wood to Whelan, Sept. 2, 1862, vol. 4 (Sept.–Oct.) for 1862, box 12, LRB; Whelan to Solomon Sharp, Nov. 15, 1862, vol. 22A, LSB.

14. Whelan, BUMED Report (Oct. 23, 1863), 1054; Whelan, BUMED Report (Nov. 4, 1864), 1175; Horwitz, BUMED Report (Nov. 1, 1865), 384; Horwitz, BUMED Report (Nov. 1, 1866), 195; Whelan to Wood, Feb. 22, 1864, vol. 26, LSB; Whelan to Davies, June 8, 1864, vol. 27, LSB.

15. William Whelan to Gideon Welles, Mar. 28 1862, vol. 23, LSB; Whelan, BUMED Report (Oct. 22, 1861), 510; Joseph Smith to Welles, Nov. 23, 1861, H.R. Exec. Doc. (unnumbered), 37th Cong., 2nd sess., 177–87 (1861).

16. Act of July 14, 1862, ch. 164, 12 Stat. 561, 564 (1865); Whelan memorandum, Jan. 9, 1863, vol. 24, LSB; Whelan to J.P. Hale, May 30, 1862, and to J.W. Grimes, Feb. 18, 1862, vol. 23, LSB.

17. Joseph Smith to Welles, Nov. 4, 1862, H.R. Exec. Doc. 1, 37th Cong., 3rd sess., 557–71 (1862); State of Maine, *Cong. Globe*, 38th Cong., 1st sess., 609–611 (1864); Act of Mar. 14, 1864, ch. 30, 13 Stat. 22, 26 (1866); Whelan, BUMED Report (Nov. 4, 1864), 1179–80; Naval Appropriations Bill, *Cong. Globe*, 38th Cong., 2nd sess., 850–53 (1865); Act of July 1, 1864, ch. 200, 13 Stat. 341 (1866).

18. Horwitz, BUMED Report (Nov. 1, 1865), 384, 388; Whelan, BUMED Report (Oct. 28, 1862), 897; Whelan, BUMED Report (Oct. 23, 1863), 1054; Whelan, BUMED Report (Nov. 4, 1864), 1175; Horwitz, BUMED Report (Nov. 1, 1866), 196; Entry for Navy Yard, Portsmouth, NH, p. 3, entry 41, RG 52.

19. Whelan, BUMED Report (Oct. 22, 1861), 506; Whelan, BUMED Report (Oct. 28, 1862), 897; Whelan, BUMED Report (Oct. 23, 1863), 1054; Whelan, BUMED Report (Nov. 4, 1864), 1175; Horwitz, BUMED Report (Nov. 1, 1865), 384; "Our Annapolis Letter," *Philadelphia Inquirer*, Dec. 24, 1862, 2; Whelan to Welles, May 3, 1861, roll 16, microfilm M518, RG 45.

20. Entry for Naval School, p. 222, entry 41, RG 52.

Chapter 15

1. William Whelan to R.B. Hitchcock, May 31, 1864, vol. 27, LSB; "Naval Hospital Establishment," 263–264.

2. Whelan to J.L. Fox, Jan. 23, 1862, vol. 23, LSB; Whelan to Hitchcock, May 31, 1864, vol. 27, LSB.

3. Whelan to R.B. Hitchcock, May 31, 1864, vol. 27, LSB.

4. Act of Feb. 26, 1811, ch. 26, § 3, 2 Stat. 650 (1845); Shippen, "Some Account"; Stockton, "Naval Asylum"; Navy Department, *Regulations for the Government*, 230.

5. Stockton, "Naval Asylum," 56; *Speech of Hon. S.R. Mallory*, 22; Navy Department, *Regulations for the Government*, 231; "Naval Hospital Establishment," 262.

6. Joseph Smith to Isaac Toucey, Oct. 1, 1859, H.R. Exec. Doc. (unnumbered), 36th Cong., 1st sess., 1180–95 (1860).

7. Whelan, BUMED Report (Oct. 23, 1863), 2058–59.

8. Otto, *St. Elizabeths Hospital*; Act of Aug. 31, 1852, ch. 108, 10 Stat. 76, 92 (1855); Act of Mar. 3, 1855, ch. 199, 10 Stat. 682 (1855); Act of July 1, 1916, ch. 209, 39 Stat. 262, 309 (1917). The name assigned in 1916 lacked an apostrophe after the *h* in *Elizabeths*.

9. Act of Mar. 3, 1855, ch. 199, 10 Stat. 682 (1855); Whelan, BUMED Report (Oct. 28, 1862), 899–900; Whelan, BUMED Report (Oct. 23, 1863), 1057; Whelan, BUMED Report (Nov. 4, 1864), 1179; Horwitz, BUMED Report (Nov. 1, 1865), 388; Ninth Annual Report.

10. Whelan, BUMED Report (Oct. 23, 1863), 1057; Whelan, BUMED Report (Nov. 4, 1864), 1179; Act of July 2, 1864, ch. 110, § 2, 13 Stat. 344, 348 (1866).

11. Act of July 16, 1862, ch. 182, § 6, 12 Stat. 582, 583 (1865); Hasegawa, *Mending Broken Soldiers*, 21–45.

12. Act of July 27, 1868, ch. 264, § 14, 15 Stat. 235, 237 (1869); Act of June 30, 1870, ch. 179, 16 Stat. 174 (1871); Barnes, Artificial Limbs; Hasegawa, *Mending Broken Soldiers*, 43; Horwitz, BUMED Report (Nov. 1, 1865), 387.

13. Whelan to William Selpho, Mar. 3, 1864, vol. 26, LSB; Whelan to R.B. Hitchcock, May 31, 1864, vol. 27, LSB; Barnes, Artificial Limbs.

14. Whelan, BUMED Report (Nov. 4, 1864), 1186–87; Act of July 14, 1862, ch. 166, 12 Stat. 566 (1865); Act of July 1, 1862, ch. 204 §§ 11, 13, 12 Stat. 600, 607, 608 (1865).

15. Whelan, BUMED Report (Nov. 4, 1864), 1186–87; Act of July 14, 1862, ch. 166, 12 Stat. 566 (1865); Act of July 4, 1864, ch. 247, § 5, 13 Stat. 387 (1866); Horwitz, BUMED Report (Nov. 1, 1865), 393.

16. Whelan to R.B. Hitchcock, May 31, 1864, vol. 27, LSB.

17. Stanton, Report of the Secretary, 19; Act of July 28, 1866, ch. 299, § 4, 14 Stat. 332 (1868); Act of Mar. 3, 1869, ch. 124, § 2, 15 Stat. 315, 318 (1869); Adjutant General's Office, General Orders No. 16, Mar. 10, 1869, and No. 17, Mar. 15, 1869, H.R. Exec. Doc. 1, pt. 2, 41st Cong., 2nd sess., 235–38 (1869).

18. "Mr. Lincoln and the Disabled Soldiers," *New York Herald*, Mar. 31, 1865, 5; U.S. Sanitary Commission, advertisement, *Philadelphia Inquirer*, Dec. 1, 1865, 8.

Chapter 16

1. Horwitz, BUMED Report (Nov. 1, 1865), 385; Horwitz, BUMED Report (Nov. 1, 1866), 197; Horwitz, BUMED Report (Oct. 25, 1867), 209; *NDRs* (1861–67); J.E. Dow, "Volunteer Navy," 572.

2. William Whelan, Will, Mar. 1, 1865, Register of Wills, Washington, D.C.; Various letters, vols. 30 and 31, LSB; P.J. Horwitz to W.B. Atkinson, May 31 1865, vol. 31, LSB.

3. William Whelan to L.B. Hunter, William Johnson, David Harlan, and J.C. Palmer, June 5, 1865, vol. 31, LSB.

4. Whelan to Palmer, June 5, 1865, vol. 31, LSB.

5. Whelan to N. Pinkney, June 7, 1865, vol. 31, LSB.

6. Whelan to T. Dillard, May 26, 1865, vol. 31, LSB; Whelan to W.S.W. Ruschenberger, Aug. 28, 1861, and to B.F. Bache, Aug. 31, 1861, vol. 22, LSB.

7. Horwitz to Gideon Welles, June 12, 1865, roll 21, microfilm M518, RG 45; Death Notice, *Daily National Intelligencer* (Washington, D.C.), June 12, 1865, 3; "Late Surgeon Wm. Whelan"; "Obsequies," *Daily National Republican* (Washington, D.C.), June 16, 1865, 3.

8. "Washington News," *Alexandria (VA) Gazette*, July 12, 1865, 2; Horwitz nomination, Dec. 4, 1865, and confirmation, Jan. 22, 1866, *S. Exec. Journal*, 39th Cong., 1st sess., 14 (pt. 2):300, 485 (1887).

9. Act of Mar. 3, 1871, ch. 117, §§ 5 and 12, 16 Stat. 526, 535, 537 (1871); Navy Department, *Instructions for the Government* (1864), 47–48; Thompson, *General Orders and Circulars*, 75–77.

10. Navy Department, *Handy Book*, 302–3; Act of Mar. 3, 1899, ch. 413, § 7, 30 Stat. 1004, 1005 (1899); "Titles of Chiefs," *Evening Star*, Mar. 10, 1899 (Washington, DC), 3.

Conclusion

1. Whelan, BUMED Report (Nov. 4, 1864), 1177.

Bibliography

Archives

Abraham Lincoln Presidential Library, Springfield, IL

- George H. Bixby Papers, Call No. MS-SC2610

National Archives and Records Administration, Washington, DC, and College Park, MD

- Record Group 15: Records of the Department of Veterans Affairs
  - Microfilm M1274: Case Files of Disapproved Pension Applications of Widows and Other Dependents of Civil War and Later Navy Veterans ("Navy Widows' Certificates")
- Record Group 19: Records of the Bureau of Ships
  - Alphabetical Series of Ship Engineering Drawings, 1789–1967
- Record Group 24: Records of the Bureau of Naval Personnel
  - Entry 118: Logbooks of U.S. Navy Ships, ca. 1801–1940
  - Entry 132: Muster Rolls of Ships, Jan. 1, 1860–June 9, 1900
  - Microfilm M330: Abstracts of Service Records of Naval Officers ("Records of Officers")
  - Microfilm M1953: Weekly Returns of Enlistments at Naval Rendezvous ("Enlistment Rendezvous"), Jan. 6, 1855–Aug. 8, 1892
- Record Group 29: Records of the Bureau of the Census
  - Microfilm M653: Eighth Census of the United States, 1860
- Record Group 45: Naval Records Collection of the Office of Naval Records and Library
  - Entry 164: Registers of Volunteer (Acting) Officers, May 1861–ca. 1880
  - Entry 502: Subject File of the U.S. Navy, 1775–1910
  - Microfilm M89: Letters Received by the Secretary of the Navy from Commanding Officers of Squadrons ("Squadron Letters"), 1841–86
  - Microfilm M148: Letters Received by the Secretary of the Navy from Commissioned Officers below the Rank of Commander and from Warrant Officers ("Officers' Letters"), 1802–84
  - Microfilm M480: Letters Sent from the Secretary of the Navy to Chiefs of Navy Bureaus, 1842–86
  - Microfilm M518: Letters Received by the Secretary of the Navy from Chiefs of Navy Bureaus, 1842–85
  - Microfilm M977: Navy Department General Orders and Circulars, 1798–1862
  - Microfilm M984: Navy Department General Orders, 1863–1948
  - Microfilm T829: Miscellaneous Records of the Office of Naval Records and Library
- Record Group 52: Records of the Bureau of Medicine and Surgery
  - Entry 1: Letters Sent ("Letter Book"), Sept. 1842–Feb. 1886

° Entry 7: Letters Received ("Letters from All Sources"), Jan. 1857–Feb. 1885
° Entry 25: Hospital Tickets and Case Papers, 1825–89
° Entry 41: List of Medical Officers, 1824–73
° Entry 43: Statements of Service of Medical Officers ("Orders of Medical Officers"), 1842–73
° Entry 44: Statements of Service of Acting Medical Officers ("Acting Medical Officers"), 1860–70
° Entry 45: Appointment Papers of Surgeon's Stewards, Apothecaries, and Nurses, 1861–64
° Entry 45A: Compiled List of Names of Surgeon's Stewards and a List of Documents Concerning Them
• Record Group 125: Records of the Office of the Judge Advocate General (Navy)
° Microfilm M273: Records of General Courts-Martial and Courts of Inquiry of the Navy Department, 1799–1857

National Library of Medicine, Bethesda, MD
• Examination Papers Collection, 1831–60, U.S. Navy Department, Bureau of Medicine and Surgery

Navy Department Library, Washington, DC
• ZB (Personnel) Files

Nimitz Library, Special Collections and Archives, United States Naval Academy, Annapolis, MD
• Daniel D.T. Nestell Papers, Call No. MS 310

U.S. Army Heritage and Education Center, Carlisle, PA
• Civil War Photograph Collection, Military Order of the Loyal Legion of the United States, Massachusetts Commandery

Articles, Books, and Online Sources

Adams, George Worthington. *Doctors in Blue.* Baton Rouge: Louisiana State University Press, 1952.

Austin, H.W. "Historical Sketch of the United States Marine-Hospital Service, at Boston, Mass." In *Annual Report of the Supervising Surgeon-General of the Marine-Hospital Service of the United States for the Fiscal Year 1896*, 267–76. Washington, DC: Government Printing Office, 1896.

Barnes, J.K. Artificial Limbs Furnished to Soldiers, May 11, 1866. H.R. Exec. Doc. 108, 39th Cong., 1st sess. (1866).

Bartlett, Elisha. *The History, Diagnosis, and Treatment of the Fevers of the United States.* 4th ed. Philadelphia: Blanchard and Lea, 1865.

Batten, John M. *Reminiscences of Two Years in the United States Navy.* Lancaster, PA: Inquirer, 1881.

Beale, J. Report of the Bureau of Medicine and Surgery, Nov. 1, 1875. In *Annual Report of the Secretary of the Navy on the Operations of the Department for the Year 1875*, 100–104. Washington, DC: Government Printing Office, 1876.

Billings, John S. "Medical Reminiscences of the Civil War." *Transactions of the College of Physicians of Philadelphia* 27 (1905): 115–21.

Bollet, Alfred Jay. *Civil War Medicine: Challenges and Triumphs.* Tucson: Galen, 2002.

Bollet, Alfred Jay. "Rheumatic Diseases among Civil War Troops." *Arthritis and Rheumatism* 34, no. 9 (Sept. 1991): 1197–1203.

Boyer, Samuel Pellman. *Naval Surgeon: Blockading the South 1862–1866.* Edited by Elinor Barnes and James A. Barnes. Bloomington: Indiana University Press, 1863.

Bradshaw, Watson. *The Anatomy of Dyspepsia.* London: George Philip and Son, 1864.

Bumstead, Freeman J. *The Pathology and Treatment of Venereal Diseases.* Philadelphia: Blanchard and Lea, 1861.

Callahan, Edward W., ed. *List of Officers of the Navy of the United States and of the Marine Corps from 1775 to 1900.* New York: L.R. Hamersly, 1901.

Catalogue of the Medical Graduates of the University of Pennsylvania. Philadelphia: Lydia R. Bailey, 1838.

"Changes in Navy Uniform," *Army Navy Journal* 1, no. 13 (Nov. 21, 1863): 199.

Channing, William F. "The Alkaline Treatment of Rheumatism." *Boston Medical and Surgical Journal* 52, no. 17 (May 31, 1855): 235–36.

Chatelain, Neil P. "Turnover and Turmoil Off Charleston." *Naval History* 38, no. 4 (Aug. 2024): 44–49.

Churchman, John W. "The Use of Quinine During the Civil War." *Bulletin of the Johns Hopkins Hospital* 17, no. 183 (June 1906): 175–81.

Condy, Henry Bollmann. *Disinfection and the Prevention of Disease.* London: John W. Davies, 1862.

Confederate States Navy. *Regulations for the Navy of the Confederate States, 1862.* Richmond: Macfarlane and Fergusson, 1862.

Cotton, Richard Payne. *On Consumption: Its Nature, Symptoms, and Treatment.* 2nd ed. London: John Churchill, 1858.

Death Notice for William Whelan. *Boston Medical and Surgical Journal* 72, no. 21 (June 22, 1865): 433.

Derby, George. "The Use of Quinine in Malarious Districts." *Boston Medical and Surgical Journal* 69, no. 9 (Oct. 1, 1863): 169–71.

Dixon, Ben F. "The 'White Lily.'" *Hospital Corps Quarterly* 18, no. 7 (July 1945): 2–21.

Dodson, C. Marion. "The Apothecary in our Navy." *American Druggist and Pharmaceutical Record* 26, no. 3 (Aug. 10, 1895): 65–66.

Dow, J.E. "Volunteer Navy." In *A Naval Encyclopaedia: Comprising a Dictionary of Nautical Words and Phrases; Biographical Notices, and Records of Naval Officers,* 569–72. Philadelphia: L.R. Hamersly, 1884.

Dudley, William S. *Going South: U.S. Navy Officer Resignations & Dismissals on the Eve of the Civil War.* Washington, DC: Naval Historical Foundation, 1981.

Dunglison, Robley. *Medical Lexicon: A Dictionary of Medical Science.* Philadelphia: Blanchard and Lea, 1860.

Dunham, Carroll. "Homoeopathy in the Army: Appeal to the People." In *Transactions of the Homeopathic Medical Society of the State of New York for the Year 1864.* Albany, NY: Comstock and Cassidy, 1864.

Earp, Charles Albert, ed. *Yellow Flag: The Civil War Journal of Surgeon's Steward C. Marion Dodson.* Baltimore: Maryland Historical Society, 2002.

Ellis, Benjamin. *The Medical Formulary.* Philadelphia: Blanchard and Lea, 1854.

Ericsson, John. "The Monitors." *Century Magazine* 31, no. 2 (Dec. 1885): 280–99.

Farenholt, A. "Historical Sketch of the U.S. Naval Hospital, Mare Island, Calif." *United States Naval Medical Bulletin* 15, no. 1 (Jan. 1921): 1–10.

Farquharson, R.S. "Scurvy in the Navy." *American Medical Times* 7 (July 25, 1863): 35–37; 7 (Aug. 8, 1863): 61–62, and 66 (editors' note).

Field, Marilyn J. *Dental Education at the Crossroads: Challenges and Change.* Washington, DC: National Academy Press, 1995.

Flint, Austin. "Conservative Medicine." *North American Medico-Chirurgical Review* 5, no. 6 (Nov. 1861): 1038–59.

Foltz, Charles S. *Surgeon of the Seas: The Life of Surgeon General Jonathan M. Foltz.* Indianapolis: Bobbs-Merrill, 1931.

Forman, J.G. *The Western Sanitary Commission: A Sketch.* St. Louis: R.P. Studley, 1864.

Fowler, William M., Jr. "Relief on the River: The Red Rover." *Naval History* 5, no. 3 (Fall 1991): 14–19.

Freedley, Edwin T. *Leading Pursuits and Leading Men: A Treatise on the Principal Trades and Manufactures of the United States.* Philadelphia: Edward Young, 1854.

Fuller, Henry William. *On Rheumatism, Rheumatic Gout, and Sciatica.* 3rd ed. London: John Churchill, 1860.

Garratt, Alfred C. *Medical Electricity: Embracing Electro-Physiology and Electricity as a Therapeutic.* 3rd ed. Philadelphia: J.B. Lippincott, 1866.

Gatewood, J.D. "William Longshaw, Jr., Assistant Surgeon, United States Navy (1839–1865)." *United States Naval Medical Bulletin* 7, no. 4 (Oct. 1913): 503–17.

"Gen. Butler on Yellow Fever." *Medical and Surgical Reporter* 17, no. 3 (July 20, 1867): 61–62.

Gradijan, Leanne. "Navy Surgeons in the Civil War: A Statistical Report." *Grog: A Journal of Navy Medical History and Culture* 6, no. 3 (Summer 2011): 28–29.

Griffith, R. Eglesfeld. *A Universal Formulary.* Philadelphia: Blanchard and Lea, 1859.

Hammond, W.A. Circular No. 6, May 4, 1863. *American Medical Times* 6, no. 21 (May 23, 1863): 252.

Harris, Chapin A. *A Dictionary of Medical Terminology, Dental Surgery, and the Collateral Sciences.* Philadelphia: Lindsay and Blakiston, 1854.

Harris, Thomas. Report of the Bureau of Medicine and Surgery, Nov. 6, 1846. H.R. Exec. Doc. 4, 29th Cong., 2nd sess., 590–94 (1846).

Harris, Thomas. Report of the Bureau of Medicine and Surgery, Oct. 30, 1848. H.R. Exec. Doc. 1, 30th Cong., 2nd sess., 935–39 (1848).

Hasegawa, Guy R. *The Confederate Navy Medical Corps: Organization, Personnel and Actions.* Jefferson, NC: McFarland, 2024.

Hasegawa, Guy R. *Matchless Organization: The Confederate Army Medical Department.* Carbondale: Southern Illinois University Press, 2021.

Hasegawa, Guy R. *Mending Broken Soldiers: The Union and Confederate Programs to Supply Artificial Limbs.* Carbondale: Southern Illinois University Press, 2012.

Hasegawa, Guy R. "'We Got Up and Began to Pack Our Medicines': What Dr. Fulton Prescribed." In *Civil War Medicine: A Surgeon's Diary,* edited by Robert D. Hicks, 288–301. Bloomington: Indiana University Press, 2019.

Hepworth, George H. *The Whip, Hoe, and Sword; or, The Gulf-Department in '63.* Boston: Walker, Wise, 1864.

Hill, Jim Dan. *The Civil War Sketchbook of Charles Ellery Stedman, Surgeon, United States Navy.* San Rafael, CA: Presidio, 1976.

Holden, Edgar. "The First Cruise of the 'Monitor' Passaic." *Harper's New Monthly Magazine* 27, no. 161 (Oct. 1863): 577–95.

Holden, Edgar. "An Inquiry in the Causes of Certain Diseases on Ships of War." *American Journal of the Medical Sciences,* n.s., 51, no. 101 (Jan. 1866): 75–84.

Homans, Benjamin. *Register of the Commissioned and Warrant Officers of the Navy of the United States, Including Officers of the Marine Corps. Corrected from Authentic Sources to the 15th September 1842.* Washington, DC: Alexander and Barnard, 1842.

Horner, G.R.B. *Diseases and Injuries of Seamen: With Remarks on Their Enlistment, Naval Hygiene, and the Duties of Medical Officers.* Philadelphia: Lippincott, Grambo, 1854.

Horwitz, P.J. Report of the Bureau of Medicine and Surgery, Nov. 1, 1865. H.R. Exec. Doc. 1 39th Cong., 1st sess., bureau reports, 383–426 (1865).

Horwitz, P.J. Report of the Bureau of Medicine and Surgery, Nov. 1, 1866. In *Report of the Secretary of the Navy,* 194–219. Washington, DC: Government Printing Office, 1866.

Horwitz, P.J. Report of the Bureau of Medicine and Surgery, Oct. 25, 1867. In *Report of the Secretary of the Navy,* 207–302. Washington, DC: Government Printing Office, 1867.

Hospital Surgeon of Philadelphia. "Hints and Observations on Military Hygiene, Relating to Diet, Dress, Exercise, Exposure, and Best Means of Preventing and Curing Medical and Surgical Diseases in the Army." *Medical and Surgical Reporter* 6, no. 11 (June 15, 1861): 241–44; no. 12 (June 22, 1862): 263–68.

Howard, Horton. *Improved System of Botanic Medicine.* Cincinnati: Kost, Bigger and Hart, 1854.

Hunter, Alvah H. *A Year on a Monitor and the Destruction of Fort Sumter.* Edited by Craig L. Symonds. Columbia: University of South Carolina Press, 1987.

Keen, W.W. "Surgical Reminiscences of the Civil War." *Transactions of the College of Physicians of Philadelphia* 27 (1905): 95–114.

Kennedy, Joseph C.G. *Population of the United States in 1860; Compiled from the Original Returns of the Eighth Census.* Washington, DC: Government Printing Office, 1864.

Kenney, Edward C. "From the Log of the Red Rover, 1862–1865: A History of the First U.S. Navy Hospital Ship." *Missouri Historical Review* 60, no. 1 (Oct. 1965): 31–49.

Langley, Harold D. *A History of Medicine in the Early U.S. Navy.* Baltimore: Johns Hopkins University Press, 1995.

"The Late Surgeon Wm. Whelan, U.S.N." *Army Navy Journal* 2, no. 45 (July 1, 1865), 711.

Lee, Charles A. "Remarks on Disinfectants." *Medical Record* 1 (May 1, 1866): 126–29.

Lieber, Francis. *Instructions for the Government of Armies of the United States.* Washington, DC: Government Printing Office, 1898.

Lyman, George H. *Historical Sketch of the Obstetrical Society of Boston in the War of the Rebellion.* Boston: David Clapp, 1887.

McQuillen J.H. "Dentists in the Army and Navy of the United States." *Dental Cosmos,* n.s., 3, no. 5 (Dec. 1861): 268–69.

The Medical and Surgical History of the War of the Rebellion. 3 vols. Washington, DC: Government Printing Office, 1870–88.

"Medical News." *American Medical Times* 2, no. 20 (May 18, 1861): 330.

Meigs, M.C. *Report of the Quartermaster General of the United States Army to the Secretary of War, for the Year Ending June 30, 1865.* Washington: Government Printing Office, 1865.

Merritt, J. King. "Quinine as a Prophylactic in Malarious Regions." *American Medical Times* 3, no. 19 (Nov. 9, 1861): 305–306.

Mills, Robert. *Guide to the Capitol and to the National Executive Offices of the United States.* Washington, DC: J.C. Greer, 1854.

Mitchell, S. Weir, George R. Morehouse, and William W. Keen. *Gunshot Wounds and Other Injuries of Nerves.* Philadelphia: J.B. Lippincott, 1864.

Moss, Sandra W. *Edgar Holden, M.D., of Newark, New Jersey: Provincial Physician on a National Stage.* N.p.: Xlibris, 2014.

Munden, Kenneth W., and Henry Putney Beers. *The Union: A Guide to Federal Archives Relating to the Civil War.* Washington, DC: National Archives and Records Administration, 1986.

"The Naval Hospital Establishment." *United States Service Magazine* 2, no. 3 (Sept. 1864): 256–65.

"Naval Medical Board." *American Medical Times* 3, no. 23 (Dec. 7, 1861): 380.

Navy Department. *Allowances Established for Vessels of the United States Navy.* Washington, DC: Government Printing Office, 1865.

Navy Department. A Code of Regulations for the Government of the Navy. H.R. Exec. Doc. 2, 35th Cong., 2nd sess., 24–424 (1858).

Navy Department. *Dictionary of American Naval Fighting Ships.* 8 vols. Washington, DC: Navy Department, 1959–81.

Navy Department. *General Regulations for the Navy and Marine Corps of the United States, 1841.* Washington, DC: J. and G.S. Gideon, 1841.

Navy Department. *Handy Book for the Hospital Corps.* Washington, DC: Government Printing Office, 1917.

Navy Department. *Instructions for the Government of the Medical Officers of the Navy of the United States.* Washington, DC: Alexander and Barnard, 1844.

Navy Department. *Instructions for the Government of the Medical Officers of the Navy of the United States.* Washington, DC: A.O.P. Nicholson, 1857.

Navy Department. *Instructions for the Government of the Medical Officers of the Navy of the United States.* Washington, DC: Government Printing Office, 1864.

Navy Department. *Official Register of the Officers and Midshipmen of the United States Naval Academy.* Newport, RI: Frederick A. Pratt, 1864.

Navy Department. *Ordnance Instructions for the United States Navy.* Washington, DC: Government Printing Office, 1864.

Navy Department. *Register of the Commissioned and Warrant Officers of the Navy of the United States, Including Officers of the Marine Corps, and Others, for the Year 1848.* Washington, DC: C. Alexander, 1848.

Navy Department. *Register of the Commissioned and Warrant Officers of the*

Navy of the United States, Including Officers of the Marine Corps, and Others, for the Year 1853. Washington, DC: C. Alexander, 1853.

Navy Department. *Register of the Commissioned and Warrant Officers of the Navy of the United States. Including Officers of the Marine Corps, and Others, for the Year 1859.* Washington, DC: William A. Harris, 1859.

Navy Department. *Register of the Commissioned and Warrant Officers of the Navy of the United States, Including Officers of the Marine Corps and Others, for the Year 1860.* Washington, DC: n.p., 1860.

Navy Department. *Register of the Commissioned and Warrant Officers of the Navy of the United States, Including Officers of the Marine Corps and Others, for the Year 1861.* Washington, DC: George W. Bowman, 1861.

Navy Department. *Register of the Commissioned and Warrant Officers of the Navy of the United States, Including Officers of the Marine Corps and Others, to August 31, 1861.* Washington, DC: Government Printing Office, 1861.

Navy Department. *Register of the Commissioned, Warrant, and Volunteer Officers of the Navy of the United States, Including Officers of the Marine Corps and Others, to September 1, 1862.* Washington, DC: Government Printing Office, 1862.

Navy Department. *Register of the Commissioned, Warrant, and Volunteer Officers of the Navy of the United States, Including Officers of the Marine Corps and Others, to January 1, 1863.* Washington, DC: Government Printing Office, 1863.

Navy Department. *Register of the Commissioned, Warrant, and Volunteer Officers of the Navy of the United States, Including Officers of the Marine Corps and Others, to January 1, 1864.* Washington, DC: Government Printing Office, 1864.

Navy Department. *Register of the Commissioned, Warrant, and Volunteer Officers of the Navy of the United States, Including Officers of the Marine Corps and Others, to January 1, 1865.* Washington, DC: Government Printing Office, 1865.

Navy Department. *Register of the Commissioned, Warrant, and Volunteer Officers of the Navy of the United States, Including Officers of the Marine Corps and Others, to January 1, 1866.* Washington, DC: Government Printing Office, 1866.

Navy Department. *Register of the Commissioned, Warrant, and Volunteer Officers of the Navy of the United States, Including Officers of the Marine Corps and Others, to January 1, 1867.* Washington, DC: Government Printing Office, 1867.

Navy Department. *Register of the Commissioned, Warrant, and Volunteer Officers of the Navy of the United States, Including Officers of the Marine Corps and Others, to July 1, 1867.* Washington, DC: Government Printing Office, 1867.

Navy Department. *Register of the Commissioned, Warrant, and Volunteer Officers of the Navy of the United States, Including Officers of the Marine Corps and Others, to July 1, 1879.* Washington, DC: Government Printing Office, 1879.

Navy Department. *Register of the Commissioned, Warrant, and Volunteer Officers of the Navy of the United States, Including Officers of the Marine Corps and Others, to July 1, 1881.* Washington, DC: Government Printing Office, 1881.

Navy Department. *Regulations for the Government of the United States Navy, 1865.* Washington, DC: Government Printing Office, 1865.

Navy Department. *Regulations of the U.S. Naval Academy.* Washington: Geo. W. Bowman, 1860.

Navy Department. *Uniform for Officers of the United States Navy as Prescribed in Regulations for the Uniform of the U.S. Navy, Jan. 28, 1864.* New York: Tomes, Melvain, 1864.

Negus, Samuel. "'Conduct Unbecoming of an Officer': Fraudulent Enlistment Practices at U.S. Navy Recruitment Rendezvous during the American Civil War." *Northern Mariner* 22, no. 1 (Jan. 2012): 27–52.

Newman, Harry Wright. *The Smoots of Maryland and Virginia.* Washington, DC: Harry Wright Newman, 1936.

Ninth Annual Report of the Board of Visitors, and the Tenth Annual Report of the Superintendent of Construction, Government Hospital for the Insane, for the Year 1863–'64. H.R. Exec. Doc. 1, 38th Cong., 2nd sess., 714–726 (1864).

Official Records of the Union and Confederate Navies in the War of the Rebellion. 30 vols. in 2 ser. Washington, DC: Government Printing Office, 1884–1922.

Otto, Thomas. *St. Elizabeths Hospital: A History.* Washington, DC: General Services Administration, 2013.

Paoli, G.C. "Double Pneumonia, with Chronic Bronchitis, Cured by Sugar of Lead and Sulphate of Quinine." *Chicago Medical Examiner* 6, no. 1 (Jan. 1865): 36–38.

Parton, James. *Life and Times of Benjamin Franklin,* vol. 2. New York: Mason Brothers, 1864.

Paullin, Charles Oscar. "A Half Century of Naval Administration in American, 1861–1911." Pts. 1–3. *United States Naval Institute Proceedings* 38, no. 4 (Dec. 1912): 1309–36; 39, no. 1 (Mar. 1913): 165–95; 39, no. 2 (June 1913): 735–60.

Paullin, Charles Oscar. "Naval Administration, 1842–1861." *Proceedings of the United States Naval Institute* 33, no. 4 (Dec. 1907): 1435–77.

"Philadelphia School of Anatomy: A Change." *Medical and Surgical Reporter* 10, no. 1 (May 2, 1863): 11–12.

Porter, David D. *Incidents and Anecdotes of the Civil War.* New York: D. Appleton, 1886.

Porter, David D. *The Naval History of the Civil War.* New York: Sherman, 1886.

Portrait and Biographical Record of Randolph, Jackson, Perry, and Monroe Counties, Illinois. Chicago: Biographical Publishing, 1894.

"Position of the Society with Regard to the Introduction of the Homoeopathic Practice into the Army: Resolutions Adopted at the Tenth Annual Meeting." In *Transactions of the Homoeopathic Medical Society of the State of New York, for the Year 1864.* Albany, NY: Comstock and Cassidy, 1864.

Pray, Ezra. *Civil War Journal of Acting Assistant Surgeon Ezra Pray.* Washington, DC: Navy Historical Foundation, n.d. https://archive.org/details/PrayJournalsmaller/Pray%20Journal%20%28smaller%29/.

"Proceedings of Societies: New York Academy of Medicine." *New York Medical Times* 5, no. 1 (Oct. 1855): 54–61.

"Professor Morgan's Plan of Preserving Meat." *Scientific American,* n.s., 10, no. 24 (June 11, 1864): 372.

Provost Marshal General's Office. Circular No. 13, Mar. 25, 1864. *Army & Navy Official Gazette* 1, no. 39 (Mar. 29, 1864): 624.

"Recruiting for the Navy." *Frank Leslie's Illustrated Newspaper* 12, no. 288 (May 25, 1861): 22, 27.

"Regulations for Admission and Promotion in the Medical Department of the Navy." *New York Medical Press* 2, no. 14 (Oct. 1, 1859): 662–63.

Reidy, Joseph P. "Black Men in Navy Blue during the Civil War." *Prologue* 33, no. 3 (Fall 2001): 155–67.

Report of the Board of Visitors of the Government Hospital for the Insane, Oct. 1, 1861. H.R. Exec. Doc. (unnumbered), 37th Cong., 2nd sess., 890–98 (1861).

Report of the Board of Visitors of the Government Hospital for the Insane, Oct. 1, 1862. H.R. Exec. Doc. 1, 37th Cong., 3rd sess., 619–27 (1862).

Report of the Western Sanitary Commission for the Year Ending June 1st, 1863. St. Louis: Western Sanitary Commission, 1863.

Review of *Incidents and Anecdotes of the Civil War,* by David D. Porter, *Nation* 42, no. 1071 (Jan. 7, 1886), 16.

Roberts, John C. "What Is a 'Naval Station'?" *JAG Journal* (Apr. 1951): 14–16.

[Ruschenberger, W.S.W.] *A Brief History of an Existing Controversy on the Subject of Assimilated Rank in the Navy of the United States.* Philadelphia: C. Sherman, 1850.

Ruschenberger, W.S.W. "The Naval Laboratory—Error Corrected." *Journal of the American Medical Association* 1, no. 9 (Sept. 8, 1883): 279–80.

Ruschenberger, W.S.W. "Oakum as a Substitute for Lint, in Gunshot and Other Suppurating Wounds." *Boston Medical and Surgical Journal* 67, no. 10 (Oct. 9, 1862): 192–96.

[Ruschenberger, W.S.W.] Review of *Outlines of Naval Surgery,* by John Wilson. *American Journal of Medical Sciences,* n.s., 12, no. 24 (Oct. 1846): 407–25.

Salter, Henry Hyde. *On Asthma: Its Pathology and Treatment.* London: John Churchill, 1860.

Sansom, Arthur Ernest. *Chloroform: Its Action and Administration.* Philadelphia: Lindsay and Blackiston, 1866.

Sayre, Lewis A. "Oakum as a Substitute for Lint." *American Medical Times* 5, no. 6 (Aug. 9, 1862): 82.

Selfridge, Thomas O. "The Navy at Fort Fisher." In *Battle and Leaders of the Civil War,* vol. 4, edited by Robert Underwood Johnson and Clarence Clough Buel, 655–61. New York: Century, 1884–88.

Sherman, William T. *Memoirs of General William T. Sherman.* Vol. 2. London: Henry S. King, 1875.

Shippen, Edward. "Some Account of the Origin of the Naval Asylum at Philadelphia." *Pennsylvania Magazine of History and Biography* 7, no. 2 (1883): 117–42.

Slawson, Robert G. "Medical Training in the United States Prior to the Civil War." *Journal of Evidence-Based Complementary and Alternative Medicine* 7, no. 1 (Jan. 1, 2012): 11–27.

Smith, Daniel B. "On Certain Compounds of Carburetted Hydrogen." *Journal of the Philadelphia College of Pharmacy* 4, no. 2 (July 1832): 114–21.

Smith, George Winston. *Medicines for the Union Army.* Madison, WI: American Institute of the History of Pharmacy, 1962.

Smith, Joseph. Report of the Chief of Bureau of Yards and Docks, Oct. 17, 1863. H.R. Exec. Doc. 1, 38th Cong., 1st sess., 612–760 (1863).

Snyder, Thomas L. *Mare Island Naval Hospital: A History, 1864–1957.* Jefferson, NC: McFarland, 2025.

Sobocinski, André B. "Dr. Bache and the Founding of the U.S. Navy Laboratory; or Looking Back at the Navy's own 'Benjamin Franklin.'" *Logistically Speaking* (Jan.–Mar. 2018), 18–21.

Speech of Hon. S.R. Mallory, of Florida, on the Law of 1855, for Promoting the Efficiency of the Navy. Washington, DC: Congressional Globe Office, 1856.

Stanton, Edwin M. Report of the Secretary of War, Nov. 22, 1865. H.R. Exec. Doc. 1, 39th Cong., 1st sess., 1–48 (1866).

Statistics of the United States (Including Mortality, Property, &c.) in 1860; Compiled from the Original Returns and Being the Final Exhibit of the Eighth Census. Washington, DC: Government Printing Office, 1866.

Stockton, Charles H. *The Laws and Usages of War at Sea: A Naval War Code.* Washington, DC: Government Printing Office, 1900.

Stockton, Charles H. "The Naval Asylum and Service Pensions for Enlisted Men." *Proceedings of the United States Naval Institute* 12, no. 2 (1886): 53–67.

Tenney, W.J. *The Military and Naval History of the Rebellion in the United States.* New York: D. Appleton, 1865.

Thompson, M. S., comp. *General Orders and Circulars Issued by the Navy Department from 1863 to 1887.* Washington, DC: Government Printing Office, 1887.

Thompson, Robert Means, and Richard Wainwright, eds. *Confidential Correspondence of Gustavus Vasa Fox.* 2 vols. New York: Naval History Society, 1918.

Thurm, Richard H. *For the Relief of the Sick and Disabled: The U.S. Public Health Service Hospital at Boston, 1799–1969.* Washington, DC: Government Printing Office, 1972.

Tily, James C. *The Uniforms of the United States Navy.* New York: Thomas Yoseloff, 1964.

Toll, Larry, Alan Chilton, Jeffrey Patrick, and Brooks C. Place. "George Holmes Bixby, MD, USS *Red Rover*: Photographer on the Western Rivers." *Civil War Navy—The Magazine* 7, no. 2 (Fall 2019): 4–17.

True, Rowland Stafford. "Life Aboard a Gunboat." *Civil War Times Illustrated* 9, no. 10 (Feb. 1971): 36–43.

Tryon, J.R. "Naval Architecture and Sanitation." *Cassier's Magazine* 18, no. 2 (June 1900): 129–45.

War Department. *Revised United States Army Regulations, of 1861, with an Appendix Containing the Changes and Laws Affecting Army Regulations and Articles of War to June 25, 1863.* Washington, DC: Government Printing Office, 1863.

Warner, John Harley. *The Therapeutic Perspective: Medical Practice, Knowledge, and Identity in America, 1820–1885.* Princeton, NJ: Princeton University Press, 1997.

Watson, Thomas. *Lectures on the Principles and Practice of Physic.* Philadelphia: Blanchard and Lea, 1858.

Welles, Gideon. *Diary of Gideon Welles.* 3 vols. Boston: Houghton Mifflin, 1911.

Welles, Gideon. General Order No. 36, May 16, 1864. *United States Service Magazine* 2, no. 1 (July 1864): 111–12.

Welles, Gideon. *Report of the Secretary of the Navy,* July 4, 1861. S. Exec. Doc. 1, 37th Cong., 1st sess., 85–98 (1861).

Welles, Gideon. *Report of the Secretary of the Navy,* Dec. 2, 1861. S. Exec. Doc. 1, 37th Cong., 2nd sess., 3–23 (1861).

Welles, Gideon. *Report of the Secretary of the Navy,* Dec. 1, 1862. H.R. Exec. Doc. 1, 37th Cong., 3rd sess., 3–46 (1862).

Welles, Gideon. *Report of the Secretary of the Navy, with an Appendix, Containing Reports from Officers. December, 1864.* Washington, DC: Government Printing Office, 1864.

Welles, Gideon. *Report of the Secretary of the Navy, with an Appendix, Containing Reports from Officers. December, 1865.* Washington, DC: Government Printing Office, 1865.

Whelan, William. Report of the Bureau of Medicine and Surgery, Oct. 19, 1860. S. Exec. Doc. 1, 36th Cong., 2nd sess., 371–81 (1860).

Whelan, William. Report of the Bureau of Medicine and Surgery, June 10, 1861. H.R. Exec. Doc. (unnumbered), 37th Cong., 1st sess., 107–8 (1861).

Whelan, William. Report of the Bureau of Medicine and Surgery, Oct. 22, 1861. H.R. Exec. Doc. (unnumbered), 37th Cong., 2nd sess., 505–14 (1861).

Whelan, William. Report of the Bureau of Medicine and Surgery, Oct. 28, 1862. H.R. Exec. Doc. 1, 37th Cong., 3rd sess., 896–901 (1862).

Whelan, William. Report of the Bureau of Medicine and Surgery, Oct. 23, 1863. H.R. Exec. Doc. 1, 38th Cong., 1st sess., 1053–70 (1863).

Whelan, William. Report of the Bureau of Medicine and Surgery, Nov. 4, 1864. H.R. Exec. Doc. 1, 38th Cong., 2nd sess., 1174–93 (1864).

"William Whelan." *United States Naval Medical Bulletin* 32, no. 4 (Oct. 1934): 535.

Wilson, Joseph. *Naval Hygiene.* Washington, DC: Government Printing Office, 1870.

Wineberger, J.A. *Department Directory and Register of Officers in the Service of the United States in the City of Washington.* Washington, DC: C. Bohn, 1862.

Wood, George B. *A Treatise on the Practice of Medicine.* 5th ed. 2 vols. Philadelphia: J.B. Lippincott, 1858.

Wood, George B. *A Treatise on Therapeutics, and Pharmacology or Material Medica.* 2 vols. Philadelphia: J.B. Lippincott, 1856.

Wood, George B., and Franklin Bache. *The Dispensatory of the United States of America.* 11th ed. Philadelphia: J.B. Lippincott, 1858.

Woodward, Joseph Janvier. *The Hospital Steward's Manual.* Philadelphia: J.B. Lippincott, 1862.

Woolsey, Theodore S. "The Naval War Code." *Columbia Law Review* 1, no. 5 (May 1901): 298–301.

Yeoman, T.H. *Catarrh, Influenza, Bronchitis, and Asthma.* London: Sampson Low, 1849.

Index

Numbers in ***bold italics*** refer to pages with illustrations

www.ingramcontent.com/pod-product-compliance
Lightning Source LLC
La Vergne TN
LVHW022203200926
848481LV00006B/1830